Physiopathology of the Cardiovascular System

Physiopathology of the Cardiovascular System

Joseph S. Alpert, M.D.
Professor of Medicine and Director,
Division of Cardiovascular Medicine,
University of Massachusetts Medical School,
Worcester, Massachusetts

Foreword by
DeWitt S. Goodman, M.D., Series Editor
Professor of Medicine and Chief,
Division of Metabolism and Nutrition,
Columbia University College of Physicians
and Surgeons, New York

Little, Brown and Company   Boston/Toronto

Library of Congress Catalog Card No. 83-81578

ISBN 0-316-03504-1

Printed in the United States of America

HAL

Second Printing

To Niels A. Lassen, Lewis Dexter, and James E. Dalen,
who sparked my interest in cardiovascular pathophysiology

Contents

Contributors

Andrew J. Cohen, M.D.
Assistant Professor of Medicine and Physiology, Division of Renal
Medicine, University of Massachusetts Medical School; Acting Chief,
Division of Renal Medicine, University of Massachusetts Medical Center,
Worcester, Massachusetts
Chapter 9

Robert J. Goldberg, Ph.D.
Assistant Professor of Medicine and Epidemiology, Department of
Medicine, University of Massachusetts Medical School, Worcester,
Massachusetts
Chapter 4

Joel M. Gore, M.D.
Assistant Professor of Medicine, University of Massachusetts Medical
School; Associate Director, Coronary Care Unit, University of Massachusetts
Medical Center, Worcester, Massachusetts
Chapter 4

Roger B. Hickler, M.D.
Lamar Soutter Distinguished Professor of Medicine and Director, Division of
Geriatric Medicine, University of Massachusetts Medical School; Director,
Division of Geriatric Medicine, University of Massachusetts Hospital,
Worcester, Massachusetts
Chapter 10

Richard S. Irwin, M.D.
Associate Professor of Medicine, University of Massachusetts Medical
School; Director, Division of Pulmonary Medicine, University of
Massachusetts Medical Center, Worcester, Massachusetts
Chapter 8

Emil R. Smith, Ph.D
Associate Professor of Pharmacology, University of Massachusetts Medical
School, Worcester, Massachusetts
Chapter 14

Carl Teplitz, M.D.
Professor of Medical Sciences, Division of Biology and Medicine, Brown
University Program in Medicine; Director, Division of Surgical Pathology,
Rhode Island Hospital, Providence, Rhode Island
Chapter 8

Foreword by the Series Editor

The goal of the Little, Brown Physiopathology Series is to provide textbooks that describe and illustrate the scientific foundations underlying the current practice of clinical medicine. The concept of this series developed from curricular changes that occurred in American medical schools during the early 1970s. These changes resulted in increased emphasis in the teaching of normal and abnormal human biology, usually to second-year medical students, as the bridge between the traditional basic science courses and the clinical clerkships. A need existed for textbooks in this "bridge" area; this series was designed to address this need.

Each book in this series deals with a different medical subspecialty. Each book aims to provide a clear and solid discussion of the basic scientific concepts and principles on which the clinical subspecialty is built. This discussion includes selected aspects of normal and abnormal physiology, biochemistry, morphology, cell biology, and so on, as appropriate. The discussion of the basic science material is usually presented in the context of the approach to the study of clinical material. Major clinical phenomena and disease processes are, in turn, analyzed in terms of normal and abnormal human biology. Thus, the books show how the art of modern clinical medicine involves firm scientific knowledge and the scientific approach in order to be effective.

Although designed for second-year medical students, this series will, we hope, be useful as well to more advanced students and practitioners as a readable and up-to-date review of the scientific basis for clinical practice in a given area.

DeWitt S. Goodman

Preface

Nothing in clinical medicine is as exciting as that moment when one understands the pathophysiology of the patient's condition and knows specific therapy that will reverse or impede the progress of that pathophysiologic process. Based on a solid understanding of both normal physiology and pathology, the pathophysiologic sequence of a particular disease is the key to understanding its natural history, its method of presentation, and the therapeutic approaches to its management.

I have tried to present in this short text a clear and concise overview of the pathophysiology of most of the common cardiovascular diseases. The myocardium is limited in the number of responses that it can make to a variety of pathological conditions: mechanical difficulties may arise resulting in heart failure, or electrical abnormalities may appear resulting in arrhythmias. The first thirteen chapters deal with heart failure and those conditions that commonly produce heart failure. Underlying renal and respiratory mechanisms in cardiac failure are discussed along with myocardial aspects. Chapter 14 is a discussion of cardiac electrical disturbances, the resultant arrhythmias, and their therapy. The last two chapters deal with peripheral cardiovascular disease and pulmonary embolism. There are three appendixes, the first of which briefly details clinical invasive and noninvasive techniques for quantitating myocardial contractile function. The second appendix is a series of questions, typical of the sort commonly given on national board examinations, dealing with the material presented in the text; the third appendix provides the answers to these questions. I believe that any student who reads this text carefully will come away with a firm understanding of the basic principles of cardiovascular pathophysiology so essential in the appropriate management of patients with these disorders.

Many individuals have aided me immeasurably in the preparation of this text. I would particularly like to acknowledge the secretarial assistance of Mrs. Marilyn Parks and Word Processing of Worcester. A number of the ideas and concepts expressed in this text were arrived at following discussions with my colleagues here at the University of Massachusetts Medical Center. The constant intelligent and incisive criticism of Lin Richter Paterson, former Medical Editor of Little,

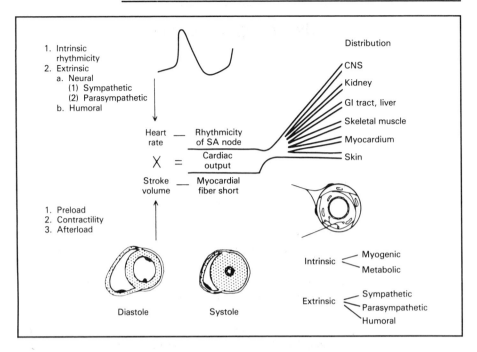

Fig. 1-1 : Schematic representation of the circulation. Cardiac output and its two determinants, heart rate and stroke volume, are central to circulatory control. Stroke volume is determined by preload, contractility, and afterload; heart rate is determined by intrinsic rhythmicity and extrinsic factors both neural and humoral. The cardiac output is distributed to a number of vascular beds. Regulation of the distribution of cardiac output depends on intrinsic and extrinsic influences on the arterioles. (From Braunwald E: Regulation of the circulation. *N Engl J Med* 290:1124–1129, 1420–1425, 1974, with permission of the author and publisher.)

Fig. 1-2 : The cardiac length-tension or Starling relationship. Any increase in preload or resting tension (up to a point) results in an increase in cardiac performance. Thus, increasing ventricular volume results in increasing stroke volume. Curve B is a Starling curve from a normal ventricle. Curve A is from a ventricle with increased myocardial contractility and Curve C is from a ventricle with depressed myocardial contractility.

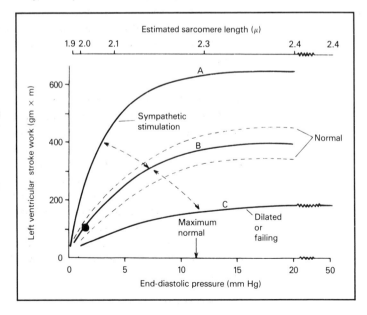

Afterload is defined as the tension in the myocardium during active contraction. This tension is determined by the resistance against which the myocardium is contracting. Thus, afterload is the work load facing the contracting myocardium. In the intact heart, afterload measurements commonly employed include ventricular systolic wall tension and ventricular systolic pressure.

Intrinsic myocardial contractility is the most difficult property of cardiac function to define. This feature of myocardial function relates to the intrinsic vigor or "oomph" of contraction of the myocardial fibers. Despite long-standing (and continuing) efforts to arrive at an ideal characterization of intrinsic myocardial contractility, no agreement has been reached on this entity. A number of variables have been suggested as truly reflecting intrinsic myocardial contractility (see Appendix A), and have been measured in clinical settings. For example, a number of measurements have been derived from recordings of the isovolumic phase of ventricular systole (rate of rise of isovolumic systolic pressure or dp/dt; maximum velocity of contraction or rate of pressure rise [V_{max}]). Unfortunately, these variables are not determined by intrinsic myocardial contractility alone, as preload and afterload exert some influence on them. Other contractility indices have been determined from analyses of ventricular wall motion obtained at the time of cardiac catheterization (see Appendix A). Variables such as ejection fraction (stroke volume/end-diastolic volume) and velocity of circumferential fiber shortening (V_{cf}) are derived in this manner. As with the indices derived from isovolumic systolic pressure recordings, ejection fraction and V_{cf} (so-called ejection phase indices) are also influenced by preload and afterload. Changes in myocardial contractility can also be demonstrated by constructing serial Starling curves. Thus, an increased myocardial inotropic state results in a movement of the Starling curve upward and to the left (Fig. 1-2). Depressed myocardial contractility results in movement of the Starling curve downward and to the right (Fig. 1-2).

None of the available measurements of myocardial contractility reflect perfectly the intrinsic state of myocardial contractility free from the influences of preload and afterload. On the other hand, each of the suggested indices reflects myocardial contractility at least in part, and most studies dealing with the state of myocardial contractility in the failing myocardium employ a number of different variables in the hope that abnormality in several of these measurements will be more meaningful than abnormality in a solitary index.

A large number of factors are capable of increasing (positively inotropic) or decreasing (negatively inotropic) myocardial contractility. As noted in Fig. 1-3, autonomic nervous stimulation, circulating catecholamines, acid-base disturbances, hypoxia, and a variety of other conditions and substances can alter myocardial contractile states.

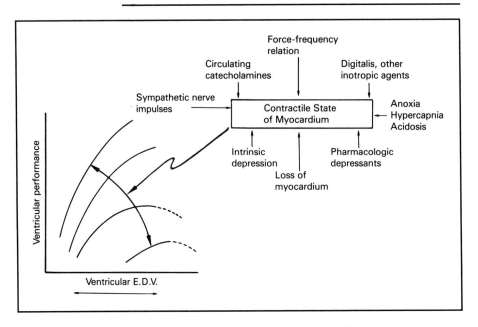

Fig. 1-3 : Factors that influence myocardial contractility. At the upper right are depicted a number of common factors that increase or decrease myocardial contractility. At the lower left are depicted the family of Starling curves that result from various levels of myocardial contractility. E.D.V. = ventricular end-diastolic volume, a measure of ventricular preload. (From Braunwald E, Ross J Jr, Sonnenblick, EH: *Mechanisms of Contraction of the Normal and Failing Heart.* Boston, Little, Brown, 1976, with permission of the authors and publisher.)

Cardiac output is determined by the product of heart rate times stroke volume. The three major variables just discussed (preload, afterload, and contractility) determine stroke volume. Heart rate is determined by properties of the cardiac cells themselves as well as by extrinsically acting influences, e.g., sympathetic and parasympathetic nerve stimulation and circulating catecholamine stimulation (Fig. 1-1). Cardiac output, systemic arterial pressure, and peripheral vascular resistance are related by the circulatory version of Ohm's law (E = IR), pressure = cardiac output $\times$ resistance. A number of factors affect peripheral vascular resistance. Metabolic by-products, or metabolites, relax vascular smooth muscle thereby producing vasodilation (Fig. 1-4). Intrinsic properties of vascular smooth muscle (myogenic factors) as well as extrinsic influences such as autonomic nerve stimulation and circulating catecholamines dilate or constrict arterioles, the major site of peripheral vascular resistance. Autonomic nerve stimulation and circulating catecholamines determine the extent to which the capacitance or storage section of the cardiovascular system, the veins, are dilated or constricted. Changes in venous capacity, in turn, result in alterations in venous return to the heart. Venous return, of course, determines preload, thereby effecting changes in stroke volume (Fig. 1-4). A number of other factors also

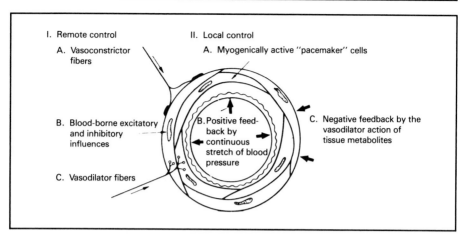

I. Remote control

  A. Vasoconstrictor fibers

  B. Blood-borne excitatory and inhibitory influences

  C. Vasodilator fibers

II. Local control

  A. Myogenically active "pacemaker" cells

  B. Positive feedback by continuous stretch of blood pressure

  C. Negative feedback by the vasodilator action of tissue metabolites

Fig. 1-4 : Factors that determine resistance of arterioles. Three local factors affect vascular smooth muscle tone (and hence vasoconstriction or vasodilatation): (1) smooth muscle pacemaker cells, (2) stretch on vascular smooth muscle from the level of the blood pressure, and (3) vasodilator metabolites. Distant factors may also affect vascular smooth muscle, e.g., sympathetic neural activity (vasoconstrictor and vasodilator fibers) and humoral influences such as catecholamines and hormones. (From Folkow B, Neil E: Principles of vascular control, in Folkow B, Neil E: *Circulation.* New York, Oxford University Press, 1971, chap. 16, pp 285–306, with permission of the authors and publisher.)

contribute to preload or the precontractile stretch of the myocardium (Fig. 1-5).

An understanding of the operation and integration of all of the controlling influences of the cardiovascular system can best be gained by observing what happens to the cardiovascular system during exercise. When exercise commences, local metabolites and sympathetic nerve stimulation (via beta-adrenergic vasodilator fibers) produce arteriolar vasodilatation in exercising skeletal muscles. Consequently, blood flow *increases* remarkably in these exercising muscles. At the same time that vasodilatation is occurring in exercising muscles, sympathetic nervous stimulation (via alpha-adrenergic vasoconstrictor fibers) produces vasoconstriction with resultant *decreases* in blood flow in a variety of other organ systems (skin, nonexercising muscle, kidneys, splanchnic bed). Beta-adrenergic stimulation of the heart results in increases in heart rate and myocardial contractility. The exercising muscles milk venous blood back towards the heart (the so-called muscle pump) thereby increasing venous return and preload. All of these influences on the heart cause an increase in cardiac output, an essential part of the circulatory system's response to exercise. The end result of these regulatory changes in cardiovascular function is a graded increase in cardiac output with increasing levels of exertion. The increased blood flow emanating from the left ventricle is distributed to the exercising muscles in order to satisfy

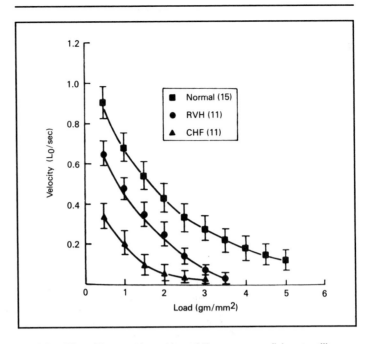

Fig. 1-7 : Effect of hypertrophy and heart failure on myocardial contractility. Force-velocity curves from three groups of cat papillary muscles. Force-velocity curves are one measure of myocardial contractility. Papillary muscles were obtained from cats with experimental right ventricular hypertrophy (RVH) and heart failure (CHF). Average values ± 1 standard error of the mean are given for each point. Note depressed myocardial function in hypertrophied and failing myocardium. (From Spann JF Jr et al: Contractile state of cardiac muscle obtained from cats with experimentally produced ventricular hypertrophy and heart failure. *Circ Res* 21:341, 1967, with permission of the authors and publisher.)

the most popular animal models of heart failure is that of pulmonary stenosis with or without tricuspid regurgitation. In such animals, the pulmonary artery is constricted by a surgical ligature. The tricuspid valve can be surgically damaged at the same time, thereby producing a regurgitant valve. These animals develop right ventricular failure. Examination of the contractile function of isolated pieces of right ventricular muscle from such animals demonstrates markedly reduced values for a variety of contractility indices (Fig. 1-7). Increments in contractility indices secondary to positive inotropic agents (for example, epinephrine) are also reduced in myocardial samples from animals with experimentally induced heart failure. Electron microscopic studies of myocardial samples from heart failure animals reveal no abnormality in structure, implying that derangements such as overstretching are not the cause of depressed myocardial contractility. Similar results, i.e., depressed myocardial contractility despite normal ultrastructural appearance, have been demonstrated in a variety of animal models of heart failure as well as in myocardial samples taken at the time of surgery from patients with heart failure. It is of interest that abnormal contractility indices become normal or near normal if the stimulus that induced heart failure is removed (for example, removing the ligature tied around the pulmonary artery).

Abnormal contractile performance has also been documented for the intact ventricle of animals with experimental heart failure. Depressed Starling curves similar to that depicted in Fig. 1-2 have been observed in such animals. Other measures of myocardial contractility such as V_{max} (velocity of shortening) and V_{cf} (velocity of circumferential fiber shortening) are also depressed in experimentally failing animal ventricles.

In the clinical setting, depressed myocardial contractility indices have been documented in patients with clinically overt heart failure using a variety of invasive (cardiac catheterization) and noninvasive (echocardiography, phonocardiography) techniques (Fig. 1-8).* For example, depressed contractility indices are not uncommon in asymptomatic patients with clinically compensated aortic stenosis, despite the fact that such individuals may have relatively normal cardiac outputs even with exercise. Abnormal isovolumic phase indices (for example, dp/dt, V_{max}) and ejection phase indices (ejection fraction, V_{cf}) are found in patients with heart failure.

Hemodynamic Alterations in Heart Failure

Patients with heart failure usually demonstrate a number of similar hemodynamic abnormalities regardless of the etiology of heart failure. Thus, the ventricles dilate with resultant increases in end-diastolic and end-systolic volume. Cardiac output decreases as a result of a depressed stroke volume. Heart rate is frequently increased in an effort to maintain cardiac output (cardiac output = stroke volume $\times$ heart rate). The combination of a decreased stroke volume and an increased end-diastolic volume results in a depressed ejection fraction (ejection fraction = stroke volume/end-diastolic volume). Ejection fraction is usually decreased below 50% in patients with heart failure; values as low as 5–10% are occasionally seen in severe heart failure.

Ventricular compliance is also frequently reduced in a variety of conditions leading to clinically overt heart failure. As noted earlier, decreased compliance is one of the contributing factors that elevate ventricular diastolic pressure. Increasing end-diastolic volume (the Starling mechanism) also contributes to elevation of the ventricular diastolic pressure (Fig. 1-6).

Biochemical Alterations in the Failing Myocardium

As we have already noted, the failing myocardium is characterized by depressed intrinsic contractility. Considerable effort has been expended on determining the subcellular mechanism for this decrease in contractile function. Consequently, numerous studies have exam-

*See Appendix A for a discussion of the various ways to measure contractility indices.

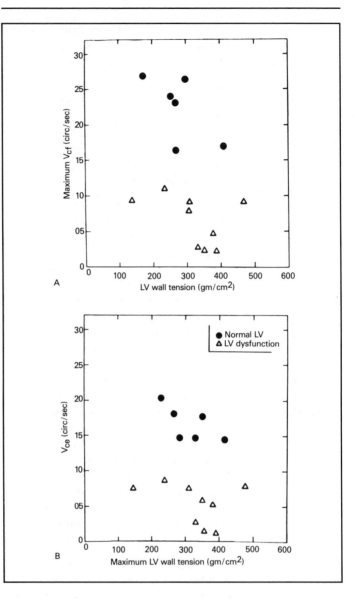

Fig. 1-8 : Myocardial contractility indices in patients with normal left ventricular function (normal LV) and abnormal left ventricular function (LV dysfunction). Two indices of myocardial contractility are depicted: (A) maximum velocity of circumferential fiber shortening (V_{cf}) and (B) velocity of the contractile elements (V_{ce}). Both contractility indices are plotted against corresponding levels of left ventricular wall tension expressed as grams per square centimeter (gm/cm²). circ/sec = circumferences/second. Note the abnormal values for V_{cf} and V_{ce} obtained from patients with left ventricular dysfunction. (From Gault JH, Ross J Jr, Braunwald E: Contractile state of the left ventricle in man: Instantaneous tension-velocity-length relations in patients with and without disease of the left ventricular myocardium. *Circ Res* 22:451, 1968, with permission of the authors and publisher.)

ined various aspects of myocardial metabolism, energy production, and contractile protein function in the failing myocardium. An occasional, unusual form of heart failure such as beriberi heart disease is associated with decreased adenosine triphosphate (ATP) production. In beriberi heart disease, depressed ATP production is the result of abnormally low myocardial levels of the co-factor, thiamine, resulting in impaired citric acid cycle (oxidative metabolic) function.

Depressed myocardial function may be the result of inadequate delivery of oxygen and substrates to myocardial cells, i.e., coronary artery disease. However, many diseases that result in heart failure develop despite completely normal coronary arteries and adequate myocardial nutritional blood flow. A number of investigators have demonstrated that mitochondrial oxidative phosphorylation, i.e., energy production, is abnormal in the experimentally and clinically failing myocardium. However, depressed mitochondrial energy production appears to be a very late finding in the failing myocardium. Therefore, this abnormality cannot explain the finding of depressed myocardial contractility early in the course of heart failure. In addition, normal levels of ATP and creatine phosphate have been documented in myocardium samples from animals with experimentally induced heart failure. Thus, in most forms of heart failure abnormal energy production is *not* the cause of reduced myocardial contractility.

Actin, myosin, and the structure of the assembled contractile protein apparatus are also normal in the failing myocardium. However, levels of the enzyme ATPase are reduced in myofibrils obtained from the failing myocardium of patients with clinical heart failure and from animals with experimentally induced heart failure. Despite this reduction in contractile protein-associated ATPase, the conversion of chemical energy to mechanical work in the failing myocardium is not inefficient. Indeed, recent work supports the hypothesis that the major abnormality in the failing myocardium is impairment of intracellular calcium (Ca^{2+}) regulation by the sarcoplasmic reticulum. Decreased reuptake of Ca^{2+} by the sarcoplasmic reticulum after each systole results in a greater than normal accumulation of Ca^{2+} in myocardial mitochondria. Such intracellular abnormalities in Ca^{2+} transport and binding interfere with normal myocardial cell excitation-contraction coupling. This latter abnormality combined with reduced myofibrillar ATPase activity would seem to be the molecular causes of the depression in myocardial contractility observed in the failing myocardium.

Alterations in the Autonomic Nervous System in Heart Failure

Norepinephrine concentration is markedly reduced in myocardial samples from animals with experimental heart failure and from patients with clinical heart failure (Fig. 1-9). Conversely, circulating and urinary excretion of norepinephrine is increased in patients with heart failure (Fig. 1-10). Thus, contractile function is supported by circulating rather than by endogenous norepinephrine in the failing myocardium.

Exercise leads to minimal changes in plasma norepinephrine levels in normal subjects. In patients with heart failure, however, exercise results in marked increases in plasma norepinephrine levels. Increased quantities of circulating norepinephrine in individuals with heart failure reflect increased adrenergic activity in the adrenal medulla and peripheral sympathetic nervous system.

The failing myocardium with depleted norepinephrine stores is hy-

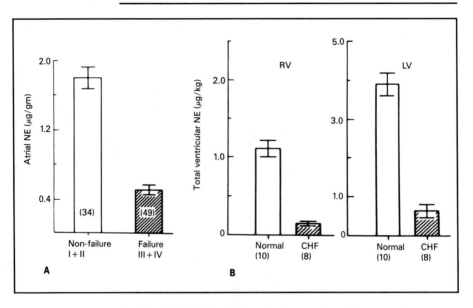

Fig. 1-9 : Effect of heart failure on cardiac norepinephrine stores. A. Concentration of norepinephrine (NE) in biopsies of atrial muscle obtained at open heart surgery from patients with heart failure (clinical classes III and IV) and without heart failure (clinical classes I and II). B. Total norepinephrine content of the right and left ventricles in normal dogs and in dogs with experimental heart failure. All graphs depict average values ± 1 standard error. Note depressed norepinephrine levels in failing myocardium. (From Braunwald E, Ross J Jr, Sonnenblick EH: *Mechanisms of Contraction of the Normal and Failing Heart.* **Boston, Little, Brown, 1976, with permission of the authors and publisher.)**

persensitive to the effects of infused exogenous norepinephrine. Thus, the failing myocardium exhibits a hypersensitive response to norepinephrine similar to that observed in the denervated myocardium. Levels of the enzyme, tyrosine hydroxylase, an enzyme employed in the synthesis of norepinephrine, are also reduced in samples of myocardium from animals with experimental heart failure. Apparently, reduced synthetic activity accounts for the reduced myocardial levels of norepinephrine in a failing heart muscle. Reversal of experimental heart failure is associated with replenishment of myocardial norepinephrine stores.

Despite increased levels of circulating norepinephrine in animals and humans with heart failure, maneuvers that are associated with acceleration in heart rate (mediated by cardiac sympathetic nerve stimulation) produce less cardioacceleration than normal in the face of heart failure. Thus, stimulation of the sympathetic cardioaccelerator nerve in animals with experimental heart failure results in a much smaller increase in heart rate than is observed in animals without heart failure. Parasympathetic nervous stimulation of the heart also produces less than the expected decrease in heart rate in patients with heart

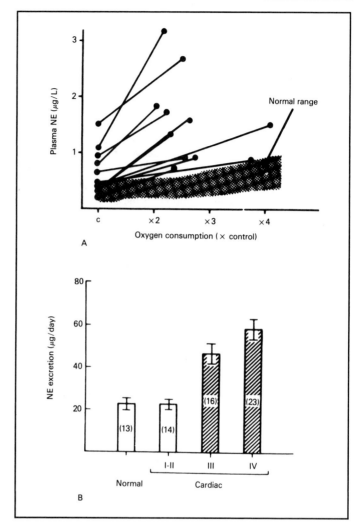

Fig. 1-10 : Plasma and urinary norepinephrine concentrations in patients with heart failure and in normal individuals. A. Plasma norepinephrine concentrations during exercise in patients with heart failure plotted against oxygen consumption levels obtained during exercise. Oxygen consumption during exercise is expressed as multiples of the resting oxygen consumption (c = resting value for oxygen consumption). The normal range of plasma norepinephrine values is demonstrated by the stippled area. B. Daily urinary norepinephrine excretion in normal individuals and in patients with heart failure (clinical classes III and IV) and without heart failure (clinical classes I and II). All graphs depict average values ± 1 standard error. (From Braunwald E, Ross J Jr, Sonnenblick EH: *Mechanisms of Contraction of the Normal and Failing Heart.* Boston, Little, Brown, 1976, with permission of the authors and publisher.)

Higgins CB et al: Effects of experimentally produced heart failure on the peripheral vascular response to severe exercise in conscious dogs. *Circ Res* 31:186–194, 1972.

Shepherd AP et al: Local control of tissue oxygen delivery and its contribution to the regulation of cardiac output. *Am J Physiol* 225:747–755, 1973.

Johnson PC: The microcirculation and local and humoral control of the circulation, in Jones CE, Guyton AC (eds): *Cardiovascular Physiology,* Physiology Series I: vol I. Baltimore, University Park Press, 1974.

Guyton AC, Coleman TG, Granger HJ: Circulation: Overall regulation. *Annu Rev Physiol* 34:13–46, 1972.

Ross J Jr, Braunwald E: Studies on Starling's law of the heart: IX. The effects of impeding venous return on performance of normal and failing human left ventricle. *Circulation* 30:719–727, 1964.

Katz AM: The descending limb of the Starling curve and the failing heart. *Circulation* 32:871–875, 1965.

Spann JF Jr et al: Contractile performance of the hypertrophied and chronically failing cat ventricle. *Am J Physiol* 223:1150–1157, 1972.

Zelis R et al: Peripheral circulatory control mechanisms in congestive heart failure. *Am J Cardiol* 32:481–490, 1972.

Epstein SE et al: Characterization of the circulatory response to maximal upright exercise in normal subjects and patients with heart disease. *Circulation* 35:1049–1062, 1967.

Zelis R, Mason DT, Braunwald E: Partition of blood flow to the cutaneous and muscular beds of the forearm at rest and during leg exercise in normal subjects and in patients with heart failure. *Circ Res* 24:799–806, 1969.

Higgins CB et al: Effects of experimentally produced heart failure on the peripheral vascular response to severe exercise in conscious dogs. *Circ Res* 31:186–194, 1972.

Spann JF Jr et al: Contractile state of cardiac muscle obtained from cats with experimentally produced ventricular hypertrophy and heart failure. *Circ Res* 21:341–354, 1967.

Spann JF Jr: Cardiac norepinephrine stores and the contractile state of heart muscle. *Circ Res* 19:317–325, 1966.

Kaufmann RL, Homburger H, Wirth H: Disorder of excitation contraction coupling of cardiac muscle from cats with experimentally produced right ventricular hypertrophy. *Circ Res* 28:346–357, 1971.

Cooper G IV et al: Normal myocardial function and energetics after reversing pressure-overload hypertrophy. *Am J Physiol* 226:1158–1165, 1974.

Chidsey CA et al: Norepinephrine stores and contractile force of papillary muscle from the failing human heart. *Circulation* 33:43–51, 1966.

Ross J Jr: Adaptations of left ventricle to chronic volume overload. *Circ Res* 35(suppl 2):64–69, 1974.

Dodge HT: Hemodynamics of cardiac failure, in Braunwald E (ed): *The Myocardium: Failure and Infarction.* New York, Hospital Practice, 1974, chap 7, pp 70–79.

Gault JH, Ross J Jr, Braunwald E: Contractile state of the left ventricle in man: Instantaneous tension-velocity-length relations in patients with and without disease of the left ventricular myocardium. *Circ Res* 22:451–463, 1968.

Mason DT: Regulation of cardiac performance in clinical heart disease: interactions between contractile state, mechanical abnormalities and ventricular compensatory mechanisms. *Am J Cardiol* 32:427–448, 1973.

Hugenholtz PG et al: Myocardial force-velocity relationships in clinical heart disease. *Circulation* 41:191–202, 1970.

Schwartz A et al: Abnormal biochemistry in myocardial failure. *Am J Cardiol* 32:407–422, 1973.

Katz AM: Biochemical "defect" in the hypertrophied and failing heart. *Circulation* 47:1076–1079, 1973.

Katz AM: Congestive heart failure—Role of altered myocardial cellular control. *N Engl J Med* 293:1184, 1975.

Wikmann-Coffelt J et al: Mechanism of impaired contractile protein function in aortic stenosis: Alterations in myosin ATPase activity in the chronically pressure overloaded canine left ventricle. *Am J Cardiol* 35:177, 1975.

Dhalla NS et al: Role of mitochondrial calcium transport in failing heart, in Dhalla NS (ed): *Recent Advances in Cardiac Structure and Metabolism*. Baltimore, University Park Press, 1975, vol 5.

Owens K et al: Fragmented sarcoplasmic reticulum of the cardiomyopathic Syrian hamster: Lipid composition Ca^{++} transport and Ca^{++} stimulated ATPase, in Dhalla NS (ed): *Myocardial Biology: Recent Advances in Studies on Cardiac Structure and Metabolism*. Baltimore, University Park Press, 1974, vol 4, pp 541–550.

Sordahl LA et al: Mitochondria and sarcoplasmic reticulum function in cardiac hypertrophy and failure. *Am J Physiol* 224:497–502, 1973.

Kim ND, Harrison CE: $^{45}Ca^{2+}$ accumulation by mitochondria and sarcoplasmic reticulum in chronic potassium depletion cardiomyopathy, in Dhalla NS (ed): *Myocardial Biology*. Baltimore, University Park Press, 1972, vol 4, pp 551–562.

Rutenberg HL, Spann JF Jr: Alterations in cardiac sympathetic neurotransmitter activity in congestive heart failure. *Am J Cardiol* 32:472–480, 1973.

Braunwald E, Chidsey CA: The adrenergic nervous system in the control of the normal and failing heart. *Proc R Soc Med* 58:1063–1066, 1965.

Thomas JA, Marks BH: Plasma norepinephrine in congestive heart failure. *Am J Cardiol* 4:233, 1978.

Eckberg DL, Drabinsky M, Braunwald E: Defective cardiac parasympathetic control in patients with heart disease. *N Engl J Med* 285:877–883, 1971.

Zelis R et al: Peripheral circulatory control mechanisms in congestive heart failure. *Am J Cardiol* 32:481, 1973.

Cohn JN: Vasodilator therapy for heart failure: The influence of impedance on left ventricular performance. *Circulation* 48:5–8, 1973.

Bristow MR et al: Decreased catecholamine sensitivity and β-adrenergic receptor density in failing human hearts. *N Engl J Med* 307:205, 1982.

2 : Myocardial Ischemia

Ischemic heart disease is the commonest cause of death in the United States. Coronary atherosclerosis can restrict myocardial blood flow with resultant inadequate myocardial nutritional blood flow (ischemia). Ischemia produces a number of biochemical and physiologic alterations in the myocardium. These alterations often lead to symptoms and disordered myocardial function that are recognized by physicians as the clinical expressions of coronary heart disease.

Myocardial Metabolism

Energy, in the form of adenosine triphosphate (ATP), is required by myocardial cells for the process of contraction. In the normal heart, these high-energy phosphate compounds are produced by aerobic metabolic pathways (i.e., the Krebs cycle) from glucose and fatty acid precursors. Since oxygen is required for these reactions, myocardial oxygen consumption (MVO_2) is closely coupled with total cardiac energy use. Indeed, the term *MVO_2* is often used to refer to the total amount of energy utilized by the heart, although this is not strictly correct since ATP can be generated by other, anaerobic, metabolic pathways (e.g., the Embden-Meyerhof or lactic acid cycle).

Myocardial oxygen consumption can be calculated by utilizing the Fick principle (number of grams of a substance extracted by an organ equals arteriovenous difference of the substance times blood flow to the organ). If one measures the arteriovenous oxygen difference across the heart and myocardial blood flow, one can calculate the total amount of oxygen extracted by the heart per minute (MVO_2). The myocardium is quite efficient in extracting oxygen from blood. Consequently, hemoglobin in the myocardial venous blood of the coronary sinus is quite desaturated (25–30% saturated; PO_2, 18–20 mm Hg). Thus, increasing myocardial metabolic demand (increasing MVO_2) must be met by increasing coronary blood flow, since only minimal increases in myocardial extraction of oxygen from blood are possible. Normal MVO_2 in humans is approximately 8.5 ml of O_2 per 100 gm of left ventricle.

A number of different factors determine the rate of myocardial oxygen consumption (Table 2-1). MVO_2 correlates directly with myocardial wall tension, which in turn varies directly with intracardiac systolic pressure and ventricular diameter and inversely with wall

Table 2-1 : Determinants of myocardial oxygen consumption

1. Myocardial wall stress or tension (intracardiac systolic pressure, ventricular diameter, and wall thickness)
2. Myocardial fiber shortening and cardiac work (stroke volume)
3. Level of myocardial contractility or inotropic state
4. Heart rate
5. Basal metabolism
6. Activation of contractile mechanism

thickness (Fig. 2-1). The first four determinants of myocardial oxygen consumption listed in Table 2-1 are more important than the last two. That is, only a small percentage of myocardial oxygen demand is related to basal metabolism or activation of the myocardial contractile mechanism. In addition, pressure work by the myocardium requires greater energy expenditure and hence greater oxygen consumption than flow work. Consequently, the first determinant of MVO_2 listed in Table 2-1, wall stress, accounts for a greater percentage of MVO_2 than does the third determinant, fiber shortening. Heart rate is also an important factor in determining MVO_2 (Fig. 2-2). Thus, of the six factors determining myocardial oxygen demand or metabolic rate, heart rate and wall tension (which includes blood pressure) are the two most important. As noted in Fig. 2-3, heart rate and blood pressure account for almost all of MVO_2 at rest. During exer-

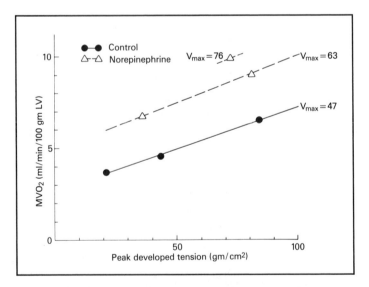

Fig. 2-1 : Myocardial oxygen consumption (MVO_2) plotted against peak developed myocardial tension in the isovolumetrically contracting isolated dog left ventricle. Solid circles show the effect on myocardial oxygen consumption of increasing tension at constant contractility (V_{max}). Triangles show the effect of increasing myocardial tension when myocardial contractility (V_{max}) is increased by norepinephrine. (From Graham TP Jr et al: The control of myocardial oxygen consumption: Relative influence of contractile state and tension development. *J Clin Invest* 47:375, 1968, with permission of the authors and publisher.)

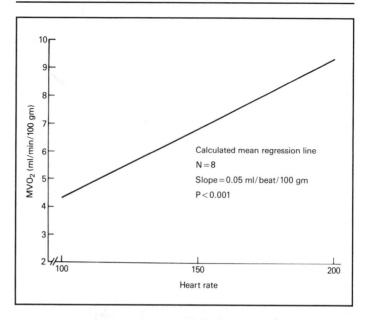

Fig. 2-2 : Effect of increasing heart rate on myocardial oxygen consumption (MVO₂) in the isovolumetrically contracting isolated dog left ventricle. The figure is the average of eight experiments. Note that doubling the heart rate results in a greater than twofold increase in myocardial oxygen consumption per minute. (From Boerth RC et al: Increased myocardial oxygen consumption and contractile state associated with increased heart rate. *Circ Res* 24:725, 1969, with permission of the authors and publisher.)

cise and isoproterenol infusion,[*] contractility accounts for an increasing portion of myocardial oxygen demand. Neosynephrine infusion produces increases in blood pressure and minimal changes in myocardial inotropic state. Thus, increases in MVO₂ during neosynephrine infusion are largely the result of increased wall tension (blood pressure). As depicted in Figure 2-3, stroke volume (myocardial fiber shortening) accounts for only a small percentage of MVO₂.

Clinicians frequently refer to the product of heart rate and blood pressure, often loosely termed the *tension time index*. This product is directly proportional to MVO₂ since it is calculated from two variables both of which are directly proportional to MVO₂.

Aerobic and anaerobic myocardial metabolism

The myocardium requires a constant supply of oxygen and nutrients in order to continue to generate sufficient ATP to sustain myocardial contraction. The heart is capable of utilizing a variety of substrates including glucose, fatty acids, lactate, pyruvate, acetate, ketone bodies and amino acids in the production of ATP. Under normal conditions, glucose and fatty acids are the major substrates that fuel myocardial production of ATP via oxidative metabolic pathways. The

[*] Isoproterenol infusion produces marked increases in heart rate and myocardial contractility.

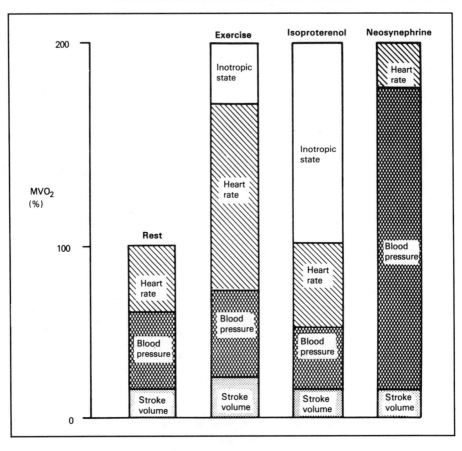

Fig. 2-3 : The various factors affecting myocardial oxygen consumption (MVO$_2$) at rest, during exercise in the normal heart, and during isoproterenol and neosynephrine infusion. Isoproterenol infusion increases myocardial contractility with minimal effect on blood pressure (afterload). Neosynephrine infusion increases blood pressure (afterload) without much effect on myocardial contractility. Note the relative contributions of systolic pressure development by the ventricle, heart rate, and increases in inotropic state on myocardial oxygen consumption. (Basal and activation oxygen consumption are not shown.) (From Ross JP Jr: *Changing Concepts in Cardiovascular Disease.* Baltimore, Williams & Wilkins, 1972, chap 4, pp 20–31, with permission of the author and publisher.)

heart prefers metabolizing free fatty acids if sufficient quantities of these substances are available. In fact, oxidative metabolism of fatty acids by the myocardium suppresses glucose utilization, particularly at rest. Under conditions of increasing MVO$_2$, both fatty acids and glucose fuel oxidative metabolic reactions leading to the production of ATP. Pyruvate and lactate are also frequently metabolized by the myocardium. Ketone bodies and amino acids, on the other hand, are only used to a minor degree.

Since large quantities of ATP are required by the myocardial contractile apparatus, it is not surprising that 36% of the total volume of cardiac muscle consists of mitochondria whose function is the production of ATP by oxidative metabolic pathways (for example, citric acid cycle).

In the presence of anoxia (perfusion with deoxygenated blood) or ischemia (cessation of perfusion), anaerobic metabolic reactions are utilized by the myocardium to produce ATP. However, only limited quantities of ATP can be produced by this route, which is capable of functioning for only brief periods of time. The anaerobic metabolic reactions (Embden-Meyerhof or lactic acid pathways) begin to produce ATP with lactic acid as a by-product when the level of oxygen tension in the myocardium falls below 5 mm Hg.

Greater resistance to the disruptive influence of anoxia or ischemia can be demonstrated in myocardial cells supplied with additional quantities of glucose and insulin during anoxic or ischemic conditions. Ischemia is not tolerated as well as anoxia because large quantities of by-products from anaerobic metabolic reactions (lactate, hydrogen ion) build up in the tissue under ischemic conditions. During anoxia, such metabolic waste products are washed out of the tissue by perfusion, albeit by deoxygenated blood. Consequently, ATP generation is much less in ischemic myocardium than it is in anoxic myocardium. Under normal conditions, myocardial cells metabolize lactate oxidatively to produce ATP and there is *extraction* of lactate by the myocardium. Under ischemic or anoxic conditions, when the myocardium is utilizing anaerobic reactions to produce ATP, lactate is *produced* by myocardial cells.

Ischemia has a profoundly negative effect on the intracellular environment of the myocardium: hydrolytic lysosomal enzymes are released into the cytoplasm, oxidation of fatty acids ceases, and these compounds accumulate in the cytoplasm resulting in intracellular lipid droplets, protein synthesis ceases while protein degradation accelerates, and membrane ion pumping mechanisms fail to maintain the normal transmembrane ionic gradients with resultant accumulation of electrolytes inside the myocardial cell. This deterioration in the internal milieu of the myocardial cell has a profound influence on the cell's ability to contract (see Alterations in Myocardial Metabolism During Ischemia.)

Regulation of Coronary Blood Flow

At rest, myocardial cells are most efficient at extracting oxygen from blood passing through the myocardial capillaries. Even at rest, myocardial cells extract almost all the oxygen possible (75–80%) from the perfusing blood. Thus, when MVO_2 is increased, by exercise, for example, the required increase in myocardial cell oxygen supply cannot be obtained by merely increasing myocardial cell oxygen extraction. Increased extraction of oxygen is commonly observed in other organs that experience sudden increases in metabolic rate, e.g., skel-

Table 2-3 : Partial list of pharmacologic agents with direct effects on coronary vascular smooth muscle

Vasodilators	Vasoconstrictors	Mixed
Isoproterenol	Digitalis glycosides	Norepinephrine (initial
Acetylcholine	Prostaglandin $F_{2\alpha}$	vasodilatation followed by
Nitrates	Angiotensin	vasoconstriction)
Dipyridamole	Propranolol and other β_2	Dopamine (initial vasoconstriction
Prostaglandins E and A	blockers	followed by vasodilatation)
Nitroprusside	Indomethacin	
Calcium channel blockers (e.g., nifedipine, verapamil)		
Bradykinin		

Apparently, there is constant, low-grade coronary vasoconstriction present under resting conditions mediated by the sympathetic nervous system. When myocardial oxygen demand is increased as it is during exercise, sympathetic alpha vasoconstriction decreases but does not cease entirely. Metabolic factors (vasodilators) oppose sympathetic alpha-receptor–mediated vasoconstriction during exercise and anoxia/ischemia. Cutaneous cold stimulation (the cold pressor response), particularly to the face, produces reflex coronary vasoconstriction.

Pharmacologic agents

A number of pharmacologic agents have direct effects on vascular smooth muscle causing either vasoconstriction or vasodilatation (Table 2-3). The various agents listed in Table 2-3 often have effects on vascular smooth muscle at different locations in the coronary vascular bed. For example, nitrates are more powerful in relaxing venous smooth muscle while nitroprusside has its major effect on arteriolar smooth muscle. In general, however, most of the agents listed affect arteriolar smooth muscle tone.

Causes and Effects of Myocardial Ischemia

In the vast majority of patients with myocardial ischemia, coronary arterial atherosclerosis is the underlying etiology. The pathophysiologic sequence that leads to coronary atherosclerosis is not fully understood. It is the subject of considerable investigation and controversy. Although it is beyond the scope of this text to include an extensive discussion of the pathogenesis of atherosclerosis, an abbreviated and simplified outline of current hypotheses is set out here.

Injury to the endothelium of medium and large arteries seems to be the initial triggering mechanism in the sequence that leads to atherosclerosis. Such endothelial injuries may be every-day occurrences in normal individuals or they may be unusual events brought on by cigarette smoking, hypertension, hyperlipidemia, or genetic predisposition.

Platelets and fibrin deposit in the area of the endothelial injury initiating a process of repair that can restore the arterial intima to normal. Under certain circumstances (for example, repeated endothelial injury or injury in the presence of hyperlipidemia or hypertension), arterial smooth muscle cells that migrate into the area of endothelial injury result in a proliferative lesion that tends to increase in size and complexity over long periods of time (months to years). Hypercholesterolemia contributes to the genesis of such proliferative lesions by increasing endothelial permeability and injury. A vicious cycle is initiated with repetitive endothelial injury, smooth muscle cell proliferation and deposition of cholesterol, other lipids, and residue from necrotic cells. This proliferating lesion thus becomes an atherosclerotic plaque (Fig. 2-4). Such early plaques are termed *fibrous* because of their highly cellular nature. With time, calcification, hemorrhage, and cell necrosis within the plaque convert it into a "complicated" lesion capable of ulceration with resultant embolization of plaque contents downstream or thrombosis at the site of the ulceration. In such a manner, complicated plaques produce significant narrowing or total obstruction of medium-sized and large arteries.

As the atherosclerotic process leads to progressive obstruction of the coronary arterial system in patients with ischemic heart disease, a compensatory mechanism, the development of collateral circulation, is set into motion. Collateral vessels are anastomotic vessels connecting coronary arteries without an intervening capillary bed. Collateral vessels exist in all normal mammalian hearts, but under normal circumstances they remain quite small. Some species are richly endowed with coronary collateral vessels, e.g., dogs, while other species have relatively few of these reserve blood vessels, e.g., pigs and man. When high-grade obstruction (90%) of a major coronary artery develops, collateral vessels rapidly increase in size and capacity in order to carry substantial amounts of blood flow. However, despite such growth, collateral vessels are rarely if ever capable of supplying normal amounts of blood flow to the involved region of myocardium. In other words, compensatory collateral blood flow in man never achieves levels that occur under normal circumstances with unobstructed coronary arteries. Collateral blood flow is frequently adequate to satisfy resting myocardial metabolic demands. At increased levels of myocardial oxygen consumption, e.g., during exercise, collateral blood flow is insufficient to meet metabolic demand, and ischemia results. Growth and development of collateral vessels is stimulated by myocardial hypoxia. Collateral circulation regresses if coronary arterial obstruction is relieved.

Alterations in myocardial metabolism during ischemia

When myocardial metabolic demand exceeds myocardial nutritional blood flow, ischemia results. A number of metabolic alterations occur in myocardial cells during periods of ischemia. Under normal circumstances, myocardial cells utilize a variety of substrates for energy production including glucose, fatty acids, lactate, pyruvate, acetate, ketone bodies, and even amino acids, although glucose and fatty acids (particularly the latter) are favored energy sources. Myocardial

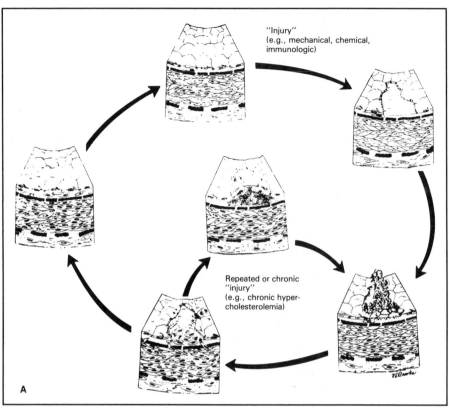

"Injury"
(e.g., mechanical, chemical, immunologic)

Repeated or chronic
"injury"
(e.g., chronic hyper-
cholesterolemia)

A

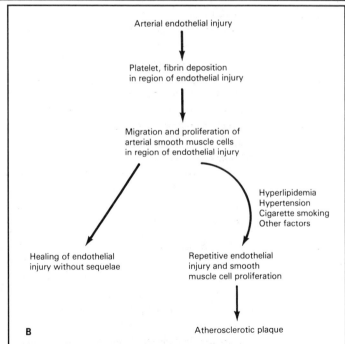

Arterial endothelial injury

Platelet, fibrin deposition
in region of endothelial injury

Migration and proliferation of
arterial smooth muscle cells
in region of endothelial injury

Hyperlipidemia
Hypertension
Cigarette smoking
Other factors

Healing of endothelial
injury without sequelae

Repetitive endothelial
injury and smooth
muscle cell proliferation

Atherosclerotic plaque

B

cells are richly endowed with mitochondria for production of high energy phosphate compounds via oxidative metabolic reactions.

Within 15 seconds of the onset of ischemia, myocardial contractile function becomes depressed, intracellular levels of high energy phosphate compounds decline, and anaerobic metabolic reactions are activated to produce ATP with lactate production as a by-product. The preferred metabolic substrate in ischemic myocardium is glucose rather than the fatty acids utilized under normal circumstances. If high levels of glucose and insulin are present in the environment surrounding ischemic myocardial cells, glucose transport into the cell is increased with resultant stimulation of anaerobic production of ATP. In addition, glycogen, stored in myocardial cells, is broken down and metabolized anaerobically under ischemic conditions. Despite these compensatory metabolic processes, normal levels of high energy phosphate compounds are *not* supplied to myocardial cells during ischemia. Anaerobic metabolic generation of ATP is associated with the production of lactate rather than the consumption of this substrate that occurs during normal oxidative metabolism.

Other metabolic alterations that occur in the myocardium during ischemia include intra- and extracellular acidosis, intracellular lipid accumulation, mitochondrial injury, depression of intracellular protein synthesis, and inhibition of the cell membrane ion pumping mechanism.

Alterations in myocardial contractile performance during ischemia

Marked depression of myocardial contractile performance occurs within 10–15 seconds of the onset of myocardial ischemia. Depression of myocardial contractility during ischemia is the result of reduced release of intracellular calcium ions from the sarcoplasmic reticulum. With in vitro preparations, the extent to which myocardial contractility is depressed during ischemia depends on the severity of the ischemia, the level of myocardial metabolic demand, and the availability of glucose and insulin in the surrounding environment. Severe ischemia results in total cessation of myocardial contraction. In the intact ventricle, ischemia produces depression or cessation of

Fig. 2-4 : A. Hypothetical cycle of events that lead to atherosclerosis. The large cycle represents what probably occurs in all persons at varying times: endothelial injury leads to desquamation, platelet adherence, aggregation, and release, followed by smooth muscle proliferation and connective tissue formation. When the injury is a single isolated event, the lesion can go on to heal and regress leaving a slightly thickened intima. The smaller inner cycle suggests the possible consequences of repeated or chronic injury to the epithelium with lipid deposition and smooth muscle proliferation continuing and leading eventually to a complicated atherosclerotic lesion containing newly formed connective tissue, lipids, and eventually calcification. It is this kind of complicated atherosclerotic lesion that leads to clinical sequelae such as thrombosis and infarction. (From Ross R, Glomset JA: The pathogenesis of atherosclerosis. *N Engl J Med* 295:420, 1976, with permission of the authors and publisher.) B. Hypothesis for generation of atherosclerotic plaques (see text).

contraction in the ischemic zone of myocardium with resultant declines in overall ventricular stroke work and contractility indices such as dp/dt or V_{max} (velocity of shortening) (Fig. 2-5). When viewed in experimental animals, ischemic regions of myocardium cease contracting, become cyanotic, and eventually bulge passively during each ventricular systole (Fig. 2-6).

Diastolic myocardial function is also impaired by ischemia since myocardial cellular relaxation is an energy-requiring process. Thus, ischemic myocardial cells relax incompletely, demonstrating depressed compliance (increased stiffness). In the intact ventricle, this translates into increased ventricular diastolic stiffness with resultant increases in ventricular diastolic (filling) pressures (Fig. 2-5). Patients with angina pectoris frequently have elevations in left ventricular diastolic pressure that resolve with relief of ischemia.

Distribution of coronary blood flow during myocardial ischemia

As noted earlier, compression of coronary blood vessels is greater in the subendocardium than in the epicardium because compressive stress in a thick-walled sphere is highest at the inner surface and falls progressively toward its outer surface. Consequently, there is a greater impediment to coronary blood flow in the subendocardium than in the epicardium; subendocardial vessels are therefore relatively dilated even under normal circumstances. Because of this relative underperfusion, the subendocardium can become ischemic with even moderate decreases in total coronary blood flow. Vasodilatation occurs in the myocardium in response to increased MVO_2. However, since the vessels in the subendocardial zone are already vasodilated, decreased coronary blood flow results in ischemia. The subendocardium is therefore said to exhibit decreased coronary vascular reserve. In patients with angina pectoris, ischemia develops first in the subendocardium.

Pathophysiology of angina pectoris

Angina pectoris is an uncomfortable sensation that patients experience during episodes of myocardial ischemia. Myocardial ischemia (and hence angina pectoris) occurs when coronary blood flow is insufficient to meet the metabolic requirements of the contracting myocardium. Two circumstances can lead to an imbalance between myocardial blood flow and myocardial oxygen demand with resultant myocardial ischemia: (1) a decrease in myocardial blood flow with constant MVO_2 (inadequate supply), and (2) an increase in MVO_2 with constant myocardial blood flow (excessive demand).

The underlying pathological state in the vast majority of patients with angina pectoris is coronary arterial atherosclerosis. Atherosclerotic lesions narrow or occlude the coronary arterial lumen with resultant depression of coronary blood flow. Under resting conditions, a reduction in the coronary arterial lumen of approximately 90% must occur before a marked decrease in coronary blood flow occurs (Fig.

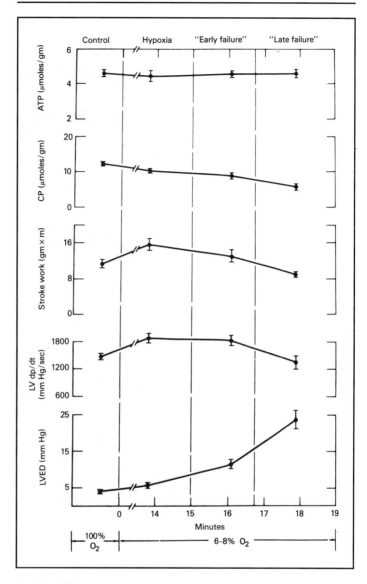

Fig. 2-5 : Effect of hypoxia on a variety of left ventricular function measurements in anesthetized open chest dogs. Three experimental periods are shown: early hypoxia, early left ventricular failure induced by continued hypoxia, and severe failure induced by continued hypoxia. It can be seen that there is a progressive deterioration in left ventricular function from early hypoxic through late hypoxic induced heart failure. ATP levels in the myocardium (ATP) do not change during this experimental protocol. However, creatine phosphate (CP) levels fall progressively during the hypoxic period. LV dp/dt = peak first derivative of the left ventricular pressure pulse, a measure of left ventricular myocardial contractility. LVED = left ventricular end-diastolic pressure. (From Pool PE et al: Myocardial high energy phosphate stores in acutely induced hypoxic heart failure. *Circ Res* 19:221, 1966, with permission of the authors and publisher.)

Tennant R, Wiggers CJ: The effect of coronary occlusion on myocardial contraction. *Am J Physiol* 112:351–361, 1935.

Braunwald E: Control of myocardial oxygen consumption: Physiologic and clinical considerations. *Am J Cardiol* 27:416–432, 1971.

Schwartz A et al: Biochemical and morphologic correlates of cardiac ischemia. *Am J Cardiol* 32:46–60, 1973.

Neely JR et al: Effects of ischemia on function and metabolism of the isolated working rat heart. *Am J Physiol* 225:651–658, 1973.

Liedtke AJ, Hughes HC, Neely JR: Metabolic responses to varying restrictions of coronary blood flow in swine. *Am J Physiol* 228:655–662, 1975.

Herman MV, Elliott WC, Gorlin R: An electrocardiographic, anatomic, and metabolic study of zonal myocardial ischemia in coronary heart disease. *Circulation* 35:834–846, 1967.

Neill WA: Myocardial hypoxia and anaerobic metabolism in coronary heart disease. *Am J Cardiol* 22:507–515, 1968.

Katz AM: Effects of ischemia on the contractile processes of heart muscle. *Am J Cardiol* 32:456–460, 1973.

Weisfeldt ML: Incomplete relaxation between beats after myocardial hypoxia and ischemia. *J Clin Invest* 53:1626–1636, 1974.

Amsterdam EA: Function of the hypoxic myocardium: Experimental and clinical aspects. *Am J Cardiol* 32:461–471, 1973.

Chatterjee K et al: Influence of direct myocardial revascularization on left ventricular asynergy and function in patients with coronary heart disease. *Circulation* 47:276–286, 1973.

Barry WH et al: Changes in diastolic stiffness and tone of the left ventricle during angina pectoris. *Circulation* 49:255–263, 1974.

Parker JO et al: Sequential alterations in myocardial lactate metabolism, S-T segments, and left ventricular function during angina induced by atrial pacing. *Circulation* 40:113–131, 1969.

Bache RJ, Cobb FR, Greenfield JC Jr: Myocardial blood flow distribution during ischemia-induced coronary vasodilatation in the unanesthetized dog. *J Clin Invest* 54:1462–1472, 1974.

Bloor CM: Functional significance of the coronary collateral circulation. *Am J Pathol* 6:562–587, 1974.

Khouri EM, Gregg DE, Lowensohn HS: Flow in the major branches of the left coronary artery during experimental coronary insufficiency in the unanesthetized dog. *Circ Res* 23:99–108, 1968.

Cannon PJ, Dell RB, Dwyer EM: Regional myocardial perfusion rates in patients with coronary artery disease. *J Clin Invest* 51:978–994, 1972.

Brazier J, Cooper M, Buckberg G: The adequacy of subendocardial oxygen delivery: The interaction of determinants of flow, arterial oxygen content and myocardial oxygen need. *Circulation* 49:968–977, 1974.

Vatner SF et al: Effects of carotid sinus nerve stimulation on the coronary circulation of the conscious dog. *Circ Res* 27:11–21, 1970.

Vatner SF et al: Coronary dynamics in unrestrained conscious baboons. *Am J Physiol* 221:1396–1401, 1971.

3 : Myocardial Infarction

As noted in the last chapter, myocardial ischemia produces severe derangement of myocardial cell function. Interruption of the delivery of oxygen and nutrients to myocardial cells results in falling intracellular levels of high-energy phosphate compounds that are required for contraction as well as for maintenance of cellular integrity. Anaerobic metabolic pathways can generate modest amounts of these high-energy compounds albeit at the expense of increasing intracellular and extracellular acidosis. At some point during ongoing ischemia even anaerobic production of ATP is not sufficient for normal cellular processes to continue and essential cellular metabolic functions cease. Shortly thereafter, irreversible changes develop in the myocardial cell which consequently undergoes necrosis. Ischemic myocardial cells demonstrate a defect in Ca^{2+} release from the sarcoplasmic reticulum. In fact, severely ischemic myocardial cells have marked binding of Ca^{2+} to the sarcoplasmic reticulum. In addition, both mitochondrial and sarcolemmal (cell membrane associated) Na^+/K^+ ATPase activity is markedly impaired.

Individual myocardial cells differ in their ability to resist ischemia. Thus, some cells may survive prolonged episodes of ischemia while others succumb after shorter episodes of inadequate substrate delivery. Irreversible disruption in myocardial cellular function is characterized by increasing permeability of the cell membrane. The Na^+/K^+ ionic gradient is no longer maintained with resultant loss of electrical polarization. Intracellular $Na+$ and water content increase resulting in cellular swelling. In addition, compounds essential to normal myocardial cellular function (e.g., creatine phosphokinase [CK]) leak out of the cell and are lost. Mitochondrial integrity is also lost and lysosomal enzymes are released into the cytoplasm resulting in further disruption of myocardial cellular structure and function. Lysosomal enzyme activation occurs relatively late in the course of myocardial necrosis—24–28 hours after the cessation of myocardial blood flow.

Other disruptive metabolic changes that develop shortly after the onset of ischemia include inhibition of protein synthesis and reduction in the intracellular level of carnitine palmital coenzyme A, a mitochondrial enzyme important in the oxidation of long-chain fatty acids. This latter alteration results in intracellular accumulation of toxic nonesterified fatty acids, thereby further hastening myocardial cellular demise.

Ultrastructural Alterations During Myocardial Necrosis

The earliest myocardial ultrastructural changes that have been observed following coronary arterial ligation consist of reduction in size and number of glycogen granules, development of intracellular edema, and swelling and distortion of the transverse tubular system, sarcoplasmic reticulum, and mitochondria. These changes are reversible with the reestablishment of myocardial blood flow. Irreversible changes start to appear 20 minutes to 2 hours after coronary ligation. In addition to worsening of the above-mentioned changes, other irreversible alterations in subcellular structure include loss of distinctness of tight junctions, swollen sacs of the sarcoplasmic reticulum, greatly enlarged mitochondria with few cristae, thinning and fractionation of the myofilaments, alterations in nuclear structure, disorientation of myofibrils, and clumping of mitochondria (Fig. 3-1). Irreversibly damaged myocardial cells are invariably swollen; the sarcolemma may even peel off the cells. Defects in the plasma membrane and fragmentation of mitochondria are also frequently noted. Deposits of calcium phosphate and other amorphous material are observed in the swollen, damaged mitochondria. It is of interest that biochemical and physiologic abnormalities can be demonstrated in ischemic myocardial cells within moments after the onset of ischemia. Ultrastructural changes in cellular architecture, however, require many minutes to hours to develop.

Changes in Myocardial Function Resulting from Myocardial Necrosis

Isolated myocardium

As noted in Chapter 2, ischemic myocardium demonstrates a marked depression in contractility. Indeed, within a few minutes of interrupting myocardial oxygenation, all myocardial contractile activity ceases. Ischemic myocardial cells also demonstrate marked impairment of diastolic myocardial function (relaxation). Studies in isolated papillary muscles reveal that myocardial diastolic function may be so severely impaired that there is incomplete relaxation of myocardial fibers even at end-diastole (end-diastolic contracture). Such incomplete relaxation results in a marked increase in myocardial stiffness (decreased compliance).

Reversal of systolic and diastolic myocardial dysfunction occurs if the myocardial oxygen supply is reestablished after a brief period of interruption. The greater the period of ischemia, the longer it takes for normal myocardial contractility and relaxation to return. Irreversible

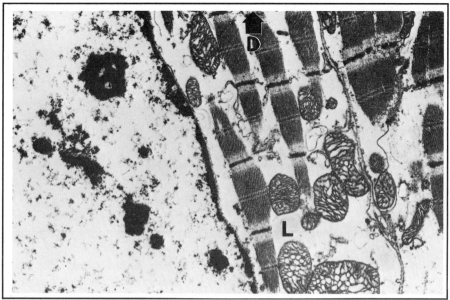

C

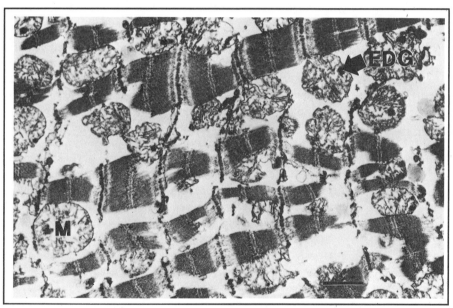

D

are vacuolated and edematous and lipid droplets (L) enlarge the cytoplasmic space. D. Myocardium subjected to 90 minutes of total ischemia and 15 minutes of reperfusion. The mitochondria (M) are swollen and frequently contain electron-dense granules (EDG) associated with irreversible myocardial cell injury. For each of these figures the bar to the lower right of B and D represents the distance of 1μ. (From Sleight P, Sobel B: *The Pathophysiology and Management of Heart Disease: Myocardial Infarction*. London, MEDI-CINE, Ltd., 1981, with permission of the authors and publisher.)

Fig. 3-2 : The vicious
cycle of myocardial
ischemia-infarction.
Ischemia or infarction
result in decreased
myocardial function
with consequent in-
creases in the deter-
minants of myocardial
oxygen demand.
Thus, myocardial oxy-
gen demand increases
in the face of decreas-
ing myocardial oxy-
gen supply.

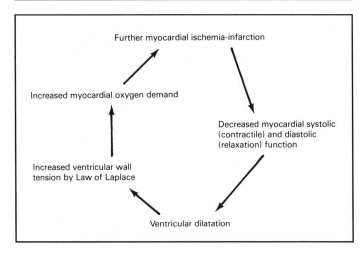

Further myocardial ischemia-infarction

Increased myocardial oxygen demand

Decreased myocardial systolic (contractile) and diastolic (relaxation) function

Increased ventricular wall tension by Law of Laplace

Ventricular dilatation

mental effects: (1) hemorrhage increases the stiffness of the infarct zone, thereby decreasing left ventricular compliance (increased stiffness) with resultant elevation in left ventricular filling pressure (pulmonary capillary pressure) and (2) hemorrhage increases the frequency and severity of certain malignant ventricular arrhythmias that are associated with the acute phase of myocardial infarction.

Acute myocardial infarction has a profound effect on left ventricular diastolic function. Both ischemia and infarction result in abnormal myocardial relaxation. Initially, ischemic myocardial zones are subjected to repetitive passive stretching because these regions are tethered to actively contracting nonischemic myocardium. This process of repetitive stretching results in a decrease in myocardial diastolic stiffness (increased compliance) in the ischemic myocardial zone. Decreased stiffness in the ischemic region results in decreased overall ventricular diastolic stiffness. In the intact ventricle, the ischemic zone of myocardium bulges passively, thereby impairing overall ventricular contractile function and leading to an increase in end-diastolic volume (Starling mechanism). Increased ventricular volume results in an increase in ventricular wall tension (by the law of Laplace), thereby increasing myocardial oxygen demand. Such augmentation in myocardial oxygen demand can be detrimental since it may lead to increases in the quantity of ischemic myocardium (Fig. 3-2).

Within hours of the onset of coronary occlusion, edema and cellular infiltration in the necrotic and ischemic zone of myocardium results in an increase in myocardial and overall ventricular stiffness. Thus, the initial transient decrease in ventricular stiffness (increased compliance) is followed by an increase in stiffness (decreased compliance). Ventricular filling pressure rises secondary to decreased compliance. Pulmonary congestion results from such increases in ventricular filling pressure (see following).

Effect of Myocardial Infarction on Cardiac Function in Man

It should come as no surprise that myocardial infarction results in ventricular dysfunction in human beings. Myocardial infarction in man predominantly affects the left ventricle, although right ventricular infarction with right ventricular dysfunction does occur. The extent of ventricular dysfunction is directly dependent on the volume of infarcted and ischemic myocardium. In other words, the larger the infarct the more severe the ventricular dysfunction.

Within hours after the onset of myocardial infarction, decreased systolic contractile function in and around the zone of myocardial necrosis results in ventricular dilatation (Starling mechanism). Cessation of regional contractile function coupled with the increase in myocardial stiffness that accompanies infarction results in increased ventricular filling pressure that is transmitted during diastole to the left atrium, pulmonary veins, and finally to the pulmonary capillaries. Increased pulmonary capillary pressure results in increased transudation of fluid into the pulmonary parenchyma, producing abnormal pulmonary compliance and blood gas exchange that are sensed by the patient as dyspnea.

Extensive myocardial necrosis in one region of the ventricle results in passive bulging (dyskinesis) of that zone of myocardium during systole when the rest of the ventricle contracts. Some of the kinetic energy imparted to the blood during systolic contraction is lost when a portion of the ventricle bulges passively during systole. Thus, a dyskinetic zone of myocardium impairs overall ventricular function in two ways: (1) the ventricle loses the contractile function of the dyskinetic zone and (2) a zone of passively bulging myocardium absorbs some of the kinetic energy meant for the blood that is being pumped into the aorta. Left ventricular dyskinesis can be identified by the examining physician. An abnormal bulging impulse is felt during precordial palpation.

A number of abnormalities of circulatory regulation develop during the acute phase of myocardial infarction (Fig. 3-3). Coronary arterial obstruction causes myocardial necrosis and ischemia with resultant systolic left ventricular dysfunction. Stroke volume falls, depressing cardiac output and peripheral perfusion. If arterial blood pressure falls secondary to the decrease in cardiac output, myocardial blood flow may also decrease with resultant expansion of the zone of myocardial ischemia and necrosis. When 40% of the left ventricle is inactivated secondary to ischemia and infarction, cardiac output falls below the level that is required to maintain perfusion of vital organs—cardiogenic shock results.

A number of compensatory circulatory mechanisms oppose the deleterious effects of a myocardial infarction. Activation of the sympathetic nervous system increases both circulating norepinephrine and cardiac sympathetic nervous stimulation, resulting in increases in

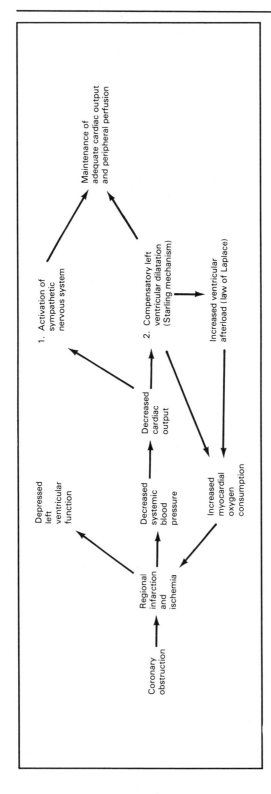

Fig. 3-3 : Circulatory regulation in patients with ischemic heart disease. Detrimental and compensatory mechanisms in patients with ischemic heart disease are shown.

myocardial contractile force, heart rate, and cardiac output. Ventricular dilatation (Starling mechanism) also opposes the decrease in cardiac output that accompanies myocardial infarction (Fig. 3-3). Unfortunately, these compensatory mechanisms may exaggerate myocardial ischemia by increasing myocardial oxygen consumption, thereby producing further ischemic myocardial dysfunction and worsening hemodynamic deterioration. Increases in heart rate, myocardial contractility, and ventricular volume (increased wall tension) all work to increase myocardial oxygen consumption. Since myocardial blood supply is already compromised, increases in myocardial oxygen consumption can accentuate and extend myocardial ischemia and necrosis. If the extent of regional myocardial dysfunction secondary to ischemia and infarction is modest, the beneficial effects of the compensatory mechanisms predominate, and circulatory homeostasis is maintained. When large quantities of left ventricular myocardium become ischemic and/or necrotic, the combination of marked left ventricular dysfunction and the deleterious effect of the compensatory mechanisms on myocardial oxygen demand combine to produce spiraling circulatory deterioration (Fig. 3-3).

Another potentially deleterious event that can occur in large myocardial infarcts is infarct expansion. Weakened, necrotic myocardial fibers are disrupted by normal systolic and diastolic wall stress. This disruption of the normal integrity of myocardial muscle bundles causes the noncontracting zone of ischemic and necrotic myocardium to expand. It is obvious that overall ventricular function suffers when a noncontracting zone of myocardium expands.

Distribution of Coronary Blood Flow in Myocardial Infarction

As noted earlier (Chap. 2, Causes and Effects of Myocardial Ischemia), resting coronary blood flow in humans with arteriosclerotic heart disease is usually adequate to maintain normal myocardial aerobic metabolism. However, if myocardial metabolic demand is increased (e.g., during exercise), the myocardial demand outstrips myocardial blood supply and ischemia develops in myocardial zones distal to obstructive coronary arterial lesions. Since obstructive coronary arterial lesions may occur in any combination of coronary arteries, marked differences in myocardial blood flow can occur during exercise (and occasionally at rest) in different myocardial zones. Thus, one zone of myocardium, supplied by a normal coronary artery, receives a normally increased quantity of blood during exercise while an adjacent zone, supplied by a markedly narrowed coronary vessel, becomes ischemic.

Following total obstruction of a coronary artery by thrombosis or coronary spasm, myocardial blood flow declines precipitously in the zone distal to the arterial obstruction and myocardial ischemia and necrosis ensue. With the development of myocardial infarction and subsequent scar formation, blood flow remains low in the infarct zone. Clinically available radioisotopic techniques can identify zones of previously infarcted myocardium by virtue of the persistently low level of blood flow in such regions. Blood flow remains low in such myocardial zones even if coronary arterial patency is reestablished, because the metabolic demand of fibrous tissue is much lower than that of myocardium.

It is essential for mean aortic blood pressure to remain above 60–70 mm Hg in patients with acute myocardial infarction, because coronary autoregulation is lost at levels of blood pressure below this point. The coronary arteries are then maximally dilated and further decline in aortic blood pressure results in a concomitant decrease in myocardial blood flow with obviously deleterious effects on myocardial function and infarct size.

Coronary vasomotor tone can be altered pharmacologically. Thus, a variety of compounds are capable of relaxing coronary arterial smooth muscle, thereby producing coronary vasodilatation. If coronary perfusion pressure remains constant, coronary vasodilatation leads to an increase in myocardial blood flow. Nitroglycerin is the best known coronary vasodilator. Increases in myocardial blood flow to ischemic zones have been demonstrated following the administration of nitroglycerin to animals with experimental infarction.

Beneficial redistribution of myocardial blood flow from normal to ischemic zones is a desirable therapeutic goal in patients with ischemic heart disease with or without myocardial infarction. Nitroglycerin produces such a redistribution of blood flow through a combination of direct effects on coronary blood vessels and indirect effects on systemic blood vessels (with resultant decrease in ventricular cavity distension and systemic blood pressure). Other pharmacologic agents such as the adrenergic beta-receptor blocker, propranolol, have also been shown to promote beneficial redistribution of myocardial blood flow from normal to ischemic myocardial zones. Propranolol promotes myocardial blood flow redistribution to ischemic zones by reducing myocardial contractility and heart rate, which, in turn, lead to decreasing myocardial metabolic demand in normal zones as well as diminished systolic extravascular compression of coronary arteries.

A number of compounds have been developed for clinical use that produce an increase in myocardial contractility (positively inotropic). Such agents *may* have a deleterious effect on the myocardial supply-demand ratio. Thus, the administration of the adrenergic beta-receptor stimulant, isoproterenol, can produce a marked increase in myocardial contractility with a concomitant increase in myocardial metabolic demand. Although coronary perfusion pressure may increase secondary to increased stroke volume, the increase in myocardial metabolic demand may actually exceed the rise in stroke volume. Thus, the end result of isoproterenol administration can be improved

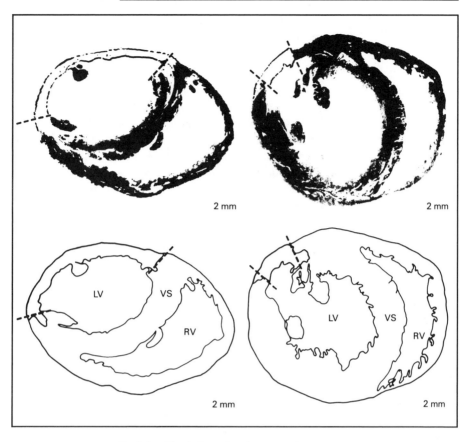

Fig. 3-4 : Histologic sections (*upper panels*) and diagrams (*lower panels*) of transverse slices of rat heart in animals killed 21 days after occlusion of the left main coronary artery. The animal on the left is a control animal that received no treatment. The animal on the right received hyaluronidase therapy. It is evident that the hyaluronidase-treated animal has a much smaller infarct than the control animal. The control animal had an infarct involving 54% of the endocardial circumference of the left ventricle while the hyaluronidase-treated animal had an infarct involving only 20% of the endocardial circumference of the left ventricle. LV= left ventricle, RV = right ventricle, VS = ventricular septum. (From Muller JE et al: *Preservation of the Ischemic Myocardium.* Kalamazoo, Mich, Upjohn Co., 1977, with permission of the authors and publisher.)

myocardial function at the expense of markedly increased myocardial metabolic demand with resultant accentuation of myocardial ischemia and possible necrosis.

A considerable effort has been made in recent years to determine if the extent or size of a particular myocardial infarct can be altered pharmacologically by applying some of the principles just discussed. For example, experimental infarct size, measured in a variety of ways in a variety of animal models, can be reduced by intravenous administration of a number of agents including nitroglycerin and propranolol (Fig. 3-4). Some pharmacologic substances decrease infarct size by depressing myocardial metabolic demand while other compounds decrease infarct size by improving substrate delivery to ischemic myocardial cells. Additional pharmacologic agents decrease experimental infarct size by other mechanisms.

It is still unclear whether pharmacologic interventions aimed at reducing infarct size are effective in humans with myocardial infarction. In experimental animal models, interventions must be performed within 2 to 6 hours after coronary occlusion in order to obtain a measurable reduction in infarct size. Many patients with myocardial infarction arrive at the hospital more than 6 hours after the onset of infarction. Such individuals probably arrive too late for any intervention to alter the size of the necrotic zone of myocardium. An unusual and as yet unproven approach to myocardial infarct size reduction is the dissolution of the coronary arterial thrombus that is the usual precipitant of myocardial infarction. Dissolution of the thrombus by infusion of the fibrinolytic agent, streptokinase, reestablishes myocardial blood flow in the ischemic-necrotic zone. If coronary arterial patency can be reestablished before extensive myocardial necrosis has occurred (within 2–4 hours after the onset of infarction), infarct size can be reduced.

Coronary Atherosclerosis, Coronary Thrombosis, and Myocardial Infarction

The vast majority of patients with acute myocardial infarction have total obstruction of the coronary artery supplying the infarcted zone. Coronary arterial obstruction is usually the result of thrombosis developing on top of extensive coronary atherosclerosis. However, many patients with extensive coronary atherosclerosis never develop thrombosis or myocardial infarction despite the presence of such coronary atherosclerotic lesions for decades. Still other individuals develop coronary arterial occlusion from coronary thrombosis *without* resultant myocardial infarction. Finally, an occasional individual develops total occlusion of a coronary artery *with* myocardial infarction as a result of coronary artery smooth muscle spasm. Clearly, the extent of coronary collateral circulation and the level of myocardial metabolic demand must play some role in determining whether myocardial infarction results from coronary occlusion. However, the relative roles played by coronary spasm, myocardial metabolic demand, and collateral coronary circulation in the ultimate pathogenesis of myocardial infarction remain unclear at the present time.

Suggested Readings

Braunwald E, Ross J Jr, Sonnenblick EH: *Mechanism of Contraction of the Normal and Failing Heart*. Boston, Little, Brown, 1976, chap 12.

Sybers HD et al: The effect of glucose-insulin-potassium on cardiac ultrastructure following acute experimental coronary occlusion. *Am J Pathol* 70:401–411, 1973.

Jennings RB, Ganote CE: Structural change in myocardium during acute ischemia. *Circ Res* 35(suppl 3):156–168, 1974.

Henry PD, Sobel BE, Braunwald E: Protection of hypoxic guinea pig heart with glucose and insulin. *Am J Physiol* 226:309–313, 1974.

Neeley JR et al: Effects of ischemia on function and metabolism of the isolated working rat heart. *Am J Physiol* 225:651–658, 1973.

Liedtke AJ, Hughes HC, Neeley JR: Metabolic responses to varying restrictions of coronary blood flow in swine. *Am J Physiol* 228:655–662, 1975.

Sobel BE: Biochemical and morphological changes in infarcting myocardium, in Braunwald E (ed): *The Myocardium: Failure and Infarction.* New York, Hospital Practice, 1974, pp 247–260.

Mueller HS et al: Propranolol in the treatment of acute myocardial infarction. *Circulation* 59:1078–1087, 1974.

Brachfeld N: Maintenance of cell viability. *Circulation* 40 (suppl 4): 209–219, 1969.

Katz AM: Effects of ischemia on the contractile processes of heart muscle. *Am J Cardiol* 32:456–460, 1973.

Weisfeldt ML et al: Incomplete relaxation between beats after myocardial hypoxia and ischemia. *J Clin Invest* 53:1626–1636, 1974.

Heyndrickx G et al: Paradoxical action of isoproterenol on regional myocardial function and injury in conscious dogs with myocardial ischemia. *Circulation* 50 (suppl. 3):359–380, 1974.

Moraski RE et al: Left ventricular function in patients with and without myocardial infarction and one, two or three vessel coronary artery disease. *Am J Cardiol* 35:1–10, 1975.

McAnulty JH et al: Improvement in left ventricular wall motion following nitroglycerin. *Circulation* 51:140–145, 1975.

Theroux P et al: Regional myocardial function during acute coronary artery occlusion and its modification by pharmacological agents in the dog. *Circ Res* 35:896–908, 1974.

Miller RR et al: Sequential alterations of left ventricular compliance following myocardial infarction: Comparison of acute, early and late recovery periods in patients with similar pump dysfunction. *Am J Cardiol* 35:157, 1975.

Hood WB Jr et al: Experimental myocardial infarction: IV. Reduction of left ventricular compliance in the healing phase. *J Clin Invest* 49:1316–1323, 1970.

Diamond G, Forrester JS: Effect of coronary artery disease and acute myocardial infarction on left ventricular compliance in man. *Circulation* 45:11–19, 1972.

Dove JT, Shah PM, Schreiner BF: Effects of nitroglycerin on left ventricular wall motion in coronary artery disease. *Circulation* 49:682–687, 1974.

Peterson DF, Bishop VS: Reflex blood pressure control during acute myocardial ischemia in the conscious dog. *Circ Res* 34:226–232, 1974.

Peterson DF, Kaspar RI, Bishop VS: Reflex tachycardia due to temporary coronary occlusion in the conscious dog. *Circ Res* 32:652–659, 1973.

Moir TW: Subendocardial distribution of coronary blood flow and the effect of antianginal drugs. *Circ Res* 30:621–627, 1972.

Bache RJ, Cobb FR, Greenfield JC Jr: Myocardial blood flow distribution during ischemia-induced coronary vasodilation in the unanesthetized dog. *J Clin Invest* 54:1462–1472, 1974.

Neill WA et al: Subendocardial ischemia provoked by tachycardia in conscious dogs with coronary stenosis. *Am J Cardiol* 35:30–36, 1975.

Maroko PR et al: Factors influencing infarct size following experimental coronary artery occlusion. *Circulation* 43:67–82, 1971.

Cannon PJ, Dell RB, Dwyer EM Jr: Regional myocardial perfusion rates in patients with coronary artery disease. *J Clin Invest* 51:978–994, 1972.

Cohen MV et al: The effects of nitroglycerin on coronary collaterals and myocardial contractility. *J Clin Invest* 52:2836–2847, 1973.

Maroko PR, Libby P, Braunwald E: Effect of pharmacologic agents on the function of the ischemic heart. *Am J Cardiol* 32:930–936, 1973.

Vatner SF et al: Effects of catecholamines, exercise and nitroglycerin on the normal and ischemic myocardium in conscious dogs. *J Clin Invest* 54:563–575, 1974.

Braunwald E et al: Effects of drugs and of counterpulsation on myocardial oxygen consumption. *Circulation* 40 (suppl 4):220–228, 1969.

Maroko PR, Braunwald E: Modification of myocardial infarct size after coronary occlusion. *Ann Intern Med* 79:720–733, 1973.

Maroko PR et al: Coronary artery reperfusion: I. Early effects on local myocardial function and the extent of myocardial necrosis. *J Clin Invest* 51:2710–2716, 1972.

Ginks WR et al: Coronary artery reperfusion: II. Reduction of myocardial infarct size at one week after the coronary occlusion. *J Clin Invest* 51:2717–2723, 1972.

Braunwald E, Maroko PR, Libby P: Reduction of infarct size following coronary occlusion. *Circ Res* 34 and 35 (suppl 3):192–201, 1974.

4 : Risk Factors and the Development of Atherosclerosis

Joel M. Gore
Robert J. Goldberg

The leading cause of death in the United States is heart disease (Fig. 4-1). Cardiovascular disorders lead to 4 deaths in every 10 and of these, 90% can be attributed to coronary heart disease (CHD). In 1978, one-third of all deaths in the United States were a direct result of CHD. There were one million deaths due to atherosclerosis and hypertension. Forty million Americans have diseases of the heart and blood vessels, and these diseases cost the United States economy more than 50 billion dollars per year in wages, lost productivity, and medical expenses.

Despite these gloomy statistics, recent trends in CHD mortality indicate a decrease in deaths due to CHD (Fig. 4-2). During the 10-year period from 1968–1978, mortality from all causes decreased in the U.S. by 19%, heart disease mortality decreased by 23%, and CHD mortality fell by 25%. The decline in CHD mortality occurred in both sexes, all races, and in all ages. No clear explanation of these encouraging trends is available. It is likely that the decline in CHD mortality is due in part to primary prevention (see below), that is, modification of coronary risk factors prior to the onset of clinical CHD. Evidence is also accumulating that shows the impact of secondary prevention (e.g., coronary care units, coronary artery bypass surgery, or emergency medical services) on this downward trend in cardiovascular mortality.

Eighty-five percent of deaths in patients suffering acute myocardial infarction, one of the clinical manifestations of CHD, occur within the first 24 hours after the onset of symptoms. The majority of these deaths occur suddenly before any medical attention can be given to the patient. Almost one quarter of all first acute coronary events are manifested as sudden death, and in the United States this amounts annually to over 400,000 individuals who die suddenly. From a public health standpoint, therefore, a large reduction in mortality from CHD may only be possible through effective primary prevention.

Concept of Epidemiology and Coronary Risk Factors

When the occurrence of disease is studied in populations, patterns can be discerned. These patterns represent variations in the frequencies or rates of occurrence of disease observed in distinguishable subgroups of a population, or in a given population over time. Such

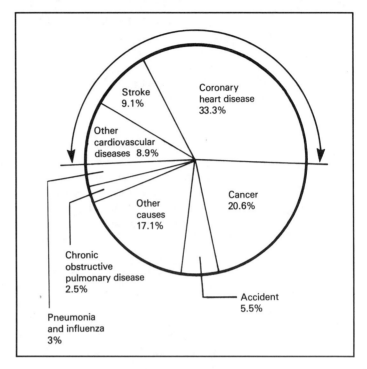

patterns, once established and properly interpreted, constitute evidence for or against various hypotheses concerning a disease and thus increase our understanding of that disease. The study of the occurrence of disease in populations is called "epidemiology." The epidemiology of CHD is concerned with both the description of rates of occurrence of CHD in different subgroups within populations and the investigation of the factors that determine its occurrence and its natural history.

There have been numerous observational and experimental studies conducted in the epidemiology of CHD. These studies have provided knowledge concerning the causes of CHD and the potential for reversibility and intervention. When populations are compared, there is a large difference in the incidence of and mortality from CHD within these populations—disease incidence generally parallels the presence of risk factors. Certain risk factor characteristics have been identified within populations that strongly relate to the future risk of CHD. All of the factors to be subsequently described are associated with the clinical manifestations of coronary atherosclerosis. However, they may or may not cause CHD, but their presence allows us to predict the likelihood or probability that a person has or will develop CHD within a defined limit of time. Correspondingly, it should not be inferred that individuals free of these identified risk factors to date are immune from the risk of developing CHD. In the United States, there

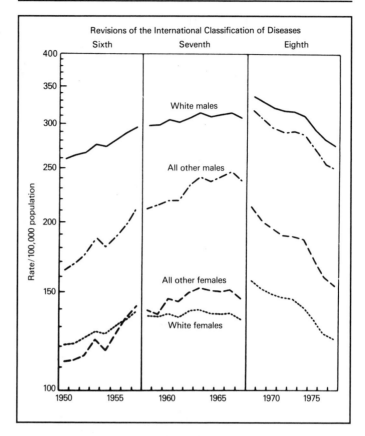

Fig. 4-2 : Age-adjusted death rates for ischemic heart disease by race and sex in the United States, 1950–1976.

exist many individuals who have none of the presently identified risk factors present, yet the incidence of CHD in groups of such individuals is much higher when compared to the incidence in groups of similar individuals in other parts of the world. One possible explanation for this phenomenon is the existence of as yet unidentified risk factors. Many of these presently known risk factor characteristics are present in childhood and persist through the adult years. When a member of a given population migrates into another population, this individual soon adopts the risk factor characteristics of the new population. Subpopulation studies show that levels of risk factors can be significantly modified in a favorable direction thereby resulting in changes in CHD morbidity and mortality.

Concept of Risk Factors

Risk factors are characteristics that are associated with a greater than average probability of developing a particular disease. It is generally acknowledged that CHD is a multifactored disease: that is, a variety of factors are involved in the development and clinical manifestations of this disease. A number of risk factors (see Table 4-1) have been shown to be related to CHD risk, but none has been found to be strictly causative. Certain hereditary, physiologic, or environmental

---

Table 4-1 : Risk factors

Hypertension
Smoking
Diabetes
Hyperlipidemia
Family history
Personality type
Menopause/birth control pills
Alcohol
Gout
Obesity
Trace metals
Physical activity

---

characteristics predispose an individual to the development of cardio-vascular disease. These characteristics as a group are referred to as "cardiovascular risk factors."

The risk factors most consistently linked to subsequent cardiovascular disease are hypertension, smoking, elevated serum cholesterol, diabetes, obesity, lack of exercise, psychosocial traits, age, sex, and heredity. Other characteristics that may be related to CHD include menopause, use of oral contraceptives, gout, alcohol and coffee consumption, soft water, and deficiencies in certain trace elements.

Individual Risk Factors

Hypertension

Elevation of blood pressure, both systolic and diastolic, is highly correlated with the development of CHD. For therapeutic and clinical purposes, when the resting adult arterial pressure is above 150/90 mm Hg, hypertension is said to be present. However, there is no sharp dividing line between normal and elevated blood pressure, and the distinction between normal and elevated blood pressure is arbitrary. Most patients with hypertension are asymptomatic and the blood pressure abnormality is usually discovered as an incidental finding. Approximately twenty-five million American adults have hypertension, ten million have definite hypertension, and fifteen million have borderline hypertension.

Elevated blood pressure, either systolic or diastolic, is predictive of an increased risk of developing CHD (Fig. 4-3). The risk of morbidity and mortality from CHD has a direct relationship to the level of blood pressure. There is no cutoff point at which risk suddenly changes from a low to a high value.

Several large scale studies, including the Framingham Heart Study, have shown a strong and stepwise relationship between diastolic and systolic blood pressure levels and cardiovascular related events (myocardial infarction, for example) and deaths. These epidemiologic studies also reveal that hypertension increases with age, and the rate

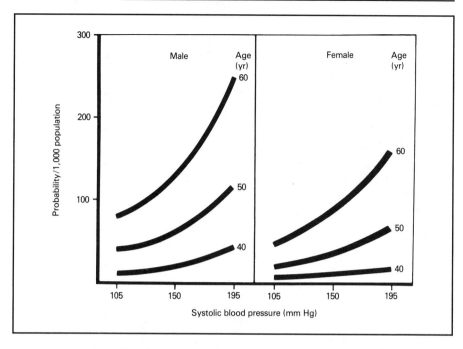

Fig. 4-3 : Independent risk of developing cardiovascular disease within 8 years according to level of systolic blood pressure in men and women by age. (From Kannel WB et al: Hypertension as an ingredient of a cardiovascular risk profile. *Br J Hosp Med* 11:508, 1974, with permission of the authors and publisher.)

of increase is higher among men than among women. There is also a marked racial difference in the prevalence of hypertension, with black males having the highest prevalence.

Cultural comparisons suggest that hypertension by itself does not explain the wide variation in CHD incidence found between populations, despite the fact that within populations it is significantly related to CHD risk. Elevated blood pressure is clearly related to the atherosclerotic process and the individual risk of CHD. Control of blood pressure has improved in the United States in recent years. The trends in the improvement of blood pressure control parallel those for improved CHD mortality rates. Certain changes that are presently occurring in the United States, for example, increased involvement in exercise, more attention to weight control, and increased awareness of and decreased consumption of salt all minimize the risk in the population for developing high blood pressure.

Cigarette smoking Cigarette smoking is unique among all risk factors in coronary heart disease. Unlike hypercholesterolemia or hypertension where doubt remains about the potential efficacy of their alteration, there seems to be no reservation about the importance of smoking cessation. It has

Fig. 4-4 : Relation of
relative risk of myo-
cardial infarction to
cigarette smoking
habits in young
women under the age
of 50. (From Sloan D:
Relation of cigarette
smoking to myocar-
dial infarction in
young women. *N Engl
J Med* 798:1273,
1978, with permis-
sion of the author and
publisher.)

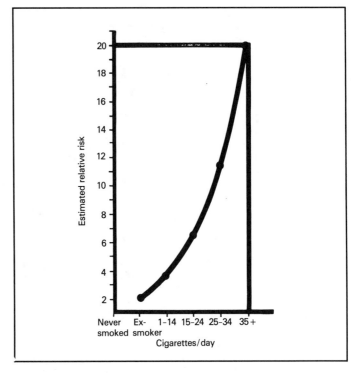

been well established that smoking cigarettes increases one's risk of coronary heart disease (Fig. 4-4), that the habit can be altered, and that abandoning cigarettes will reduce the risk of CHD.

Available data indicate that total mortality (death from all causes) is about twice as high among cigarette smokers as among nonsmokers. The majority of these excess deaths are due to mortality from cardiovascular diseases, particularly sudden death and myocardial infarction. Cigarette smoking significantly enhances the effect of other coronary heart disease risk factors. For any level of risk, smoking at least doubles that risk.

It is important to be aware that those people who stop smoking assume a lesser risk than those who continue. The excess risk in ex-smokers seems to decline within a year or two of the discontinuation of smoking but tends to remain slightly greater than the risk assumed by someone who has never smoked.

Cigarette smoke probably results in increased heart rate and myocardial oxygen demand and decreased oxygen carrying capacity of the blood because of carboxyhemoglobin formation. It does not appear that the tobacco industry's efforts to make "safer" cigarettes has had any direct effect on cardiovascular risk. There is a direct relationship between the number of cigarettes smoked and the risk of cardiac disease: the more one smokes the greater the risk.

Unlike the risk of smoking and lung cancer, for which risk appears to be cumulative and expressible in pack-years of smoking, the risk of coronary artery disease seems to be related to the current level of smoking and to be reversible when smoking is discontinued, at least in those individuals under age 65. It appears that pipe and cigar smoking, as long as the smoke is not inhaled, does not significantly increase one's risks for developing coronary disease.

Of all the major risk factors for cardiovascular disease, cigarette smoking is such a predominant factor, so highly prevalent, and so potentially correctible that it deserves the utmost attention as a preventive measure to control cardiovascular disease.

Diabetes

Despite major advances in the understanding and treatment of diabetes, it continues to contribute to excess rates of cardiovascular complications including coronary heart disease, stroke, and congestive heart failure. Clinically apparent diabetes mellitus has long been recognized as a precursor of atherosclerotic vascular disease. In men, diabetes increases the risk for CHD by approximately twofold whereas in women it triples the risk with a fourfold risk in younger women. Interestingly, diabetes in young individuals appears to be associated with renal disease whereas adult onset diabetes is associated with cardiac disease. The increased risk of cardiovascular disease related to diabetes is thought to be due to alterations that the disorder gradually brings about in the vascular system. The exact mechanism whereby diabetes causes these changes is unknown.

In diabetics, the incidence of coronary heart disease is similar for both sexes. In addition, in autopsy series, patients with diabetes have an increased frequency and severity of myocardial infarction as compared to age- and sex-matched patients without diabetes. The relation of diabetes to CHD is most strongly pronounced in affluent Western societies. In underdeveloped countries, other factors seem to affect the influence of diabetes on CHD.

Diabetes is often associated with hypertension and hyperlipidemia. It is possible that the increased risk of CHD in patients with diabetes is related to other risk factors. However, multivariate analysis of studies has verified the independent effect of diabetes. Diabetics also have alterations in platelet function and this may be involved in the CHD risk. Thus, it would appear that a number of mechanisms may be involved separately or in concert in diabetic patients.

Lipids

Of all risk factors, none has provoked as much controversy as the role of lipids in relation to cardiovascular disease. The lipid hypothesis, based on available epidemiologic data relating the level of serum

Fig. 4-5 : Risk of developing a heart attack in 10 years according to serum cholesterol level, in men 30–59 years at entry. Framingham Heart Study. (From Dawber TR: An approach to longitudinal studies in a community: The Framingham Study. *Ann NY Acad Sci* 107:534, 1963, with permission of the author and publisher.)

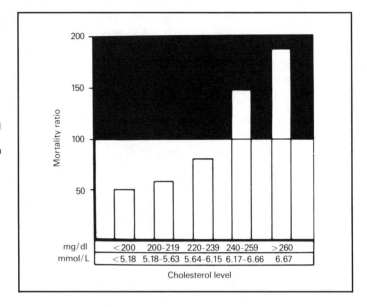

cholesterol to the incidence of coronary heart disease, maintains that reducing the level of an individual's serum cholesterol will lead to a reduction in his risk for CHD (Fig. 4-5). Studies remain inconclusive concerning the importance of serum triglycerides as a coronary risk factor. The accuracy of predicting the risk of CHD from serum cholesterol concentrations is greatest in the population under 65 years of age. The Keys study of the 1950s was the first multinational study to show the relation between CHD and cholesterol. Comparing sample populations from seven different countries, Keys found a high correlation between serum cholesterol levels and 5-year incidence rates for CHD. Multiple other prospective studies have confirmed these results in different population settings. In the Framingham Heart Study, both young males and females showed a linear association between the serum cholesterol level and the risk of CHD. This indicates that there is no such thing as a "safe" level of cholesterol below which the risk of CHD is negligible. For older individuals, and particularly for males, cholesterol levels do not predict the risk for CHD nearly as well as in younger individuals.

It appears that the contribution of lipids to cardiovascular risk is determined by partition of cholesterol into its various lipoprotein fractions. The major plasma lipids, including cholesterol and triglycerides, do not circulate freely in solution in the blood but rather are transported by lipoprotein complexes. The major lipoproteins include chylomicrons, very low-density lipoproteins (VLDL), low density lipoproteins (LDL), and high-density lipoproteins (HDL). While LDL has been shown to be associated with an increased risk for arteriosclerotic disease, the role of VLDL and triglycerides in atherosclerotic complications is as yet uncertain. HDL, which accounts for about 25% of total serum cholesterol, is thought to exert a protective effect against atherosclerotic morbidity. Several investigators have found that HDL cholesterol has the strongest relationship to CHD in men and women older than the age of 50 years. Since HDL normally composes 20–25% of total cholesterol, a favorable ratio of HDL to total cholesterol is 4.5 or less to 1.

The existence of an association between cholesterol and CHD does not of itself, however, establish causality or even indicate that intervention for modifying the lipid risk factor is feasible. There have been several large-scale studies in which a reduction in mean cholesterol was achieved without altering outcome in terms of reduction of CHD mortality. Thus, a major question has not been satisfactorily answered: does lowering of serum cholesterol reduce CHD mortality rates? Many methodologic problems will have to be overcome before an accurate answer to this question can be given.

Although the information available makes universal changes in diet or drug use for the reduction of cholesterol premature, the absence of hard data does not justify abandonment of concern for hyperlipidemia. Especially in patients with multiple risk factors, vigorous attempts should be made to lower blood cholesterol levels.

Family history

A family history of early coronary artery disease (before the age of 50) is a risk indicator. However, this does not provide conclusive evidence as to the role of genetic influence as families share not only genes but also environmental, social, and ethnic characteristics. Familial and genetic factors probably play an important role in the determination of some major risk factors, for example, hypertension, diabetes, and cholesterol levels. Genetic studies to date have failed to elucidate a relationship between social, cultural, and environmental variables and inherent factors related to metabolic and pathological components of arterosclerosis. Whether there is any particular familial or genetic predisposition to CHD, independent of other known risk factors, remains to be seen.

Psychosocial factors

The concept of the CHD-prone behavior has been advanced for several decades. Freidman in the late 1950s introduced the concept of behavioral and social characteristics related to CHD and of the type A and type B personalities. Type A personalities are typically characterized as aggressive, ambitious, and competitive. They are often preoccupied with deadlines and are very work-oriented. These individuals are, in general, very impatient and usually have a strong sense of time urgency, constantly striving to complete tasks within a deadline.

In contrast, the individual with a type B personality usually has no pressing conflict with either time or other persons; such individuals are free of any sense of time urgency. Unfortunately, the environ-

Fig. 4-6 : Eight-year incidence rates of myocardial infarction (MI) among men by personality type and age. Framingham Heart Study. (From Haynes SG: Relationship of psychosocial factors to coronary heart disease in the Framingham Study. III. Eight-year incidence of coronary artery disease. *Am J Epidem* 3:37, 1980, with permission of the author and publisher.)

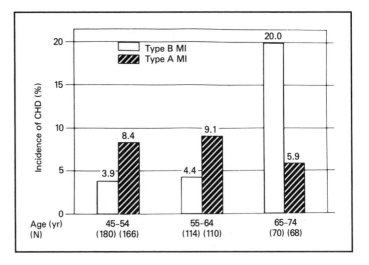

ment of the 1980s generally encourages type A behavior because it rewards those who function rapidly and aggressively.

In one study involving only men, type A personality was associated with a twofold increase in the incidence rates of CHD as compared to type B personality (Fig. 4-6). In addition to acting as an independent risk factor, there are associations between type A behavior and smoking and eating patterns. Additional psychosocial factors associated with the occurrence of CHD include stressful life events, sociocultural mobility, and status incongruity. It is not yet known if one can change psychosocial characteristics in such a way that CHD risk characteristics or disease rates can be altered.

Menopause and birth control pills

The excess CHD risk in white men is well documented throughout modernized affluent Western societies. However, the sex difference in CHD mortality is not so readily apparent in nonwhite populations and in areas of the world where the risk for CHD is low. Relative female protection from CHD risk is assumed to be the result of hormonal factors; however, the specific hormone(s) responsible has yet to be established. Among women, both the onset of menopause and the use of birth control pills are related to an increased risk for developing CHD. The marked increase in CHD risk in the white male population prompted the Coronary Drug Project to perform a controlled trial of exogenous estrogen administration in white males. To the surprise of many people, those males receiving the estrogen preparations had an increase in the incidence rates of CHD as compared to placebo patients; the trial was abruptly terminated. When a woman undergoes menopause, her risk for developing CHD increases approximately three times as compared to a woman of the same age who is still menstruating. It is unclear at this time what factor or factors occur during the menopause that are responsible for this increased risk.

The excess risk of thromboembolism, stroke, and myocardial infarction in women who are taking birth control pills is well known. It is particularly important to be aware of the extremely high risk associated with the combination of birth control pills and cigarette smoking. Birth control pills also tend to produce an increase in blood pressure and an unfavorable alteration in serum lipoproteins.

The effect of estrogen replacement in post-menopausal females is much less clear than the effect in males. It appears that estrogen replacement in older women has little influence on the risk of CHD. Young females receiving noncontraceptive estrogens are at increased risk for developing CHD. To date, the sexual difference in the incidence of cardiovascular disease cannot be adequately explained on the basis of known effects of estrogens alone. It is apparent that estrogens or other hormones are playing an as yet unidentified role in the etiology of CHD. Delineation of the responsible agent or agents for the marked sexual difference in CHD risk may have profound public health importance.

Alcohol consumption

One of the most conflict-filled areas of cardiovascular risk factor research involves the role of alcohol. It has recently been reported that regular alcohol intake of up to two drinks a day is, in fact, protective against coronary artery disease, possibly as a result of alcohol's peripheral vasodilating effect or its ability to increase serum HDL levels. Other reports indicate that alcohol has no protective influence on coronary heart disease. Further studies will be required before any definitive conclusions can be drawn about the relationship of CHD and alcohol. In the presence of unimpaired cardiac function or functionally insignificant coronary artery disease, the major concern about alcohol is its contribution to caloric excess and its encouragement of unhealthy life-style habits such as smoking, overeating, and underactivity.

Gout

There appears to be a weak but consistent association between gouty arthritis and cardiovascular disease risk. Elevated levels of uric acid appear to be associated with obesity, hypertension, and hyperlipidemia and thus make the independent effect of uric acid and gout on CHD difficult to interpret. Further understanding of the complex nature of these metabolic abnormalities would greatly assist in explaining the relationship of gout and other factors and CHD.

Obesity

Irrespective of its physiologic or psychologic effects, obesity is generally believed to increase one's risk both for generally poorer health and for cardiovascular disease in particular. It is a commonly held myth that excess weight puts an added strain on the heart. Epidemiologic studies, however, have shown that although fat people have more high blood pressure and diabetes than thinner individuals, they do not have more coronary disease if other risk factors, such as smoking, hypertension, age, and serum cholesterol are controlled for. Relative obesity appears to offer little explanation for significant population differences in CHD incidence and, within high-risk cultures, little independent contribution to individual risk of CHD.

When obesity is considered a metabolic abnormality associated with other metabolic abnormalities, including diabetes, hypertension, and hyperlipidemia, its relation to CHD risk becomes more apparent. These metabolic abnormalities are amenable to correction by weight loss and/or increased physical activity. Thus, though obesity does not appear to be an independent risk factor for CHD, it should not be ignored and concerted efforts should be made to educate patients in proper ways of weight reduction and maintenance.

Coffee

There is no definitive proof that the consumption of coffee or tea in any way increases the risk for cardiovascular disease. However, coffee drinking in excessive amounts (≥ 6 cups per day) may act as a triggering agent for the clinical manifestations of the atherosclerotic process.

Trace metals and water hardness

Minerals and trace elements are subjects of current research because of an epidemiologic association between soft water, hypertension, and CHD mortality. Most studies relating data on water hardness to causes of death show an inverse relationship between water hardness and CHD death rates. Several investigators have even suggested that "the harder the water, the softer the arteries." Hardness of water is not due to a single specific chemical element but is characterized by a myriad of elements, most notably calcium and magnesium. Efforts to isolate individual elements in water and relate them to CHD mortality rates have been unsuccessful. The evidence is as yet insufficient for public health action.

Physical activity

Studies examining the association of physical activity and subsequent development of CHD have been consistently fraught with controversy. However, there appears to be growing evidence that physical activity can prevent the development of coronary heart disease. As a matter of fact, there appears to be an epidemic of Americans who are exercising for the sake of cardiovascular fitness. There are many questions still unanswered such as to the type, duration, and regularity of exercise that is required in order to provide a protective effect on developing CHD. There is no agreement about whether exercise improves myocardial function and coronary circulation directly or whether its protective effect acts through the alteration of other risk factors. It is important to remember that exercise itself can be hazardous. Many physicians recommend that individuals over the age of 35 or those less than 35 with strong risk factors for CHD should undergo an exercise treadmill test before beginning an exercise program that represents a major increase in physical activity.

Risk markers

Unlike risk factors, which are potentially reversible variables that are related to the risk of developing coronary heart disease, risk markers

Table 4-2 : Risk markers

Age
Sex
Race
Geography
Blood Type

are nonmodifiable characteristics that are related to risk of CHD (Table 4-2). These markers identify patient subgroups at greater than average probability of developing CHD. Some risk markers have been well established, while others are only clinical impressions.

It is important for the patient and physician to differentiate between risk factors and risk markers. Risk markers simply label the person as being at increased risk; they are typically not amenable to alteration.

AGE. The mortality from coronary heart disease has a strong relationship to age in both sexes. CHD still remains an uncommon disease in patients under the age of 35. By age 35–45, CHD has become an important cause of morbidity and mortality in the population, especially in males. By age 55, almost 50% of all deaths in the United States are related to CHD.

SEX. The excess CHD risk in white men is documented throughout Western society. However, the sex difference is less prominent in nonwhite populations and in areas of the world where the incidence of CHD is normally low. The sex difference is also much greater at younger ages than at older ages. Essentially, CHD mortality rates for females lag many years behind those of males. There appears to be a significant increase in CHD mortality in females after the menopause at which time females seem to "catch up" to males.

RACE. There appears to be an increased incidence of CHD in whites as compared to nonwhites in the male population. In females, it would seem that nonwhites have a slightly higher incidence than whites. Both black and white males have a greater rate of CHD than females, although the difference is much more pronounced prior to the menopause. Migrant and ethnic group studies have identified certain subgroups with a lower than expected incidence rate for CHD as compared with the population as a whole. Two such groups are Japanese-Americans and Puerto Ricans. Interestingly, although Japanese-Americans have a lower incidence rate of CHD as compared to their fellow Americans, they have a much higher incidence of CHD when compared to Japanese still living in Japan. Migrant population studies, which in part control for major gene effects, show that risk characteristics and disease incidence rapidly approach levels of the adopted culture.

GEOGRAPHY. There are marked regional variations in CHD mortality within the United States. The mortality from CHD is highest in the

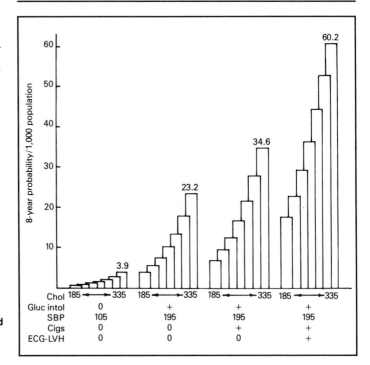

Fig. 4-7 : Eight-year risk of cardiovascular disease by serum cholesterol levels and combinations of other risk factors among men aged 35 years. Framingham Heart Study. Chol = cholesterol; Gluc intol = glucose intolerance; SBP = systemic blood pressure; Cigs = cigarette smoking; LVH = left ventricular hypertrophy by ECG. (From Kannel WB: Cholesterol in the prediction of atherosclerotic disease. New perspectives based on the Framingham Study. *Ann Intern Med* 90:85, 1979, with permission of the author and publisher.)

southeastern Atlantic Coast states and in southern Alabama and Georgia. It is relatively high in the Northeast and Midwest. In comparison, the mortality rate in the Great Plains and Mountain states is relatively low. The reasons for these regional differences are not readily apparent.

The weather, particularly the invasion of cold fronts, snowfall, and rapid falls in barometric pressure, have also been correlated with new hospital admissions and the likelihood of coronary events. Also, high atmospheric inversions and air pollution are related to hospitalization and death rates from cardiovascular and pulmonary disease.

OTHER RISK MARKERS. Numerous other variables are said to be risk markers for CHD. For the most part these are reflected in isolated reports that have not been verified. For example, there have been reports that people with blood type O have a lower risk of CHD as compared to individuals with blood type A. A frequently made clinical observation is that patients with rheumatoid arthritis have a lower than expected incidence of CHD. It has been speculated that the ingestion of large amounts of aspirin has a protective effect for these patients. For a while, a widely held myth was that people with ear lobe creases had a much higher risk of CHD.

Multiple Risk Factors

The discussion up to now has indicated that there are many attributes in individuals that are clearly related to risk of CHD. What happens when an individual has one or more risk factors present (Fig. 4-7)? The greater the number of risk factors present in an individual the more apt that individual is to manifest signs of CHD. The effects of these risk factors appear to be additive, as individuals with hyperlipidemia, hypertension, and smoking have an age adjusted rate of first CHD events more than eight times that of individuals with no risk factors. When two of these risk factors are present, the rate of CHD events was increased by more than fourfold. These findings reinforce the need for preventive measures in high-risk individuals with multiple risk factors as the risk of CHD clearly increases in an exponential fashion.

Undoubtedly, other risk factors for CHD exist. The search for additional risk factors or for new relationships among existing ones continues. The identification of the major risk factors for atherosclerotic disease is the scientific foundation for prevention. It is apparent that coronary heart disease is a multifactored illness.

Suggested Readings

Borhani NO: Primary prevention of coronary heart disease: A critique. *Am J Cardiol* 40:251–259, 1977.

Hypertension Detection and Follow-up Program Cooperative Group: Five-year findings of the hypertension detection and follow-up program. I. Reduction in mortality of persons with high blood pressure, including mild hypertension. *JAMA* 242:2562–2571, 1979.

Hillis LD, Braunwald E: Myocardial ischemia. *N Engl J Med* 296:971–978, 1034–1041, 1093–1096, 1977.

Jenkins CD: Psychologic and social precursors of coronary disease. *N Engl J Med* 284:244–255, 307–317, 1971.

Kannel WB, McGee DL: Diabetes and glucose tolerance as risk factors for cardiovascular disease: The Framingham Study. *Diabetes Care* 2:120–126, 1979.

Kannel WB: Some lessons in cardiovascular epidemiology from Framingham. *Am J Cardiol* 37:269–282, 1976.

Kannel WB: Preventive cardiology. What should the clinician be doing about it? *Post Grad Med* 61:74–85, 1977.

Multiple Risk Factor Intervention Trial Research Group: Multiple risk factor intervention trial. *JAMA* 748:1465–1477, 1978.

Stamler J: Research related to risk factors. *Circulation* 60:1575–1587, 1979.

Stern MP: The recent decline in ischemic heart disease mortality. *Ann Intern Med* 91:630, 1979.

5 : Valvular Heart Disease

Approximately 20% of individuals who visit a cardiologist have some form of valvular heart condition. The category, ''valvular heart disease,'' includes a number of different entities, each with its own pathophysiologic sequence. Some of these diseases, such as mitral stenosis, aortic stenosis, and mitral regurgitation, are quite common, while others, such as pulmonic regurgitation and tricuspid stenosis, are quite rare. In this chapter, the pathophysiology of each of these forms of valvular heart disease will be discussed following some general introductory remarks concerning the pathogenesis of valvular disorders.

Valvular disease can consist of either isolated stenosis or regurgitation (also termed *insufficiency* or *incompetence*) of a single valve or mixed stenosis and regurgitation affecting one or more valves. Certain patterns of valvular pathology are associated with different causes of valvular disease. For example, atherosclerosis can affect the aortic valve in elderly individuals producing mild to marked aortic stenosis with no or only mild aortic regurgitation. Other valves are unaffected and function normally. Rheumatic heart disease, on the other hand, often affects more than one valve. The combination of mitral stenosis and aortic regurgitation is frequently observed in individuals who have had acute rheumatic fever during childhood or adolescence.

A large number of pathological processes are associated with damage to one or more cardiac valves (Table 5-1). Some of these entities are relatively common, e.g., rheumatic heart disease, while others are fortunately unusual, e.g., amyloidosis. Cardiac valves can be injured in a variety of different ways. Rheumatic fever and the collagen vascular diseases produce inflammatory lesions and even inflammatory cellular infiltration in heart valves. In bacterial endocarditis, collections of bacteria, fibrin, and inflammatory cells disrupt valvular function by means of mechanical injury to the valvular apparatus. A third example of a disease process affecting valvular function is myxomatous degeneration of the valve in which the normal supporting histologic architecture of the valve dissolves over a number of years rendering the valve incompetent. Many valvular pathologic entities are slow processes requiring years to express themselves, rheumatic

Table 5-1 : Potential causes of valvular heart disease

Degenerative changes, aging
  General, nonspecific degeneration (normal aging)
  Pathologic degeneration
    Mitral anular calcification
    Aortic valvular calcification: tricuspid valve, congenitally bicuspid valve
  Myxomatous degeneration
Infiltration and storage diseases
  Amyloid
  Mucopolysaccharidoses
    Type I: Hurler syndrome, Scheie syndrome
    Type II: Hunter syndrome
  Glycogen storage: type II Pompe disease
  Hyperlipoproteinemia type II
  Sarcoidosis
  Gout
Heritable disorders of connective tissue
  Marfan syndrome
  Homocystinuria
  Ehlers-Danlos syndrome
  Pseudoxanthoma elasticum
Rheumatic heart disease
  Acute rheumatic fever
  Chronic rheumatic valvular disease
Rheumatoid arthritis, syphilis, and collagen vascular disease
  Rheumatoid arthritis
  Ankylosing spondylitis
  Reiter syndrome
  Syphilitic aortitis
  Relapsing polychondritis
  Systemic lupus erythematosus
Tumors and miscellaneous conditions
  Myxoma
  Papillary tumors; Lambl's excrescences
  Carcinoid disease
  Methysergide-induced fibrosis
Infective
  Bacterial
  Fungal
  Rickettsial
  Parasitic
  Viral

heart disease, for example, while other diseases, such as bacterial endocarditis, disrupt valvular function acutely within hours or days. Some valvular disease entities are congenital, such as pulmonic stenosis and bicuspid aortic valve, while other conditions, rheumatic heart disease, for one, are acquired. Finally, more than one form of valvular heart disease can coexist in the same patient. Thus, patients with previous injury to a heart valve resulting from any of the pathological conditions listed in Table 5-1 are at an increased risk of developing a bacterial infection (bacterial endocarditis) on the affected valve.

Mitral Stenosis

Most patients with mitral stenosis have had acute rheumatic fever in childhood or adolescence. Decades then pass before clinical symptoms appear. Indeed, the mitral valve develops slowly progressive stenotic changes over this period of years. The explanation for the long latency period between the episode(s) of acute rheumatic fever and the development of adult mitral stenosis is largely unknown. However, the most reasonable pathophysiologic sequence is the following: acute rheumatic fever leads to mitral valve inflammation that in turn results in abnormal flow patterns across the mitral valve. These abnormal flow patterns place increased and/or abnormal stress on the leaflets of the mitral valve. These increased or abnormal valvular stress patterns eventually lead to thickening, fibrosis, and even calcification of the valve with consequent stenosis.

Stenotic valves

Stenotic valves have a pressure gradient across them. An appropriate analogy is a dam across a stream: water volume, and hence pressure, builds up behind the dam in contrast to decreased volume beyond the dam. The situation is similar with mitral stenosis: pressure increases in the left atrium, behind the stenotic mitral valve (Fig. 5-1). The increase in left atrial pressure augments the amount of blood that flows across the stenotic mitral valve during diastole, thereby maintaining stroke volume and cardiac output at normal or near-normal levels until very late in the course of the disease when very severe valvular stenosis is present. The normal mitral valve has an orifice during diastole between 4.0 and 5.0 cm². No clinically detectable gradient exists across a mitral valve with such an orifice size. When the mitral valve orifice is reduced to 1.0 cm², it requires a gradient of approximately 20 mm Hg to maintain normal flow across the mitral valve. Since left ventricular diastolic pressure is commonly around 5 mm Hg, left atrial pressure must be 25 mm Hg (20 + 5 mm Hg) in order for normal cardiac output to be maintained. In other words, cardiac output is maintained at the expense of increased left atrial pressure. Since there are no valves between the left atrium and the pulmonary veins and capillaries, increases in left atrial pressure lead to similar rises in pulmonary venous and pulmonary capillary pressure (Fig. 5-1). Increased pulmonary capillary pressure leads to transudation of fluid into the pulmonary parenchyma (Starling's law of capillary filtration-reabsorption). As noted in Chapters 3 and 8, increased pulmonary parenchymal fluid leads to abnormal blood oxygenation and a sensation of dyspnea. Hemoptysis in patients with mitral stenosis results from the increased pressure in small pulmonary venules some of which actually burst and leak blood into the bronchial tree.

The right ventricle and mitral stenosis

In patients with mitral stenosis the right ventricle must bear the burden of increased work since it is responsible for pumping blood through the pulmonary vascular bed and left atrium and into the left ventricle during diastole. The work of the right ventricle gradually increases as mitral stenosis increases in severity. Indeed, the right ventricle must produce a systolic pressure that is considerably higher

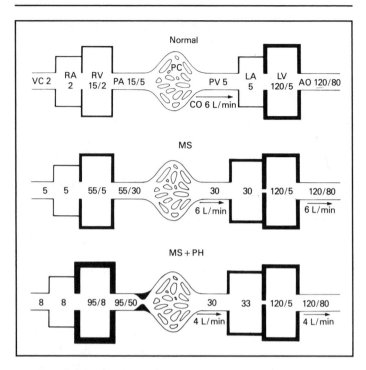

Fig. 5-1 : Pathophysiology of mitral stenosis (MS). The top panel demonstrates normal hemodynamics. The middle panel shows a patient with severe mitral stenosis but without reactive pulmonary hypertension (PH). Left atrial pressure is 30 mm Hg and there is a 25-mm gradient (30−5 mm Hg) across the mitral valve during diastole. The increased left atrial pressure is transmitted to the pulmonary capillaries (PC) and pulmonary artery (PA) and results in an increase in pulmonary arterial pressure to 55/30 mm Hg. Right ventricular systolic pressure must therefore increase to 55 mm Hg as well. There is slight dilatation and hypertrophy of the right ventricle (RV) and left atrium (LA). In the lower panel is depicted an individual with severe reactive pulmonary hypertension. Mitral stenosis is no more severe than in the patient depicted in the middle panel. However, a pulmonary hypertensive reaction has developed. The right ventricle is hypertrophied and dilated. The right ventricle has failed with right atrial and central venous pressures rising to 8 mm Hg and cardiac output falling to 4 liters/minute. VC = vena cava; RA = right atrium; PV = pulmonary veins; LV = left ventricle; AO = aorta; CO = cardiac output. (From Selzer A: *Principles of Clinical Cardiology: An Analytic Approach.* Philadelphia, Saunders, 1975, with permission of the author and publisher.)

than normal. This is the result of increased pulmonary capillary pressure that leads in turn to increased pulmonary arterial diastolic pressure. When pulmonary arterial diastolic pressure increases, systolic pressure must also increase if forward blood flow is to continue. The result is pulmonary hypertension. The right ventricle is forced to pump blood into the pulmonary artery at the increased systolic pressure (Fig. 5-1).

The increase in right ventricular work eventually leads to hypertrophy and dilatation and finally to failure of that chamber. When right ventricular failure develops, right atrial pressure rises leading to an obligatory increase in systemic venous pressure. Hepatic and mesenteric congestion and edema of peripheral tissues (commonly the soft tissues of the lower leg) develop. Cardiac output falls and the individual notes the symptoms of fatigue and malaise.

In a small number of individuals with very severe, long-standing mitral stenosis excessive degrees of pulmonary hypertension develop. In such patients, pulmonary arterial systolic pressure may even reach the same level as arterial systolic pressure. It appears that pulmonary arterial vasoconstriction is responsible for the inordinate increase in pulmonary arterial pressure in these patients.

LV work ↓

The left ventricle is spared in patients with mitral stenosis. Indeed, left ventricular filling is impaired as a result of the stenotic mitral valve and left ventricular systolic and diastolic volumes are consequently lower than normal. Left ventricular hypertrophy does not develop since left ventricular work is, if anything, diminished rather than increased. A small number of patients with mitral stenosis have reduced left ventricular function that is apparently not related to the extent or severity of mitral stenosis. The etiology of left ventricular dysfunction in patients with mitral stenosis is unknown.

Mitral stenosis in women

Mitral stenosis commonly affects young and middle-aged women. Consequently, pregnancy and mitral stenosis often coexist. The result is an aggravation of the hemodynamic abnormalities of mitral stenosis. In order to understand the pathophysiologic effects of pregnancy on mitral stenosis, one must first grasp a few fundamental relationships involving blood flow across narrowed cardiac valves. Blood flow through a narrowed cardiac valve is determined by three factors: (1) the pressure gradient across the valve, (2) the cardiac output, and (3) the period of time allowed for blood to flow across the valve (diastole for the mitral and tricuspid valves and systole for the aortic and pulmonic valves). In addition, the pressure gradient across a narrowed cardiac valve is directly proportional to the flow across that valve. These relationships are expressed in the formula for calculating the orifice area of a stenotic valve:

Orifice area of a stenotic valve =

$$\frac{\text{cardiac output}}{\text{heart rate} \times \frac{\text{diastolic filling time}}{\text{or}} \times \text{gradient across the narrowed valve} \times \text{constant}}$$
$$\text{systolic ejection time}$$

Pregnancy aggravates the hemodynamic abnormalities associated with mitral stenosis because it causes an increase in heart rate and cardiac output. Increases in heart rate occur at the expense of decreases in diastolic filling time since tachycardia shortens diastole proportionately more than systole. Since valve area does not change during pregnancy, increased cardiac output and heart rate and decreased diastolic filling time result in an increase in the pressure gradient across the mitral valve (see formula for valve area above). The increased pressure gradient across the mitral valve is transmitted through the left atrium to the pulmonary veins and capillaries with a resultant increase in transudation of fluid into the pulmonary parenchyma, which is sensed by the patient as increasing dyspnea. Exercise increases left atrial pressure in a similar manner: heart rate and cardiac output are augmented leading to an increase in the pressure gradient across the mitral valve.

Mitral Regurgitation

A variety of different pathological entities can lead to regurgitation or incompetence of the mitral valve. Rheumatic heart disease is still the commonest cause of the mitral regurgitation followed by myxomatous degeneration, ischemic heart disease, and infective endocarditis. Each of these entities affects the mitral valve apparatus in a different fashion but the end-result is the same: regurgitation of blood during systole from the left ventricle through the incompetent mitral valve and into the left atrium. The amount of backwards systolic flow across the mitral valve is dependent on five factors: (1) size of the mitral valve orifice during systole (often called the "regurgitant orifice"), (2) left ventricular systolic pressure, (3) left atrial pressure during ventricular systole, (4) left ventricular systolic ejection time, and (5) heart rate. The first three factors are of greatest importance. Clearly, the larger the regurgitant orifice, the greater will be the systolic regurgitant flow from left ventricle to left atrium. Similarly, mitral regurgitant flow is increased if the systolic gradient across the mitral valve (left ventricular systolic pressure minus simultaneous left atrial pressure) increases. Increases in systolic ejection time and heart rate can result in modest increases in the quantity of mitral regurgitant flow per minute.

The left ventricle in mitral regurgitation

In patients with mitral regurgitation, the left ventricle ejects blood via two routes: (1) through the aortic valve to the systemic circulation and (2) through the mitral valve into the left atrium. Since left atrial pressure is lower than aortic pressure (Fig. 5-2), the left ventricle empties itself more rapidly than normal into the left atrium during early systole. There is a rapid fall in left ventricular systolic wall tension, and much of the increased work of the left ventricular myocardium is expended in shortening at normal or less than normal levels of wall tension. This means that the left ventricle is not as greatly "stressed" by the volume overload imposed by mitral regurgitation as by the pressure overload of certain other lesions (see below, Aortic Stenosis).

In order for the left ventricle to maintain normal systemic cardiac output in the face of mitral regurgitation, more complete systolic emptying of the ventricle is required (reduced end-systolic volume).

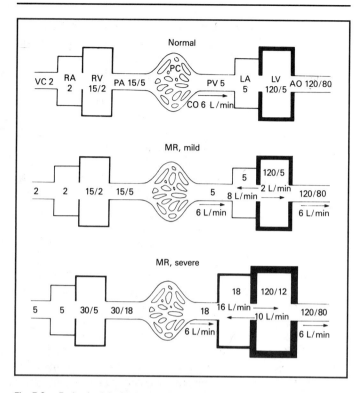

Fig. 5-2 : Pathophysiologic changes in patients with mitral regurgitation (MR). Normal hemodynamics are demonstrated in the top panel. The middle panel demonstrates mild mitral regurgitation. It can be seen that there is a regurgitant flow across the mitral valve of 2 liters/minute. Consequently, during diastole 8 liters/minute flow into the left ventricle (6 liters/minute represents right ventricular cardiac output [CO] arriving in the left atrium and 2 liters/minute represents the regurgitant flow that has entered the left atrium during left ventricular systole). Left-sided pressures are still normal. In the lower panel, a patient with severe mitral regurgitation is depicted. In this individual, 10 liters/minute flow from the left ventricle (LV) to the left atrium (LA) during systole. Left atrial and pulmonary venous pressures are increased to 18 mm Hg. Consequently, right ventricular systolic and pulmonary arterial pressures must also rise. Left ventricular end-diastolic pressure is slightly increased because of left ventricular hypertrophy and dilatation. VC = vena cava; RA = right atrium; RV = right ventricle; PA = pulmonary artery; PC = pulmonary capillaries; PV = pulmonary veins; AO = aorta. (From Selzer A: *Principles of Clinical Cardiology: An Analytical Approach.* Philadelphia, Saunders, 1975, with permission of the author and publisher.)

However, over many years, the additional burden imposed by mitral regurgitation on the myocardium leads to dilatation (increased end-diastolic volume) and hypertrophy of the left ventricle. Eventually, after many decades, left ventricular failure develops (see Chap. 1).

During each left ventricular contraction, a bolus of blood is delivered to the left atrium expanding that chamber's capacity. During the subsequent diastolic filling period the left atrium empties into the left ventricle. Left ventricular filling volume is increased at this point since the left atrium delivers the regurgitant blood volume *plus* the normal forward moving bolus of blood. Thus, the left ventricle must pump an increased stroke volume during each systole (part into the aorta and part into the left atrium), hence, the term, *volume over-load.* Whether or not this volume overload of the left ventricle leads to increased left ventricular filling pressures, and thereby pulmonary congestion, depends on two factors: (1) left ventricular systolic function and (2) left ventricular diastolic function. If left ventricular systolic function is abnormal, the ventricle dilates and filling pressure rises (Starling mechanism).

Diastolic function of the myocardium has already been discussed in Chapters 1 and 3. Abnormal diastolic function of the left ventricular myocardium often develops in patients with valvular heart disease. Such abnormal diastolic function is usually the result of myocardial hypertrophy, failure, and/or interstitial fibrosis secondary to the long-standing burden imposed by the valvular lesion. Patients with long-standing mitral regurgitation frequently manifest abnormal diastolic function of the left ventricular myocardium (decreased compliance = increased stiffness). Increased myocardial stiffness leads to elevated left ventricular diastolic pressure that in turn leads to pulmonary congestion.

Pathophysiology of mitral regurgitation

Several pathophysiologic features of mitral regurgitation should be emphasized. First, mitral regurgitation tends to perpetuate itself: regurgitation leads to left atrial dilatation, which pulls the posterior mitral leaflet further away from the anterior leaflet. In this manner, the amount of mitral regurgitation increases with time (Fig. 5-3). Second, marked left ventricular dilatation or hypertrophy can lead to mitral regurgitation since both these processes can displace the mitral valve papillary muscles from their usual position in the left ventricular cavity. The result is abnormal traction on the mitral valve leaflets with resultant valvular regurgitation (Fig. 5-4). In the past it was thought that left ventricular dilatation commonly led to dilatation of the mitral valve anulus. Dilatation of the mitral anulus was said to produce mitral regurgitation. Currently, it is felt that mitral anular dilatation infrequently occurs and that such dilatation is a very uncommon cause of mitral regurgitation.

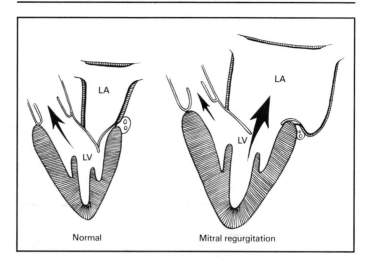

Normal   Mitral regurgitation

Fig. 5-3 : The mechanism of the increasing degrees of mitral regurgitation that result from left atrial enlargement. Dilatation of the left atrium (LA) does not affect the position or function of the anterior mitral valve leaflet. This leaflet is anchored to the root of the aorta. The posterior leaflet, however, is directly affected: as the left atrium enlarges, its posterior wall is displaced posteriorly and downward. Because of the continuity of the left atrial endocardium and the posterior mitral valve leaflet, this displacement exerts tension on the posterior mitral valve leaflet. The posterior leaflet is displaced with accentuation of the mitral regurgitant orifice. Thus, left atrial enlargement results in increasing degrees of mitral regurgitation. LV = left ventricle. (From Perloff JK, Roberts WC: The mitral apparatus: Functional anatomy of mitral regurgitation. *Circulation* 46:227, 1972, with permission of the authors and publisher.)

Finally, the size and compliance of the left atrium is important in determining whether mitral regurgitation produces pulmonary congestion and hence symptoms. Mitral regurgitation into a small left atrium or a left atrium with a hypertrophied, noncompliant wall results in a marked increase in left atrial pressure (Fig. 5-5). Large, high-pressure regurgitant waves (so-called V waves) appear in the left atrial, pulmonary venous, and pulmonary capillary pressure tracing. Such high-pressure waves in the pulmonary capillaries produce increased transudation of fluid into the pulmonary interstitium with resultant dyspnea. Patients who develop mitral regurgitation acutely, e.g., infectious endocarditis or myocardial infarction with papillary muscle necrosis, usually present with this form of pathologic physiology. Mitral regurgitation into a large left atrium or a left atrium with a thin, compliant wall results in little or no increase in left atrial pressure (Fig. 5-5). Large regurgitant (V) waves are *not* seen, and such individuals are frequently asymptomatic. This pattern of pathologic physiology is commonly observed in patients with chronic, long-standing mitral regurgitation. Chronic mitral regurgitation causes left atrial dilatation with resultant diminution in the size of mitral waves.

[handwritten margin notes: acute ↑ LA pressure → dyspnea; chronic LA dilates not ↑ pressure]

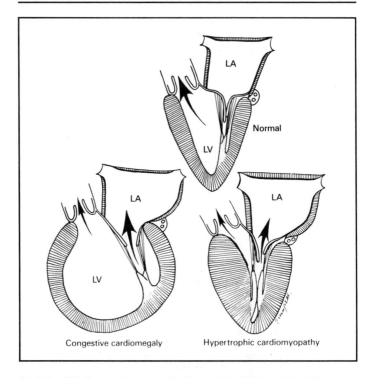

Fig. 5-4 : Mitral regurgitation resulting from a dilated left ventricle (LV). A patient with congestive cardiomyopathy may develop mitral regurgitation secondary to left ventricular dilatation, which pulls the mitral valve papillary muscles laterally and caudally, thereby disturbing mitral valvular function and producing mitral regurgitation. Patients with hypertrophic cardiomyopathy may also have disturbed mitral valve function and mitral regurgitation secondary to distortion or bending of the papillary muscles, which in turn results from the severe, disproportional hypertrophy of the ventricular septum. The normal left ventricle is shown above for comparison. As noted in the figure, the normal axes of the papillary muscles are more or less parallel to the major axis of the left ventricular cavity. LA = left atrium. (From Roberts WC, Perloff JK: Mitral valvular diseases. *Ann Int Med* 77:939, 1972, with permission of the authors and publisher.)

Aortic Stenosis

Aortic valvular stenosis is usually the result of a congenital abnormality of the valve that leads in time to fibrosis and calcification of the valve. Rheumatic valvular injury can also lead to aortic stenosis. The presumed mechanism that leads from a congenitally bicuspid (as opposed to the normal tricuspid) valve or a rheumatically injured valve to aortic stenosis involves abnormal flow patterns and increased wall stress within the aortic valve leaflets themselves. Such increased leaflet stress leads to excessive wear and tear of the leaflet with eventual fibrosis and calcification.

Aortic stenosis results in a gradient across the aortic valve; left ventricular systolic pressure is commonly 50–100 mm Hg higher than systemic systolic pressure. For example, if brachial arterial pressure is 120/80 mm Hg and there is an 80 mm Hg gradient across the

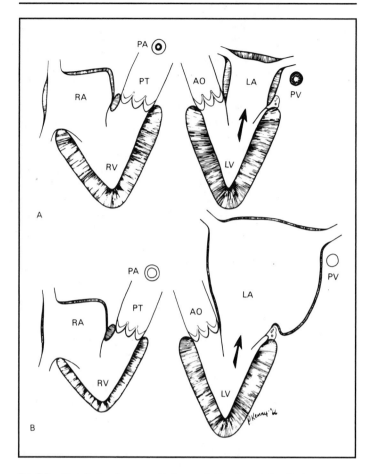

Fig. 5-5 : Two forms of severe mitral regurgitation, i.e., acute mitral regurgitation with a small, high-pressure left atrium (A) and chronic mitral regurgitation with a large, low-pressure left atrium (B). When severe mitral regurgitation develops suddenly in individuals with previously normal or near normal hearts, the left atrium (LA) is relatively small and the high pressure within it is transmitted to the pulmonary vessels and the right ventricle (RV). The left atrium and right ventricle hypertrophy in response to this sudden increase in pressure work. Marked intimal proliferation and medial hypertrophy of pulmonary veins (PV) and arteries (PA) result. In patients with severe chronic mitral regurgitation, the left atrium dilates over time and is therefore capable of "absorbing" the regurgitant flow without elevating the pressure in the pulmonary vessels and right heart. Consequently, there is no intimal proliferation or medial hypertrophy of the pulmonary veins or arteries and the right ventricular wall is not hypertrophied. PT = main pulmonary artery; AO = aorta; RA = right atrium; LV = left ventricle. (From Perloff JK, Roberts WC: The mitral apparatus: Functional anatomy of mitral regurgitation. *Circulation* 46:227, 1972, with permission of the authors and publisher).

aortic valve, then left ventricular systolic pressure is 200 mm Hg. With exercise or pregnancy, cardiac output is augmented, increasing the magnitude of the aortic valve gradient and the systolic pressure that the left ventricle must generate. The situation parallels that of patients with hypertension or coarctation of the aorta in which resistance to left ventricular ejection is located not in the aortic valve but in the systemic arterioles and aortic arch respectively. The increased pressure work (hence the term *pressure overload*) demanded of the left ventricle leads to compensatory left ventricular hypertrophy that is frequently marked. Eventually, pressure overload leads to left ventricular failure. Left ventricular diastolic pressure rises in patients with aortic stenosis as a result of (1) the Starling mechanism and (2) decreased myocardial compliance (increased stiffness). Altered myocardial compliance in aortic stenosis is commonly the result of marked left ventricular hypertrophy. Elevated left ventricular diastolic pressure is transmitted to the left atrium, pulmonary veins, and pulmonary capillaries resulting in increased pulmonary interstitial fluid and the sensation of dyspnea (Fig. 5-6).

The left ventricle in aortic stenosis

Overall left ventricular function as gauged by the ejection fraction (stroke volume/end-diastolic volume) is usually normal in patients with aortic stenosis or other pressure overload conditions. Moreover, left ventricular volumes (end-systolic, end-diastolic volume) are usually also normal. Volume overload, such as that occurring in mitral regurgitation or aortic regurgitation, leads to ventricular dilatation often with reduced ejection fraction. For example, a typical patient with long-standing aortic stenosis has normal left ventricular ejection fraction and left ventricular volumes, markedly increased left ventricular wall thickness, and increased left ventricular diastolic pressure; a typical patient with mitral regurgitation has a reduced left ventricular ejection fraction, markedly increased left ventricular volumes, moderately increased left ventricular diastolic pressure, and normal or slightly increased left ventricular wall thickness (Table 5-2.)

Left atrial systole is important to the maintenance of hemodynamic compensation in patients with aortic stenosis. An appropriately timed atrial systole or "atrial kick" helps to maintain left ventricular end-diastolic volume at the level necessary for effective left ventricular contraction. The thickened, noncompliant left ventricular wall resists diastolic filling. If atrial systole is lost (for example, in atrial fibrillation), left ventricular end-diastolic filling is incomplete and left ventricular stroke volume (pumped through the stenotic aortic valve) declines. Thus, patients with severe aortic stenosis may develop marked clinical deterioration if they develop atrial fibrillation.

Angina pectoris

Patients with aortic stenosis may manifest the symptom of angina pectoris despite the *absence* of coronary arterial obstruction. As

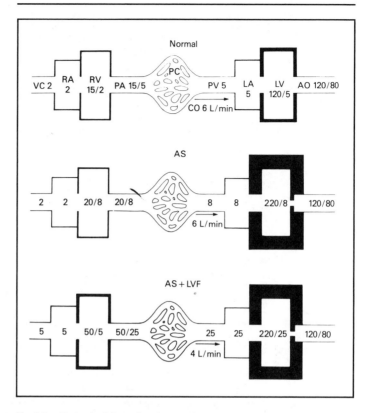

Fig. 5-6 : Pathophysiology of patients with aortic stenosis (AS). The top panel demonstrates normal hemodynamics for comparison. The middle panel demonstrates a patient with severe aortic stenosis and a well-compensated left ventricle (LV). The left ventricle is hypertrophied in response to the increase in pressure work. Left ventricular systolic pressure is 220 mm Hg and aortic systolic pressure is 120 mm Hg. Thus, there is a 100-mm gradient across the aortic valve. Left ventricular diastolic pressure is slightly increased at 8 mm Hg and this small increase in left ventricular diastolic pressure is transmitted to the pulmonary capillaries (PC). Cardiac output (CO) is normal at 6 liters/minute. In the lower panel is depicted a patient with severe aortic stenosis and left ventricular failure (LVF). The gradient across the aortic valve is the same as in the middle panel. However, the left ventricle in the lower panel has failed with resultant elevation in left ventricular diastolic pressure to 25 mm Hg. Consequently, left atrial, pulmonary venous, and pulmonary capillary pressures also rise to 25 mm Hg. Left ventricular stroke volume falls and systemic cardiac output is reduced to 4 liters/minute. There is a secondary rise in pulmonary arterial and right ventricular pressures as a result of the increase in pulmonary venous pressure. VC = vena cava; RA = right atrium; RV = right ventricle; PA = pulmonary artery; PV = pulmonary veins; LA = left atrium; AO = aorta. (From Selzer A: *Principles of Clinical Cardiology: An Analytic Approach.* Philadelphia, Saunders, 1975, with permission of the author and publisher.)

**Table 5-2 : Comparison of pathophysiologic features
of pressure and volume overload of the left ventricle**

Feature	Left ventricular pressure overload (example: aortic stenosis)	Left ventricular volume overload (example: aortic regurgitation)
Ejection fraction	Normal	↓
Volumes	Normal (nondilated)	↑↑ (dilated)
Diastolic pressure	↑↑	↑
Systolic pressure	↑↑	Normal or slightly ↑
Wall thickness	↑↑	Normal or ↑
Compliance	↓↓	Normal or ↓

↑ = modestly increased; ↑↑ = markedly increased; ↓ = modestly decreased; ↓↓ = markedly decreased.

noted in Chapter 2, angina pectoris can occur when myocardial metabolic demand exceeds supply. Such an imbalance of myocardial supply and demand usually develops as a result of obstructive coronary arterial stenoses that impair delivery of oxygen and nutrients to the myocardium despite increasing metabolic demand such as that occurring with exercise. In aortic stenosis, myocardial metabolic demand can outstrip supply even if normal coronary arteries are present. Markedly thickened left ventricular myocardium together with the increased pressure work of aortic stenosis result in such a large increase in myocardial metabolic demand that myocardial ischemia (and hence angina pectoris) develops despite normal coronary arterial supply. Three other factors probably play a minor role in producing myocardial ischemia in patients with aortic stenosis and normal coronary arteries: (1) systolic constriction of intramural coronary arteries during contraction of the hypertrophied left ventricular wall, (2) increased distance between capillaries in the hypertrophied left ventricular wall resulting in a greater than normal diffusion distance for myocardial cell nutrients, and (3) decreased aortic diastolic pressure (the major determinant of coronary arterial perfusion pressure) in some patients with severe aortic stenosis. Of course, angina pectoris may be the result of associated atherosclerotic coronary artery disease.

Syncope

Patients with aortic stenosis may experience episodes of syncope or fainting spells. Such episodes are the result of transient decreases in cerebral blood flow secondary to decreased cardiac output. Two mechanisms are involved in these episodes of transient depression of left ventricular cardiac output: (1) the episodic occurrence of arrhythmias such as atrial fibrillation with the attendant loss of atrial kick can result in a sudden decline in stroke volume that can depress systemic blood pressure and cerebral blood flow, thereby leading to syncope, and (2) the onset of reflex or exercise-induced vasodilatation results in decreased left ventricular filling with a consequent reduction in stroke volume, systemic blood pressure, and cerebral blood flow.

Occasional patients with severe aortic stenosis have marked depression of left ventricular function as manifested by low ejection fraction and a dilated left ventricle. Since stroke volume (aortic valve flow) is low in such individuals, the aortic valve gradient is also low (see Mitral Stenosis in Women, above, for discussion of valve area, gradient, and flow). Such patients may be mistakenly thought to have mild aortic stenosis because of the small aortic valve gradient.

Aortic Regurgitation

Regurgitation of blood back through the aortic valve during diastole occurs as a result of a number of different pathological entities: rheumatic heart disease, bicuspid aortic valve, infectious endocarditis, and myxomatous degeneration to mention only a few. Each of these pathological entities affects the aortic valve so that the leaflets fail to coapt during diastole. Blood flow regurgitates from the aorta into the left ventricle. The volume of regurgitant blood flow increases with rises in aortic diastolic pressure since increased aortic diastolic pressure augments the regurgitant pressure gradient (aortic diastolic pressure minus left ventricular diastolic pressure) across the aortic valve. Bradycardia also increases aortic regurgitant flow by increasing the period of time during which regurgitation occurs, the diastolic filling time. Conversely, tachycardia decreases aortic regurgitant flow. Of course, the extent to which the aortic leaflets fail to coapt, i.e., the area of the regurgitant orifice, is also a determinant of the volume of aortic regurgitant flow: the larger the regurgitant orifice, the greater the flow. In patients with severe aortic regurgitation, regurgitant flow equals or even exceeds forward, systemic flow.

Aortic regurgitation produces a volume overload of the left ventricle; each contraction must eject the normal stroke volume *plus* the regurgitant volume. Left ventricular end-diastolic volume is increased by the quantity of regurgitant blood flow. Thus, the left ventricle is dilated at end-diastole and uses Starling's mechanism to eject the increased volume of blood present at that phase of the cardiac cycle (Table 5-2). Initially, compensatory left ventricular hypertrophy and dilatation maintain cardiovascular homeostasis. Over a period of many years, however, left ventricular function deteriorates and signs and symptoms of heart failure ensue. Left ventricular diastolic pressure rises and is transmitted to the pulmonary capillaries producing pulmonary congestion and the sensation of dyspnea (Fig. 5-7). Increased left ventricular and aortic systolic pressure result from the larger than normal stroke volume; decreased aortic diastolic pressure results from the large run-off of blood backwards into the left ventricle.

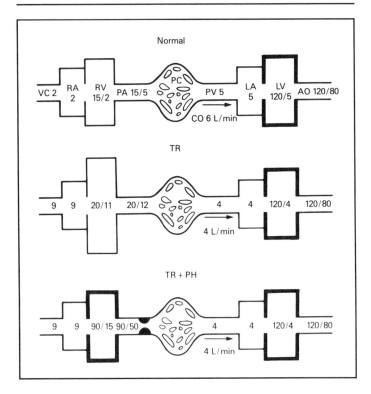

Fig. 5-8 : Pathophysiology of tricuspid regurgitation (TR). The top panel depicts normal hemodynamics for comparison. The middle panel demonstrates the hemodynamic measurements obtained in a patient with tricuspid regurgitation but without pulmonary hypertension (PH). In this individual there is severe regurgitation across the tricuspid valve during right ventricular systole. Consequently, right atrial and central venous pressures are elevated. Right ventricular diastolic pressure increases, the right ventricle (RV) dilates, and forward cardiac output (CO) is reduced to 4 liters/minute. In the lowest panel is depicted a patient with tricuspid regurgitation secondary to pulmonary hypertension. A variety of conditions can result in pulmonary hypertension with secondary tricuspid regurgitation. As noted here, severe pulmonary hypertension is present, and the right ventricle has dilated and hypertrophied in response to the remarkable increase in pulmonary arterial pressure. Severe tricuspid regurgitation results with consequent elevation in central venous and right atrial pressures. Forward cardiac output is reduced to 4 liters/minute. Left heart pressures are unaltered. VC = vena cava; RA = right atrium; PA = pulmonary artery; PC = pulmonary capillaries; PV = pulmonary veins; LA = left atrium; LV = left ventricle; AO = aorta.

right atrial pressures are both elevated secondary to volume overload of the right ventricle. Note that left-sided pressures (left ventricular, left atrial, pulmonary venous, and pulmonary capillary) are at the lower limits of normal reflecting decreased right ventricular stroke volume. Compensatory dilatation of the right ventricle usually develops as a result of tricuspid regurgitation, regardless of etiology. The second series of right heart pressures recorded in Figure 5-8 (labeled 2) are typical of an individual with secondary tricuspid regurgitation. Severe pulmonary hypertension of any etiology (see Chap. 16) produces pressure overload of the right ventricle. The right ventricle dilates and fails more readily than the left ventricle when it is subjected to increased pressure work. Presumably, this is a reflection of the thinner wall and crescentic architecture of the right ventricle. The right ventricle is capable of handling increased volume work with greater ease than increased pressure work. The second example (2) in Figure 5-8 demonstrates the hemodynamic consequences of severe pulmonary hypertension such as that resulting from primary pulmonary hypertension or recurrent pulmonary embolism (see Chap. 16). Right ventricular systolic pressure is markedly increased reflecting the level of pulmonary arterial pressure. The dilated right ventricle has abnormal systolic and diastolic function; right ventricular diastolic and right atrial pressures are increased. Dilatation of the right ventricle combined with the markedly increased level of right ventricular systolic pressure render the tricuspid valve incompetent. Since the valve itself is structurally sound, this form of tricuspid regurgitation is called "secondary." Secondary tricuspid regurgitation is invariably caused by either pulmonary hypertension or right ventricular dilatation and failure. Left ventricular, left atrial, and pulmonary venous and capillary pressures are usually normal.

The regurgitant bolus of blood entering the right atrium results in a marked increase in pressure in that chamber. A recording of right atrial pressure from a patient with tricuspid regurgitation demonstrates the same large regurgitant waves (V waves) as occur in the left atrial pressure recording of patients with mitral regurgitation.

Tricuspid valve disease and mitral regurgitation

Mitral regurgitation is almost always the result of a structural abnormality of the valve, i.e., secondary mitral regurgitation is rare. The anulus of the tricuspid valve is far flimsier in construction than the mitral valve anulus rendering the former prone to dilatation with resultant tricuspid regurgitation.

Tricuspid stenosis

Tricuspid stenosis is a rare entity. It almost always occurs in association with mitral stenosis in patients with rheumatic heart disease. The pathophysiology of tricuspid stenosis is similar to that of mitral stenosis except, of course, that it occurs on the right side of the heart rather than the left (Fig. 5-9). An interesting pathophysiologic feature of combined mitral and tricuspid stenosis is that pulmonary edema

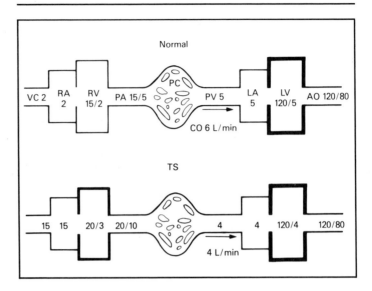

Fig. 5-9 : Pathophysiology of tricuspid stenosis (TS). The upper panel demonstrates normal hemodynamics for comparison. The lower panel demonstrates the situation in a patient with severe tricuspid stenosis. During diastole there is a 12-mm gradient (right atrial pressure of 15 mm Hg − right ventricular pressure of 3 mm Hg) across the tricuspid valve. The marked increase in right atrial pressure is transmitted to the central veins. Pulmonary arterial and left-sided pressures are normal. The stenotic lesion results in a decrease in right ventricular filling with a resultant decrease in forward cardiac output (CO) to 4 liters/minute. VC = vena cava; RA = right atrium; RV = right ventricle; PA = pulmonary artery; PC = pulmonary capillaries; PV = pulmonary veins; LA = left atrium; LV = left ventricle; AO = aorta.

almost never occurs in these individuals despite very severe mitral stenosis. Tricuspid stenosis reduces the volume of blood in the pulmonary circulation thereby decreasing pulmonary capillary pressure and transudation of fluid into the pulmonary interstitium.

Pulmonic Valve Disease

Pulmonic valve disease is relatively uncommon in adults. Pulmonic stenosis is invariably congenital and as such represents one of the commonest congenital cardiac anomalies. Pulmonic regurgitation is an exceedingly rare entity except in patients who have undergone repair of some form of congenital heart disease. These individuals have pulmonic regurgitation as a result of mechanical disruption of the valve at the time of surgery.

The pathophysiology of pulmonic stenosis is similar to that observed with aortic stenosis except, of course, that the gradient occurs across the pulmonic valve (Fig. 5-10). Severe, long-standing pulmonic stenosis leads to marked right ventricular hypertrophy and eventually right ventricular failure with systemic venous congestion. Patients with right ventricular failure can have peripheral edema, hepatic enlargement (secondary to engorgement of the liver with blood), asci-

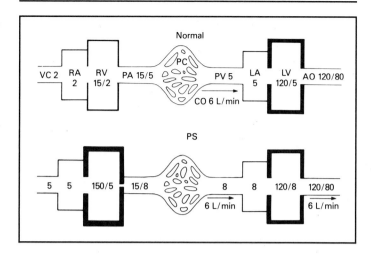

Fig. 5-10 : Pathophysiology of pulmonic stenosis. The upper panel demonstrates the normal situation for comparison. The lower panel demonstrates the situation in a patient with severe pulmonic stenosis (PS). There is a 135-mm gradient across the pulmonic valve (right ventricular systolic pressure of 150 mm Hg – pulmonary arterial systolic pressure of 15 mm Hg). This remarkable increase in right ventricular pressure work results in dilatation and hypertrophy of that chamber. There is a modest increase in right ventricular diastolic pressure (5 mm Hg), which is transmitted to the right atrium (RA) and central vein. Left-sided pressures are normal. The right ventricle (RV) has not failed and therefore forward cardiac output (CO) remains nomal at 6 liters/minute. VC = vena cava; PA = pulmonary artery; PC = pulmonary capillaries; PV = pulmonary veins; LA = left atrium; LV = left ventricle; AO = aorta. (From Selzer A: *Principles of Clinical Cardiology: An Analytic Approach.* Philadelphia, Saunders, 1975, with permission of the author and publisher.)

tes, and malabsorption of nutrients from the bowel (secondary to edema of the bowel wall). Left heart pressures (pulmonary capillary, pulmonary venous, left atrial, and left ventricular) are usually low normal in patients with severe pulmonic stenosis because of the reduced volume of blood that is pumped to the left heart chambers through the stenotic pulmonic valve.

Pulmonic regurgitation

As noted above, pulmonic regurgitation secondary to a primary valvular abnormality is a rare entity. Figure 5-11 records the pathophysiology for two forms of pulmonic regurgitation, primary (1) and secondary (2). In the rare primary pulmonic regurgitation, pulmonary arterial pressure is nearly normal: systolic pressure is modestly increased and diastolic pressure is low normal so that the mean pressure is normal. The right ventricle is dilated secondary to the volume overloaded state analogous to that which occurs with aortic regurgitation. Right ventricular failure essentially never occurs as a result of primary pulmonic regurgitation. Secondary pulmonic regurgitation is usually the result of pulmonary hypertension (Fig. 5-11, Ex. 2). Marked degrees of pulmonary hypertension result in pulmonic valve anular dilatation with resultant pulmonic regurgitation. Right ven-

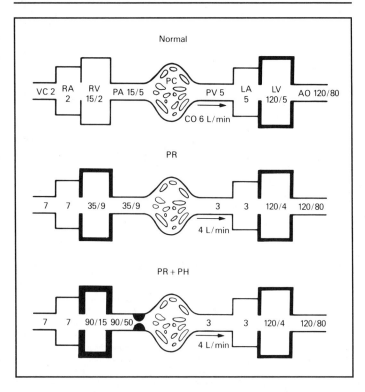

Fig. 5-11 : Pathophysiology of pulmonic regurgitation (PR). The uppermost panel demonstrates normal hemodynamic data for comparison. The middle panel depicts a patient with pulmonic regurgitation without pulmonary hypertension (PH). Right ventricular diastolic and pulmonary artery (PA) diastolic pressures are equal because of communication between these two chambers during diastole as a result of pulmonic regurgitation. There is moderate dilatation and hypertrophy of the right ventricle (RV) with subsequent elevation in right ventricular diastolic pressure. Increased right ventricular diastolic pressure is transmitted to the right atrium (RA) and central veins. Right ventricular systolic output and pressure are increased because of the increase in diastolic filling that results from the regurgitation. Left-sided pressures are normal. There is a modest decrease in forward cardiac output (CO). The lowest panel depicts pulmonic regurgitation secondary to severe pulmonary hypertension. A variety of conditions may result in such severe pulmonary hypertension. Marked right ventricular hypertrophy and dilatation result from the marked pressure and volume overload. The pulmonic valve is insufficient as a result of the marked increase in pulmonary artery pressure. Right ventricular diastolic pressure is elevated and this elevation is transmitted to the right atrium and central veins. Left-sided pressures are normal. Forward cardiac output is reduced as a result of the reduction in right ventricular stroke volume. **VC** = vena cava; **PC** = pulmonary capillaries; **PV** = pulmonary veins; **LA** = left atrium; **LV** = left ventricle; **AO** = aorta.

tricular failure with attendant systemic venous congestion often results from chronic pulmonary hypertension since the right ventricle tolerates such pressure overload poorly. Thus, secondary pulmonic regurgitation may be accompanied by signs and symptoms of right ventricular failure. However, right ventricular failure is the result of pulmonary hypertension and not pulmonic regurgitation. Left heart pressures are usually quite low in patients with pulmonic regurgitation secondary to pulmonary hypertension (Fig. 5-11).

Suggested Readings

Roberts WC, Perloff JK: Mitral valvular disease. *Ann Intern Med* 77:939, 1972.

Selzer A, Cohn KE: Natural history of mitral stenosis: A review. *Circulation* 45:878, 1972.

Gorlin R, Gorlin SG: Hydraulic formula for calculations of the area of the stenotic mitral valve, other cardiac valves, and central circulatory shunts. *Am Heart J* 41:1, 1951.

Rapaport E: Natural history of aortic and mitral valve disease. *Am J Cardiol* 35:221, 1975.

Ward C, Hancock BW: Extreme pulmonary hypertension caused by mitral valve disease. *Br Heart J* 37:74, 1975.

Selzer A: Nonrheumatic mitral regurgitation. *Mod Concepts Cardiovasc* 48:25, 1979.

Selzer A, Katayama F: Mitral regurgitation: Clinical patterns, pathophysiology and natural history. *Medicine* (Baltimore) 51:337, 1972.

Tyrrell MJ et al: Correlation of degree of left ventricular volume overload with clinical course in aortic and mitral regurgitation. *Br Heart J* 32:683, 1970.

Braunwald E: Mitral regurgitation: Physiologic, clinical and surgical considerations. *N Engl J Med* 281:425, 1969.

Perloff JK, Roberts WC: The mitral apparatus: Functional anatomy of mitral regurgitation. *Circulation* 46:227, 1972.

Bulkley BR, Roberts WC: Dilatation of mitral anulus: A rare cause of mitral regurgitation. *Am J Med* 59:457, 1975.

Heikkila J: Mitral incompetence complicating acute myocardial infarction. *Br Heart J* 29:162, 1976.

Bartle SH, Hermann HJ: Acute mitral regurgitation in man. *Circulation* 36:839, 1967.

Bolen JL, Aldermann EL: Ventriculographic and hemodynamic features of mitral regurgitation of cardiomyopathic, rheumatic and nonrheumatic etiology. *Am J Cardiol* 39:177, 1977.

Sanders CA et al: Etiology and differential diagnosis of acute mitral regurgitation. *Prog Cardiovasc Dis* 14:129, 1971.

Roberts WC: Aortic valve stenosis and the congenitally malformed aortic valve, in Roberts WC (ed): *Congenital Heart Disease in Adults*. Philadelphia, Davis, 1979, pp 416–426.

Roberts WC: Anatomically isolated aortic valvular disease. The case against its being of rheumatic etiology. *Am J Med* 49:151, 1970.

Stein PD, Sabbah HN, Pitha JV: Continuing disease process of calcific aortic stenosis: Role of microthrombi and turbulent flow. *Am J Cardiol* 39:159, 1977.

Roberts WC, Perloff JK, Constantino T: Severe valvular aortic stenosis in patients over 65 years of age. A clinicopathologic study. *Am J Cardiol* 27:497, 1971.

Ross J Jr, Braunwald E: Aortic stenosis. *Circulation* 38 (suppl V):61, 1968.

Flamm MD et al: Mechanism of effort syncope in aortic stenosis. *Circulation* 36 (suppl II):190, 1967.

Mark AL et al: Abnormal vascular response to exercise in patients with aortic stenosis. *J Clin Invest* 52:1138, 1973.

Johnson AM: Aortic stenosis, sudden death and left ventricular baroreceptors. *Br Heart J* 33:1, 1971.

Braunwald E et al: Congenital aortic stenosis. I. Clinical and hemodynamic findings in 100 patients. *Circulation* 27:426, 1963.

Andersen JA, Hansen GF, Lyngeborg K: Isolated valvular aortic stenosis. *Acta Med Scand* 197:61, 1975.

Kennedy JW et al: Quantitative angiocardiography. III. Relationships of left ventricular pressure, volume, and mass in aortic valve disease. *Circulation* 38:838, 1968.

Brawley RK, Morrow AG: Direct determination of aortic blood flow in patients with aortic regurgitation: Effects of alterations in heart rates, increased ventricular preload and afterload, and isoproterenol. *Circulation* 35:32, 1967.

Goldschlager N et al: The natural history of aortic regurgitation: A clinical and hemodynamic study. *Am J Med* 54:577, 1973.

Borer JS et al: Exercise-induced left ventricular dysfunction in symptomatic and asymptomatic patients with aortic regurgitation: Assessment with radionuclide cineangiography. *Am J Cardiol* 42:351, 1978.

Judge TP et al: Quantitative hemodynamic effect of heart rate in aortic regurgitation. *Circulation* 44:355, 1971.

Lewis RP, Bristow JD, Griswold HE: Exercise hemodynamics in aortic regurgitation. *Am Heart J* 80:171, 1970.

Fischl SJ, Gorlin R, Herman MV: Cardiac shape and function in aortic valve disease: Physiologic and clinical implications. *Am J Cardiol* 39:170, 1977.

Rackley CE, Hood WP Jr: Quantitative angiographic evaluation and pathophysiologic mechanisms of valvular heart disease. *Prog Cardiovasc Dis* 15:427, 1973.

Morganroth J et al: Acute, severe aortic regurgitation. *Ann Intern Med* 87:223, 1977.

Salazar E, Levine HD: Rheumatic tricuspid regurgitation: The clinical spectrum. *Am J Med* 33:111, 1962.

Hansing CE, Rowe GG: Tricuspid insufficiency: A study of hemodynamics and pathogenesis. *Circulation* 45:793, 1972.

Killip T, Lukas DS: Tricuspid stenosis. Physiologic criteria for diagnosis and hemodynamic abnormalities. *Circulation* 16:3, 1957.

Keefe JF, Wolk MJ, Levine HJ: Isolated tricuspid valvular stenosis. *Am J Cardiol* 25:252, 1970.

Steelman RB et al: Congenital stenosis of the pulmonic and tricuspid valves. *Am J Med* 54:788, 1973.

Snellen HA et al: Pulmonic stenosis. *Circulation* 37,38 (suppl 5):V–93, 1968.

Alday LE, Moreyra E: Calcific pulmonary stenosis. *Br Heart J* 35:887, 1973.

Roberts WC et al: Calcific pulmonic stenosis. *Circulation* 37:973, 1968.

Silverman BK et al: Pulmonary stenosis with intact ventricular septum: Correlation of clinical and physiologic data, with review of operative results. *Am J Med* 20:53, 1956.

Moller JH, Rao S, Lucas RV: Exercise hemodynamics of pulmonary valvular stenosis: Study of 64 children. *Circulation* 46:1018, 1972.

Stone FM et al: Pre- and post-operative rest and exercise hemodynamics in children with pulmonary stenosis. *Circulation* 49:1102, 1974.

Hamby RI, Gulotta SJ: Pulmonic valvular insufficiency: Etiology, recognition, and management. *Am Heart J* 74:110, 1967.

Talbert JL et al: The incidence and significance of pulmonic regurgitation after pulmonary valvulotomy. *Am Heart J* 65:590, 1963.

Holmes JC, Fowler NO, Kaplan S: Pulmonary valvular insufficiency. *Am J Med* 44:851, 1968.

6 : Myocardial and Pericardial Disease

Myocardial Disease (Cardiomyopathy, Myocardiopathy)

A variety of disease entities can affect the heart muscle, resulting in abnormal systolic or diastolic myocardial function and/or arrhythmias. The pathophysiology of cardiomyopathy can be subdivided into four categories: hypertrophic, congestive, restrictive, and obliterative (Table 6-1). Each of these categories of cardiomyopathy is associated with a distinct pattern of abnormal physiology. A number of cardiologists also make a distinction between primary and secondary cardiomyopathy.

Primary cardiomyopathy is heart muscle disease affecting the heart alone, usually of unknown etiology. Secondary cardiomyopathy is heart muscle disease that results from a known disease process that affects other parts of the body and only ''secondarily'' involves the myocardium. However, both primary and secondary cardiomyopathy produce signs and symptoms that are the result of one of the four patterns of cardiomyopathic pathophysiology: hypertrophic, congestive, restrictive, or obliterative (Table 6-1).

Hypertrophic cardiomyopathy

This type of cardiomyopathy has acquired a bewildering array of names over the last 20 years: *asymmetric septal hypertrophy (ASH), idiopathic hypertrophic subaortic stenosis (IHSS), hypertrophic obstructive cardiomyopathy, muscular subaortic stenosis,* and *obstructive cardiomyopathy.* Abnormal *myocardial hypertrophy* is the hallmark of this condition which is inherited as an autosomal dominant trait with a high degree of penetrance. Patients develop myocardial hypertrophy, often of marked degree, involving various portions of the left ventricle. The hypertrophic process is apparently related to zones of disarrayed, disorganized, and bizarrely formed myocardial cells that work in opposition to each other rather than in concert. Patients with hypertrophic cardiomyopathy may demonstrate localized hypertrophy of the septum or free wall of the left ventricle or symmetrical hypertrophy of the entire left ventricular cavity.

The essential pathophysiologic feature of hypertrophic cardiomyopathy is abnormal myocardial diastolic function (reduced compliance or increased stiffness). This results from the marked left ventricular hypertrophy noted in many of these individuals. Increased left ventricular diastolic pressure secondary to decreased myocardial compli-

Table 6-1 : Pathophysiologic classification of cardiomyopathy

Classification	Description
I. Hypertrophic	Stiffened, thick ventricular muscle with good contractile function; can involve the heart in an asymmetric manner, e.g., asymmetric septal hypertrophy; markedly abnormal myocardial diastolic function
II. Congestive	Dilated, poorly contracting ventricle, e.g., viral or alcoholic cardiomyopathy
III. Restrictive	Stiffened ventricular muscle secondary to deposition of material between or within myocardial fibers, e.g., amyloidosis
IV. Obliterative	Obliteration of ventricular cavity; quite rare; e.g., Löffler's eosinophilic endocarditis

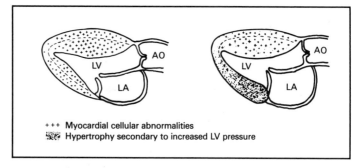

+++ Myocardial cellular abnormalities

Hypertrophy secondary to increased LV pressure

Fig. 6-1 : Pathophysiologic spectrum of hypertrophic cardiomyopathy (HOCM). In nonobstructive hypertrophic cardiomyopathy (left) abnormal, hypertrophied myocardial cells are widespread and present in both the ventricular septum and free wall. Nonuniform wall thickening in these individuals is presumably the result of these cellular abnormalities. In obstructive hypertrophic cardiomyopathy (right), however, the abnormal myocardial cells are localized largely in the ventricular septum, and uniform thickening of the free wall apparently results from the left ventricular outflow obstruction. LV = left ventricle; LA = left atrium; AO = aorta. (From Henry WL et al: Differences in distribution of myocardial abnormalities in patients with obstructive and nonobstructive asymmetric septal hypertrophy [ASH]. *Circulation* **50:447, 1974, with permission of the authors and publisher.)**

ance is transmitted to the left atrium, pulmonary veins, and capillaries. The resultant transudation of fluid into the pulmonary interstitium lies behind the sensation of dyspnea sensed by many patients with hypertrophic cardiomyopathy.

Systolic function is usually normal or supranormal in patients with hypertrophic cardiomyopathy. Late in the course of the illness patients may develop deteriorating left ventricular contractile function with associated left ventricular dilatation.

There are two pathophysiologic subcategories of hypertrophic cardiomyopathy: obstructive and nonobstructive (Fig. 6-1). In the nonobstructive form of the disease, the abnormal myocardial architecture,

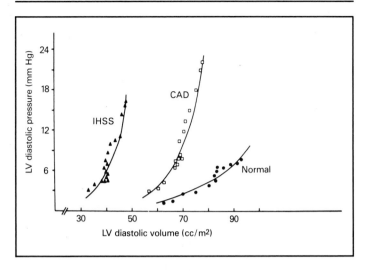

Fig. 6-2 : Left ventricular (LV) diastolic pressure in mm Hg plotted against left ventricular volume in cubic centimeters per square meter body surface area for three patients: one with hypertrophic cardiomyopathy (IHSS), one with coronary artery disease (CAD), and one with a normal heart. The patient with hypertrophic cardiomyopathy has the diastolic pressure/volume curve displaced to the left of normal. Left ventricular stiffness is three times normal in this individual. The patient with coronary artery disease also has abnormally increased left ventricular stiffness. (From Gaasch WH et al: LV compliance: Mechanisms and clinical implications. *Am J Cardiol* 38:645, 1976, with permission of the authors and publisher.)

myocardial hypertrophy, and associated fibrosis result in a marked decrease in left ventricular compliance (increased stiffness). As one can see in Figure 6-2, the pressure-volume relationship is very abnormal in patients with hypertrophic cardiomyopathy (labeled IHSS in Fig. 6-2). Thus, small increases in left ventricular diastolic volume result in large increases in diastolic pressure that are eventually transmitted to the pulmonary capillaries. Patients with ischemic heart disease (labeled CAD in Fig. 6-2) also demonstrate abnormal myocardial stiffness (see p. 30, 36). As noted earlier patients with non-obstructive hypertrophic cardiomyopathy usually have normal or supranormal systolic (contractile) function with high ejection fractions.

Patients with the obstructive form of hypertrophic cardiomyopathy have a dynamic (changing) gradient across the left ventricular outflow tract. The mechanism producing this obstructive gradient is disputed but is apparently related to marked septal hypertrophy and abnormal motion of the anterior mitral valve leaflet. Presumably, some combination of septal encroachment and anterior mitral valve leaflet displacement into the left ventricular outflow tract results in the obstruction to left ventricular emptying. Interventions that *decrease* left ventricular cavity size *increase* the degree of outflow tract

Table 6-2 : Effects of various interventions on dynamic left ventricular outflow tract obstruction in patients with hypertrophic cardiomyopathy

Interventions that decrease left ventricular volume (↑ obstruction,
   ↑ gradient, ↑ murmur)
  Valsalva maneuver
  Standing
  Nitroglycerin administration
  Hypovolemia (e.g., dehydration, hemorrhage, vasodilatation)
Interventions that increase left ventricular volume (↓ obstruction, ↓ gradient,
   ↓ murmur)
  Squatting
  Lying down with legs elevated
  Isometric handgrip
  Mueller maneuver
Interventions that increase left ventricular contractility (↑ obstruction,
   ↑ gradient, ↑ murmur)
  Exercise
  Tachycardia
  Postextrasystole
  Digitalis administration
  Isoproterenol administration
Interventions that decrease left ventricular contractility (↓ obstruction,
   ↓ gradient, ↓ murmur)
  Beta-adrenergic blockade
  General anesthesia

---

obstruction. In addition, interventions that *increase* myocardial contractility increase outflow tract obstruction (Table 6-2). Increasing outflow tract obstruction is associated with an increase in the gradient from left ventricle to aorta and with an increase in the systolic murmur that results from the obstruction (Table 6-2).

Patients with obstructive hypertrophic cardiomyopathy develop pulmonary venous and pulmonary capillary hypertension with associated transudation of fluid into the pulmonary parenchyma for two reasons: (1) decreased left ventricular compliance (as described above for nonobstructive hypertrophic cardiomyopathy) and (2) increased left ventricular volume and pressure in response to the left ventricular outflow obstruction (Starling mechanism). Systolic (contractile) left ventricular function is well preserved in obstructive hypertrophic cardiomyopathy until late in the natural history of the disease when decreasing left ventricular ejection fraction and ventricular dilatation may develop. Pulmonary congestion with attendant dyspnea worsens during this latter phase of the natural history.

Patients with hypertrophic cardiomyopathy can complain of angina, dyspnea, or syncope. Angina in the absense of obstructive coronary artery disease is the result of increased myocardial oxygen demand (increased left ventricular wall thickness; increased left ventricular systolic pressure). Dyspnea results from pulmonary venous hypertension (as described above), and syncopal episodes are secondary to episodic ventricular arrhythmias (see Chap. 14).

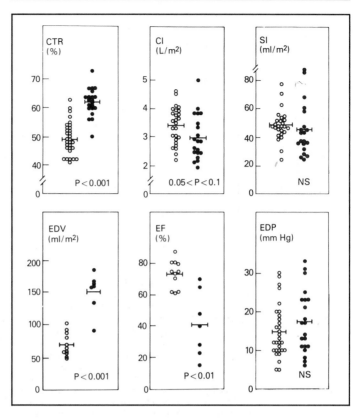

Fig. 6-3 : Comparison of a number of left ventricular functional and anatomic measurements in patients with hypertrophic cardiomyopathy to those in individuals with congestive cardiomyopathy. Patients with hypertrophic cardiomyopathy are represented by open circles; patients with congestive cardiomyopathy are represented by closed circles. CTR = cardiothoracic ratio as obtained from the standard PA chest x-ray, CI = cardiac index; SI = stroke volume index; EDV = end-diastolic volume; EF = ejection fraction of the left ventricle; EDP = left ventricular end-diastolic pressure. The horizontal bars represent mean values; P values for statistical significance are displayed at the bottom of each comparison. NS stands for nonsignificant difference. (From Kawai C, Takatsu T: Clinical and experimental studies on cardiomyopathy. *N Engl J Med* 293:592, 1975, with permission of the authors and publisher.)

Congestive
cardiomyopathy

Patients with congestive cardiomyopathy demonstrate moderate to marked *depression of left ventricular systolic (contractile) function.* Left ventricular contractility measurements of either the isovolumic phase (dp/dt, V_{max}) or the ejection phase (ejection fraction [V_{cf}]) of left ventricular systole are markedly depressed (Figs.6-3 and 6-4). The left ventricle dilates in response to the depression in myocardial contractility (Starling mechanism). Myocardial hypertrophy is absent or mild. The result is a dilated left ventricle with normal or slightly thickened walls and poor contractile function. Left ventricular ejection fraction is commonly less than 20% late in the course of the illness.

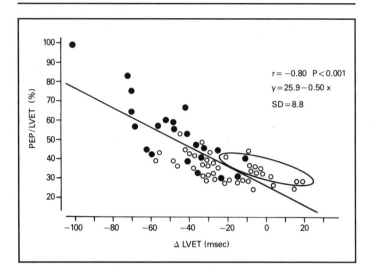

Fig. 6-4 : Left ventricular function as determined by noninvasively measured systolic time intervals. The PEP/LVET ratio (pre-ejection period/left ventricular ejection time) is plotted against deviation from the normal left ventricular ejection time (LVET) in 62 patients, 40 with hypertrophic cardiomyopathy (represented by open circles) and 22 patients with congestive cardiomyopathy (represented by closed circles). The elipse demonstrates the zone of 95% confidence limits for patients with normal left ventricular contractile function. The equation for the regression line is displayed as is standard deviation (SD) and the correlation coefficient (r). It can be seen that left ventricular contractile function is much more abnormal in patients with congestive cardiomyopathy than in patients with hypertrophic cardiomyopathy. (From Kawai C, Takatsu T: Clinical and experimental studies on cardiomyopathy. *N Engl J Med* 293:592, 1975, with permission of the authors and publisher.)

Congestive cardiomyopathy has a variety of causes: alcohol, viral or other infectious agent, hypertension, and pregnancy are among the more common. Some patients with congestive cardiomyopathy of obscure origin have an increased incidence of complement-fixing antibodies to a variety of viruses suggesting that in these individuals congestive cardiomyopathy is the result of viral myocarditis.

Patients with congestive cardiomyopathy usually have markedly dilated ventricles that are symmetrically involved by the disease process. This is in sharp contrast to the asymmetric involvement of ventricular myocardium frequently noted in patients with hypertrophic cardiomyopathy. Patients who develop dilated, failing ventricles as a result of ischemic heart disease also demonstrate asymmetric involvement of the ventricles due to regional coronary arterial obstruction. Most patients with congestive cardiomyopathy have normal coronary arteries.

Diastolic function is abnormal in patients with congestive cardiomyopathy—various measurements of myocardial stiffness are abnormally increased. However, abnormal systolic function overshadows

Table 6-3 : Etiology of acute myocarditis

Infectious	Toxic	Metabolic
Viral	Serum sickness	Nutritional deficiencies
Rickettsial	Uremia	(protein, vitamin)
Bacterial	Radiation	Endocrine (pituitary,
Fungal	Phenothiazines	thyroid)
Chagas' disease	Industrial exposure to	
(*Trypanosoma cruzi*)	toxic chemicals	
Trichinosis	Cobalt and other	
Rheumatic fever (group	heavy metals	
A beta-hemolytic		
streptococci).		

diastolic dysfunction. Abnormal systolic and diastolic function in patients with congestive cardiomyopathy leads to pulmonary venous hypertension and low cardiac output. Consequently, patients complain of dyspnea and fatigue. Left ventricular failure leads to pulmonary hypertension and eventually to right ventricular failure. Ventricular dilatation causes abnormal papillary muscle function with resultant mitral and/or tricuspid valve regurgitation that heightens pulmonary and systemic venous hypertension (Chap. 5, Pathophysiology of Mitral Regurgitation). Ventricular dilatation and hypofunction lie behind the three major fatal complications that develop in patients with congestive cardiomyopathy: (1) intractable heart failure, (2) malignant ventricular arrhythmias, and (3) arterial or venous embolism.

Acute myocarditis (inflammation of the myocardium) can present with a clinical and pathophysiologic picture that resembles congestive cardiomyopathy. A variety of agents transiently or permanently injure myocardial cells leading to diffuse systolic and diastolic myocardial dysfunction (Table 6-3). The pathophysiologic sequence may be similar to that described above for congestive cardiomyopathy. However, the timing of events is frequently different with congestive cardiomyopathy having a chronic course over years and myocarditis developing acutely. Congestive cardiomyopathy is only reversible on occasion while myocarditis is often at least partially reversible.

Restrictive and obliterative cardiomyopathy

These last two forms of cardiomyopathy are considered together since their pathophysiology is similar. *Abnormal diastolic myocardial function (increased stiffness)* is the hallmark of these two forms of cardiomyopathy. Obliterative cardiomyopathy rarely occurs in North America. This entity is characterized by progressive thrombosis and fibrosis of the left and right ventricular endocardium. Diastolic dysfunction with markedly increased ventricular filling pressures usually overshadows systolic (contractile) dysfunction. Patients manifest signs and symptoms of left (pulmonary venous hypertension) and right (systemic venous hypertension) ventricular failure.

Table 6-4 : Etiologies of restrictive cardiomyopathy

Amyloidosis
Hemochromatosis
Sarcoidosis
Neoplasm
Glycogen storage disorders
Mucopolysaccharidosis
Gaucher's disease
Whipple's disease
Fabry's disease

Table 6-5 : Etiologies of pericardial effusion

Allergic reaction: serum sickness, drug reactions
Hypersensitivity reaction: posttrauma, postpericardiotomy, postmyocardial
    infarction
Infection: viral, bacterial, fungal, parasitic
Collagen-vascular disease: rheumatoid arthritis, lupus erythematosus
Radiation
Neoplasm: metastatic involvement of the pericardium
Uremia
Hypothyroidism

Restrictive cardiomyopathy is also characterized by markedly abnormal myocardial diastolic function. The pathophysiologic sequence observed in these patients reflects the abnormal filling characteristics of the ventricles. Systolic contractile performance is often abnormal as well but is overshadowed by diastolic dysfunction. A variety of factors cause restrictive cardiomyopathy leading to abnormal diastolic function (Table 6-4).

A common feature of many of the entities listed in Table 6-4 is infiltration of the myocardium. Such infiltration leads to increased myocardial diastolic stiffness (reduced compliance) with attendant pulmonary and systemic venous hypertension. Patients complain of dyspnea (pulmonary congestion), abdominal swelling (ascites from systemic venous hypertension), and ankle edema (systemic venous hypertension). Reduced cardiac output with attendant fatigue may also be present.

Pericardial Disease   The intact pericardium functions as a restraint, preventing excessive acute ventricular dilatation. As such, it appears that the pericardium plays an important role in determining ventricular diastolic behavior (compliance). On the other hand, the pericardium does not have much effect on ventricular systolic (contractile) function. Two diseases of the pericardium have profound effects on cardiac function: cardiac tamponade and pericardial constriction.

Cardiac tamponade   A variety of pathological processes produce transudation of fluid from the epicardium and pericardium into the pericardial space (Table 6-5). Approximately 100 ml of fluid can be accommodated in the

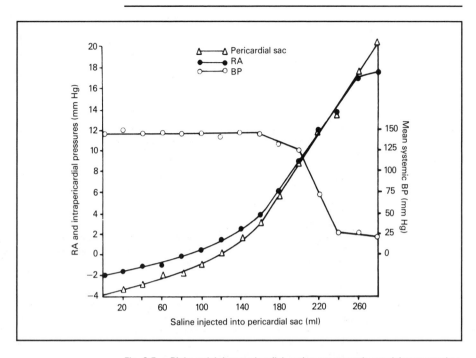

Fig. 6-5 : Right atrial, intrapericardial, and mean systemic arterial pressures in a 20.9-kg dog with experimental production of cardiac tamponade. Tamponade is produced by means of serial injections of saline solution into the pericardial sac. When more than 160 ml of saline is injected into the pericardial sac, right atrial and intrapericardial pressures rise very steeply and systemic blood pressure (BP) falls rapidly. Blood pressure in a systemic artery falls to shock levels when intrapericardial pressure exceeds 14 mm Hg. RA = right atrium. (From Fowler NO: Physiology of cardiac tamponade and pulsus paradoxus. II. Physiological, circulatory and pharmacological responses in cardiac tamponade. *Mod Conc Cardiovasc Dis* 47:115, 1978, with permission of the author and publisher.)

pericardial space without an increase in pressure. However, small amounts of additional fluid beyond that volume produce large increases in pressure in the pericardial space (Fig. 6-5). In other words, the pressure-volume curve for the pericardium and its associated space is initially flat until a volume of approximately 100 ml accumulates in the pericardial space. Thereafter, the pressure-volume curve is very steep (Fig. 6-5). Increased pericardial pressure is transmitted to the heart causing cardiac compression with resultant elevated right and left atrial pressures. Central venous and pulmonary capillary pressures rise as a result of increased right and left atrial pressures. Increased atrial pressures impede normal ventricular diastolic filling with resultant decreased ventricular systolic and diastolic volumes and stroke output. Cardiac output falls despite compensatory tachycardia mediated by increased sympathetic nervous stimulation of the heart (Fig. 6-6). Patients with pericardial effusions large enough to increase left and right atrial pressure and impair ventricular filling are said to have *cardiac tamponade.*

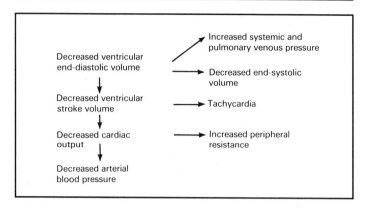

Fig. 6-6 : Pathophysiologic sequence of cardiac tamponade. (From Fowler NO: Physiology of cardiac tamponade and pulsus paradoxus. II. Physiological, circulatory and pharmacological responses in cardiac tamponade. *Mod Conc Cardiovasc Dis* 47:115, 1978, with permission of the author and publisher.)

Table 6-6 : Physical findings in cardiac tamponade

Tachycardia
Decreased systolic arterial pressure and pulse pressure
Pulsus paradoxus
Elevated jugular venous pressure
Hepatic congestion
Heart sounds faint or normal
Apical impulse not palpable

Patients with cardiac tamponade have findings on physical examination resembling those seen in individuals with heart failure because increased venous pressure and decreased cardiac output are common to both of these conditions. Table 6-6 lists the physical findings that are commonly observed in patients with cardiac tamponade. Of particular interest is the entity known as "pulsus paradoxus." The term *pulsus paradoxus* refers to an accentuation of the normal inspiratory fall in arterial blood pressure beyond the normal value of less than 10 mm Hg (Figure 6-7). Numerous experimental and clinical studies have examined the mechanism of pulsus paradoxus. Such investigations have shown that pulsus paradoxus is caused by a marked inspiratory decrease in left ventricular filling with resultant decreased stroke volume and systemic arterial blood pressure (Fig. 6-8A). The sequence of events leading to decreased left ventricular filling and stroke volume is as follows: inspiratory augmentation of negative intrathoracic pressure results in increased venous return of blood to the right heart, and this produces a shift of the ventricular septum towards the left ventricular cavity with resultant decrease in the filling capacity of that chamber (Fig. 6-8A). In other words, increased right ventricular filling occurs at the expense of decreased left ventricular filling. Decreased left ventricular filling leads to decreased stroke volume and arterial blood pressure. A second and

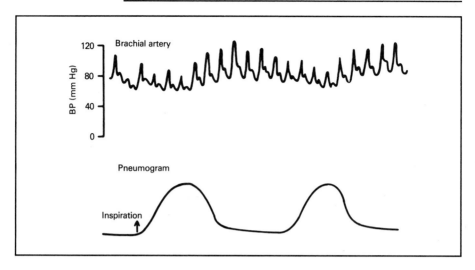

Fig. 6-7 : Demonstration of paradoxical pulse in a patient with cardiac tamponade. Note the striking inspiratory decline in brachial arterial blood pressure (BP). The pneumogram demonstrates inspiration and expiration. (From Fowler NO: *Inspection and Palpation of Venous and Arterial Pulses.* Dallas, Tex, American Heart Association, 1967, with permission of the author and publisher.)

presumably less important factor involved in the production of pulsus paradoxus is decreased inspiratory pulmonary venous return of blood to the left atrium. This is caused by an increase in pulmonary vascular capacity during inspiration (Fig. 6-8B).

All of the pathophysiologic alterations associated with cardiac tamponade are reversible if sufficient fluid is removed from the pericardial space.

Pericardial constriction

Pericardial constriction is a chronic condition of gradual onset in contradistinction to cardiac tamponade which is usually acute in onset. Constriction is the end-result of a fibrous reaction in the pericardium set into motion by an earlier episode of pericarditis. Almost any of the types of pericarditis listed in Table 6-5 can eventually lead to pericardial constriction. In such individuals, the densely adherent pericardium and associated scar tissue cause a marked decrease in myocardial compliance (increased stiffness) thereby interfering with normal ventricular diastolic function (filling). Ventricular contractile (systolic) function is normal or modestly abnormal. The pathophysiology resembles that seen with restrictive cardiomyopathy (see Restrictive and Obliterative Cardiomyopathy). The basic abnormality in both of these conditions is reduced myocardial compliance or increased myocardial stiffness. In restrictive cardiomyopathy, the myocardium itself is abnormally stiff. In pericardial constriction, however, myocardial stiffness is normal or near normal; pericardial scar tissue, tightly

Table 6-7 : Hemodynamic differentiation of constrictive pericarditis and restrictive cardiomyopathy

Parameter	Constrictive pericarditis	Restrictive cardiomyopathy
Right atrial pressure	Almost always > 15 mm Hg	Usually < 15 mm Hg if pulmonary capillary wedge pressure is normal
Right ventricular pressure	Square root sign always present End-diastolic pressure equals or exceeds one-third of systolic pressure	Square root sign may disappear with therapy
Pulmonary artery pressure	Systolic pressure usually < 40 mm Hg	Systolic pressure usually greater than 40 mm Hg
Left atrial pressure	Approximately equal to right atrial pressure	10–20 mm Hg higher than right atrial pressure
Cardiac output	Often normal	Often depressed
Resting pulmonary arterial blood oxygen saturation	Often normal	Often decreased
Respiratory variation in pressure tracings	Often absent	Often present

Pericardial constriction and pericardial tamponade usually involve the entire heart, producing elevated, equal pressures in all heart chambers during diastole. Thus, the hemodynamic hallmark of cardiac compression or constriction is right atrial pressure = right ventricular diastolic pressure = pulmonary arterial diastolic pressure = pulmonary capillary pressure = pulmonary venous pressure = left atrial pressure = left ventricular diastolic pressure. Pulsus paradoxus may be present in patients with pericardial constriction. The pathophysiologic explanation for this physical finding in individuals with constriction is the same as for patients with cardiac tamponade.

Distinguishing restrictive cardiomyopathy from pericardial constriction may be difficult since the pathologic physiology of these two entities is so similar. Table 6-7 lists a number of hemodynamic differences between these two conditions that may enable the physician to distinguish between them.

Suggested Readings

Kawai C, Takatsu T: Clinical and experimental studies on cardiomyopathy. *N Engl J Med 293:592, 1975.*

Goodwin JF: Prospects and predictions for the cardiomyopathies. *Circulation* 50:210, 1974.

Benotti JR, Grossman W, Cohn PF: Clinical profile of restrictive cardiomyopathy. *Circulation* 61:1206, 1980.

Burch GE, Tsui CY, Harb JM: Ischemic cardiomyopathy. *Am Heart J* 83:340, 1972.

Fuster V et al: The natural history of idiopathic dilated cardiomyopathy. *Am J Cardiol* 47:525, 1981.

Fowler NO: Physiology of cardiac tamponade and pulsus paradoxus, I and II. *Mod Conc Cardiovasc Dis* 48:109, 115, 1978.

Shabetai R, Fowler NO, Guntheroth WG: The hemodynamics of cardiac tamponade and constrictive pericarditis. *Am J Cardiol* 26:480, 1970.

Reddy PS et al: Cardiac tamponade, hemodynamic observations in man. *Circulation* 58:265, 1978.

Settle HP et al: Echocardiographic study of cardiac tamponade. *Circulation* 56:951, 1977.

7 : Congenital Heart Disease

Adult patients with congenital heart disease are rather uncommon since the vast majority of such defects are recognized and corrected during childhood or adolescence. However, such lesions are of interest even to cardiologists who treat adults since their pathophysiology represents some of the most interesting "experiments of nature" to be found in medicine. Five distinct entities account for more than 90% of all cases of congenital heart disease occurring in adults and more than 50% of pediatric patients with congenital heart lesions: atrial septal defect, ventricular septal defect, pulmonic stenosis, patent ductus arteriosus, and coarctation of the aorta. Pulmonic stenosis has already been discussed in Chapter 5. This chapter will consider the pathophysiology of the other four commonly occurring forms of congenital heart disease.

Atrial Septal Defect

Atrial septal defect (ASD) is the commonest form of congenital heart disease in adults if one does not classify mitral valve prolapse and bicuspid aortic valve as congenital heart defects. Atrial septal defect is often overlooked during childhood because patients are asymptomatic or nearly so and the physical findings associated with this entity are rather subtle. Consequently, ASD is first recognized in a surprisingly large number of adult patients.

It is convenient to think of the pathophysiology of ASD as if all heart chambers were in communication during diastole: both atrioventricular valves are open and the atrial septum is absent or nearly so. In this setting, systemic and pulmonary venous flow comingle in the "common atrium." Where this comingled blood goes after reaching the common atrium depends on the respective resistance to inflow of the right and left ventricles. Shortly after birth, the right ventricle is hypertrophied and hence noncompliant (stiff). This is the result of the great work load that the right ventricle faces during fetal life: the lungs are deflated and the pulmonary vascular bed has a high resistance secondary to hypertrophy of the media of the pulmonary arterioles. Moreover, the right ventricle pumps blood into the systemic circulation through the patent ductus arteriosus. Therefore, the fetal right and left ventricles present approximately equal resistances to blood flowing from the atria across the tricuspid and mitral valves during diastole. Systemic and pulmonary venous diastolic flow are thus more or less equally divided between the two ventricles in infants with ASD.

Shortly after birth, the lungs become inflated and pulmonary vascular resistance begins to decline, reaching the low value it maintains during adult life at some point during early childhood. As pulmonary vascular resistance declines, right ventricular hypertrophy regresses and right ventricular stiffness declines (increased compliance). Thus, incoming diastolic blood flow to the common atrium is faced with far less resistance across the tricuspid valve as compared with the mitral valve. Consequently, considerably more blood enters the right ventricle than arrives in the left ventricle. The result is a so-called left-to-right shunt, since essentially all of the systemic venous blood and a goodly portion of the pulmonary venous blood end up in the right ventricle (Fig. 7-1). A sample of blood taken from the right atrium, right ventricle, or pulmonary artery carries an increased amount of oxygen as compared with blood from any region proximal to (before) the shunt. Thus, the oxygen content of right atrial, right ventricular, or pulmonary arterial blood in an individual with an ASD is considerably higher than the oxygen content of blood from the inferior or superior vena cava (Fig. 7-1). Patients with an ASD are said to demonstrate an oxygen ''step-up'' at the atrial level.

The more compliant (less stiff) the right ventricle is, the greater is the amount of atrial blood that will enter the right ventricle during diastole. Conversely, the stiffer the right ventricle (less compliant), the smaller will be the left-to-right shunt. Thus, any process that results in decreased right ventricular compliance (increased stiffness) directly reduces the magnitude of the left-to-right shunt.

The commonest causes of decreased right ventricular compliance are hypertrophy and/or failure. Right ventricular hypertrophy in patients with ASD is usually the result of pulmonary hypertension that imposes an increased systolic work load on the ventricle. Pulmonary hypertension, in turn, is caused by increasing pulmonary vascular resistance secondary to the development of pulmonary vascular disease. The latter entity commonly develops in middle-aged patients with large left-to-right shunts. Pulmonary vascular disease is characterized by progressive hypertrophy and fibrosis of the medial and endothelial layers of pulmonary arterioles (Fig. 7-2). Loss of pulmonary vascular cross-sectional area occurs with a resultant increase in pulmonary vascular resistance.

Pulmonary hypertension and pulmonary vascular disease progressively worsen in patients who develop this complication of ASD: right ventricular hypertrophy increases and ventricular compliance declines as does the magnitude of the left-to-right shunt. Eventually,

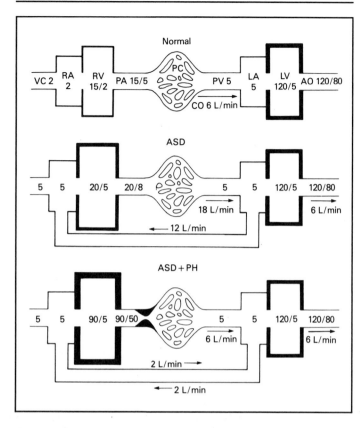

Fig. 7-1 : Pathophysiologic changes observed in patients with atrial septal defect (ASD) with normal pulmonary arterial pressures and with elevated pulmonary arterial pressures. The uppermost panel shows normal pressures and cardiac output (CO). The middle panel demonstrates the changes that occur in individuals with atrial septal defect but without pulmonary hypertension (PH). The right ventricle (RV) is dilated and modestly hypertrophied. Right ventricular compliance is greater than left ventricular compliance and consequently there is a net flow from the left atrium (LA) to the right atrium (RA) of 12 liters/minute (left-to-right shunt = 12 liters/minute). Oxygenated (red) blood shunts to the right side of the circulation where it mixes with deoxygenated (blue) blood. The resultant oxygen saturation of the blood in the right heart chambers is therefore considerably higher than normal. The right ventricle pumps the normal 6 liters/minute returning to it from the body as well as the 12 liters/minute arriving from the left-to-right shunt. Thus, there is a pulmonary blood flow of 18 liters/minute. Left heart and right heart pressures are within the normal range although right-sided pressures are slightly higher than in the normal situation. When pulmonary vascular disease develops in the patient with atrial septal defect (lower panel), right ventricular systolic and pulmonary arterial pressures rise remarkably and may even achieve systemic arterial levels. The right ventricle becomes dilated and hypertrophied and right ventricular compliance now equals left ventricular compliance. Consequently, there are small bidirectional shunts at the atrial level (2 liters/minute right-to-left and 2 liters/minute left-to-right). Forward cardiac output is maintained at 6 liters/minute. If the right or left ventricle (LV) fails, systemic cardiac output falls. VC = vena cava; PA = pulmonary artery; PC = pulmonary capillaries; PV = pulmonary veins; AO = aorta. (From Selzer A: *Principles of Clinical Cardiology: An Analytic Approach.* Philadelphia, Saunders, 1975, with permission of the author and publisher.)

Changes(s)	Grade	Morphology
Normal or thin-walled	0	
(MT)	I	
MT+IT	II	
MT+IT+ plexiform lesion	III	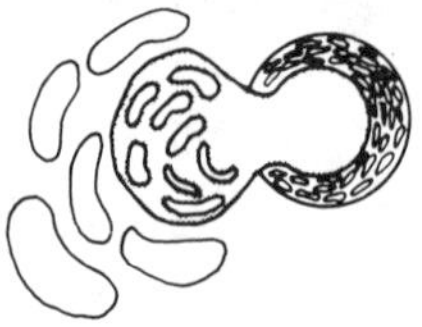

Fig. 7-2 : Changes in small pulmonary arteries with the development of pulmonary vascular disease (Eisenmenger reaction). The grading is progressive (0–III) with increasingly severe changes in the pulmonary arteries. Medial thickening (MT) is followed by intimal thickening (IT) and finally by the development of complex so-called plexiform lesions. Patients with plexiform lesions (grade III pulmonary vascular changes) frequently demonstrate pressures in the pulmonary artery that are at systemic arterial levels. (From Virmani R, Roberts WC: Pulmonary arteries in congenital heart disease: A structure-function analysis, in Roberts WC [ed]: *Congenital Heart Disease in Adults.* Philadelphia, Davis, 1979, with permission of the authors and publisher.)

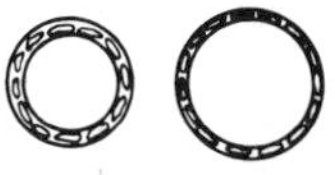

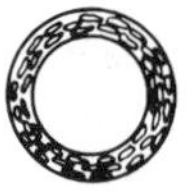

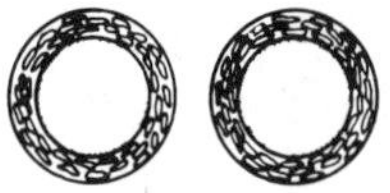

there is no or only minimal left-to-right shunting of blood, a situation described by cardiologists as "balanced shunting" since there are often small and approximately equal left-to-right and right-to-left shunts. Larger quantities of blood are shunted right-to-left when right ventricular hypertrophy causes right ventricular compliance to fall below left ventricular compliance. In other words, right ventricular hypertrophy increases the intrinsic myocardial stiffness of that ventricle to levels that exceed those of the left ventricular myocardium. Blood flow from the common atrium now prefers to cross the mitral valve as compared with the tricuspid valve: all of the pulmonary venous blood and some of the systemic venous blood enter the left ventricle (Fig. 7-1) and a net right-to-left shunt results. The oxygen content of a blood sample from the left ventricle or a systemic artery of such a patient is significantly reduced as compared with a pulmonary venous blood sample secondary to admixture of systemic venous (desaturated) blood from the right-to-left shunt. Patients with right-to-left shunting of blood secondary to pulmonary hypertension and pulmonary vascular disease are said to exhibit the "Eisenmenger reaction." Such individuals have a bluish or cyanotic tinge to their lips and nailbeds secondary to the decreased oxygen saturation of systemic arterial blood.

Right ventricular failure can also produce a marked decrease in right ventricular compliance. Failure can develop as a result of pulmonary hypertension with consequent systolic pressure overload of the right ventricle. On the other hand, right ventricular failure may develop in the absence of pulmonary hypertension. In this setting, right ventricular failure is probably the result of a large left-to-right shunt that has been present for a long time (volume overload of the right ventricle).

Right ventricular failure also produces a decrease in diastolic myocardial compliance, thereby reducing the magnitude of the left-to-right shunt. Conversely, if left ventricular failure develops (often as a result of a superimposed condition such as arteriosclerotic or hypertensive heart disease) reduced compliance develops in the left ventricle, thereby increasing the normal disparity between right and left ventricular stiffness. Increased left ventricular stiffness secondary to left ventricular failure (or other process) produces an increase in the magnitude of the left-to-right shunt. These seemingly paradoxical shifts in the size of the shunt in patients with ASD can be understood more easily if one remembers that all four cardiac chambers are in communication during diastole and that the magnitude and direction of any resulting shunt of blood flow is determined by the relative compliance (stiffness) of the two ventricles competing for their share of the diastolic blood flow.

Atrial septal defects vary greatly in size. A small patent foramen ovale may transmit a similarly small left-to-right shunt of little hemodynamic or clinical consequence. Individuals with such small defects in the atrial septum commonly demonstrate considerable difference in left and right atrial pressures. In other words, a pressure gradient exists across the small atrial septal defect. Defects whose cross-sectional area exceeds 1.0 cm^2 display no measurable gradient across the atrial septum, i.e., left and right atrial pressures are equal. As noted earlier, the magnitude and direction of any shunt flow in such individuals is the result of differences in relative ventricular compliance, *not* the result of any gradient across the atrial septum.

In patients with ASD, the right ventricle is subjected to volume overload, i.e., it must continuously pump a higher than normal cardiac output. The left ventricle, on the other hand, pumps less blood than normal since some of the pulmonary venous blood crosses the ASD and ends up in the right ventricle. Therefore, patients with ASD usually have small, "atrophic" left ventricles.

One final point concerning the pathophysiology of ASD deserves mention: the impact of the frequently associated abnormality, anomalous pulmonary venous return. In this latter entity, one or more (usually no more than two) of the pulmonary veins fails to enter the left atrium. Rather, the anomalous vein(s) drains into the right atrium or one of several sites in the systemic venous system. The pathophysiology is similar to that noted with ASD: a quantity of oxygenated blood that should have been delivered to the left atrium flows instead into the right atrium or systemic venous system: a left-to-right shunt is present. The magnitude of left-to-right shunts secondary to anomalously draining pulmonary veins is usually much smaller than left-to-right shunts that accompany atrial septal defects. Pulmonary vascular disease and pulmonary hypertension do not develop in patients with a single anomalous pulmonary vein.

Ventricular Septal Defect

Ventricular septal defect (VSD) is the commonest congenital cardiac defect in children. Such defects can range in size from very small holes of little clinical significance to large gaps involving almost the entire ventricular septum.

The hemodynamic pathophysiology of VSD during and shortly after fetal life resembles that of ASD. During uterine life and shortly after birth, resistance in the pulmonary arterioles is high secondary to hypertrophy of the smooth muscle of the medial layer. This hypertrophy gradually regresses in early childhood with resultant decrease in pulmonary vascular resistance and pulmonary arterial pressure. The right ventricle pumps blood across the high resistance, high pressure, uterine pulmonary vascular bed: high right ventricular systolic pressure and right ventricular hypertrophy are the result. The quantity of blood that flows across a defect in the ventricular system is determined by the difference in systolic blood pressure between the left and right ventricles. Thus, a large difference between left and right ventricular systolic pressure results in a large flow of blood across a VSD. Left ventricular systolic pressure is usually much higher than right ventricular systolic pressure producing a left-to-right shunt of blood flow across a VSD (Fig. 7-3). As noted in patients with ASD, the left-to-right shunt produces a step-up in blood oxygen saturation at the level of the defect. For ASD, this increased blood oxygen saturation occurs in the right atrium (Fig. 7-1). For VSD, the oxygen saturation step-up is observed in the right ventricle (Fig. 7-3).

As noted earlier, right ventricular systolic blood pressure is high during uterine life. Consequently, the systolic pressure gradient across a VSD is small during uterine life and the resultant left-to-right shunt is also minor in quantity. As pulmonary vascular resistance declines during early infancy, pulmonary arterial and right ventricular systolic

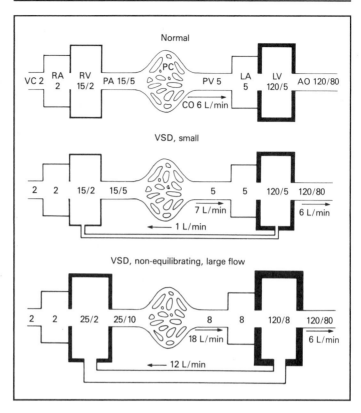

Fig. 7-3 : Pathophysiologic changes noted in patients with ventricular septal defect (VSD). The uppermost panel shows the normal situation. The middle panel demonstrates a patient with a small VSD. Pressures are unchanged as compared with normal. There is a small (1 liter/minute) left-to-right shunt from left ventricle (LV) to right ventricle (RV). Oxygenated (red) blood shunts to the right ventricle where it mixes with deoxygenated (blue) blood. The resultant oxygen saturation of the blood in the right ventricle and pulmonary arteries (PA) is therefore considerably higher than normal. The shunt results in a slight increase in pulmonary blood flow (from 6–7 liters/minute). There are no major changes in hemodynamics. The stimulus for hypertrophy of the left and right ventricles is minimal. The lower panel represents the situation in a patient with a large VSD in which considerable amounts of blood (12 liters/minute) flow from left ventricle to right ventricle. The hole in the ventricular septum is not so large that right ventricular pressure and left ventricular pressure become equal. Consequently, during ventricular systole the pressure in the left ventricle is considerably higher than that in the right ventricle and blood flows from left ventricle to right ventricle. There is a marked increase in pulmonary blood flow (18 liters/minute) representing a combination of the systemic venous return (6 liters/minute) and the left-to-right shunt (12 liters/minute). VC = vena cava; RA = right atrium; PC = pulmonary capillaries; PV = pulmonary veins; CO = cardiac output; LA = left atrium; AO = aorta. (From Selzer A: *Principles of Clinical Cardiology: An Analytic Approach.* Philadelphia, Saunders, 1975, with permission of the author and publisher.)

Patent Ductus Arteriosus

At this point, we have considered congenital lesions that produce shunts at the atrial (ASD) and ventricular (VSD) levels. Patent ductus arteriosus (PDA) causes a shunt at the level of the great vessels (aorta, pulmonary artery) (Fig. 7-5). In uterine life, oxygenation of blood occurs in the placenta and not in the lungs. Oxygenated blood reaches the systemic arterial circuit via a circuitous route: umbilical vein → inferior vena cava → right heart chambers and pulmonary artery → across the foramen ovale (atrial level) and patent ductus arteriosus (pulmonary arterial level) to the left heart and aorta. The foramen ovale and ductus arteriosus serve as "short circuits," shunting oxygenated blood to the left side of the heart before it reaches the collapsed lungs of the fetus. Both of these uterine conduits (foramen ovale, ductus arteriosus) close at the time of birth: a left atrial flap of tissue covers the foramen ovale and smooth muscle within the wall of the ductus contracts and obliterates the lumen of this vessel. Failure of the appropriate smooth muscle contractions leaves the ductus arteriosus patent during childhood and adult life.

Pulmonary vascular resistance is initially high during early infancy, and the left-to-right shunt from aorta to pulmonary artery is therefore rather small at that time. However, with falling pulmonary vascular resistance, the quantity of blood shunted left-to-right increases. The situation is analogous to that seen with VSD in that the quantity of shunt flow depends on two factors: the size of the PDA and the pulmonary vascular resistance. The size of the PDA determines the quantity of shunt blood flow when the ductus is small, thereby presenting a sizeable resistance to blood flow. Larger ducti present little or no resistance to blood flow and the volume of blood shunted through the PDA is determined by the level of pulmonary vascular resistance.

PDA and Eisenmenger syndrome

When pulmonary vascular resistance is low and the PDA is moderate or large in size, a large left-to-right shunt is present from aorta to pulmonary artery (Fig. 7-5). There is a large step-up of blood oxygen saturation between the right ventricle and the pulmonary artery. The development of pulmonary vascular disease is associated with rising pulmonary vascular resistance and pulmonary arterial pressure. As pulmonary vascular resistance increases, the volume of blood shunted left-to-right through the PDA decreases. Eventually, pulmonary vascular resistance and pulmonary arterial pressure reach levels equal to those present in the systemic arterial circuit. At this point, there is "balanced" shunting of blood through the PDA. In other words, there are only small and clinically inconsequential left-to-right and right-to-left shunts present. Further increases in pulmonary vascular resistance are associated with levels of pulmonary arterial pressure that exceed the pressure in the aorta. The result is right-to-left shunting of blood through the PDA (Eisenmenger syndrome). Patients with PDA and Eisenmenger syndrome demonstrate a finding

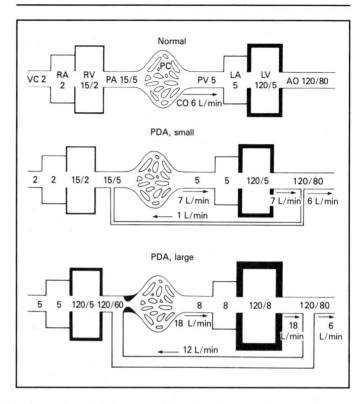

Fig. 7-5 : Pathophysiologic changes in patients with patent ductus arteriosus (PDA). The top panel shows the normal situation. The middle panel shows hemodynamic changes occurring in individuals with a small PDA. The small communication between the aorta (AO) and the pulmonary artery (PA) allows a small left-to-right shunt (1 liter/minute). This occurs because aortic pressure during systole is considerably higher than arterial pressure at that time. Oxygenated (red) blood shunts to the pulmonary artery where it mixes with deoxygenated (blue) blood. The resultant oxygen saturation of the blood in the pulmonary arteries is therefore considerably higher than normal. Pulmonary blood flow and left ventricular cardiac output are increased by 1 liter/minute to a total of 7 liters/minute. The lowest panel demonstrates a patient with a large PDA and early pulmonary vascular disease. Although pulmonary arterial and aortic systolic pressures are equal, there is still enough difference in systemic arterial (aortic) compliance and pulmonary arterial compliance to maintain a left-to-right shunt of 12 liters/minute. Pulmonary blood flow is the result of systemic venous return (6 liters/minute) and the left-to-right shunt (12 liters/minute). With worsening of this patient's pulmonary vascular disease, the left-to-right shunt will gradually disappear leaving either a net right-to-left shunt or balanced shunting. VC = vena cava; RA = right atrium; PC = pulmonary capillaries; PV = pulmonary veins; LA = left atrium; RV = right ventricle; LV = left ventricle. (From Selzer A: Principles of Clinical Cardiology: An Analytic Approach. Philadelphia, Saunders, 1975, with permission of the author and publisher.)

known as "differential cyanosis": cyanotic coloration of the toenail beds and normal color of the lips and fingernail beds. This phenomenon is easily understood if one remembers that the ductus arteriosus connects the main pulmonary artery to the descending aorta just beyond the origin of the left subclavian artery. Thus, when Eisenmenger syndrome develops in patients with PDA the desaturated blood that shunts right-to-left enters the aorta below the arteries to the arms and head. All the desaturated blood is delivered into the descending aorta resulting in cyanosis of the toenails without cyanosis of the lips and fingernails.

When pulmonary vascular resistance is low and the PDA is small or modest in size, the left-to-right shunt imposes a volume overload on the left ventricle. The right ventricle is unaffected at this point since shunted blood enters the right side of the circulation beyond the right ventricle. However, if pulmonary vascular resistance is increased, or if the PDA is large in size (thereby transmitting both increased flow and pressure to the pulmonary artery), marked pulmonary arterial hypertension will be present and the right ventricle will face a severe pressure overload. As pulmonary vascular resistance increases in patients with PDA, left-to-right shunt flow declines and the left ventricle is faced with progressively less volume overload. In patients with PDA and Eisenmenger syndrome, there is no excess load on the left ventricle but the right ventricle must achieve systolic pressure levels comparable to those present in the aorta.

Individuals with balanced shunts or Eisenmenger syndrome may become markedly cyanotic during exercise. Such patients may complain of very poor exercise tolerance. Increased cyanosis during exercise results in the following manner: metabolic demand in the exercising muscles is associated with arteriolar vasodilation with consequent reduction in systemic vascular resistance. Pulmonary vascular resistance is unaffected by exercise in these individuals. Blood flows in the direction of least resistance: since systemic vascular resistance is now lower than pulmonary vascular resistance, blood flow from pulmonary artery to aorta increases, resulting in further desaturation of systemic arterial blood (increased cyanosis).

Coarctation of the Aorta

Coarctation of the aorta is a congenital cardiac lesion that does not cause intracardiac shunting of blood even through it is often associated with other cardiac defects that do result in intracardiac shunts. A coarctation is a constricted zone of the aorta usually located just distal to the left subclavian artery in the region where the ductus arteriosus joins the aorta (Fig. 7-6). It has been suggested that the etiology of the coarctation is somehow related to the presence of the ductus arteriosus at that location in the aorta.

Fig. 7-6 : Example of a fairly severe coarctation of the aorta. Note the commonly accompanying bicuspid aortic valve and the poststenotic dilatation. Note the usual location of the coarctation in the same region as the ductus arteriosus, shown here as a small fibrotic ligamentum arteriosum. PT = main pulmonary artery; LV = left ventricle. (From Harvey WP: Auscultatory features of congenital heart disease, in Roberts WC [ed]: *Congenital Heart Disease in Adults.* Philadelphia, Davis, 1979, with permission of the author and publisher.)

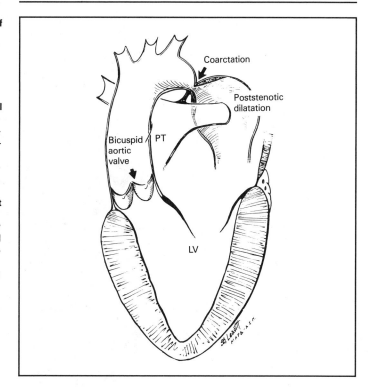

Coarctation may be mild, causing only the most minimal aortic narrowing with little or no pressure gradient present across the zone of aortic narrowing. On the other hand, coarctation may be so severe that the aortic lumen is totally occluded. Clearly, the more severe the coarctation, the greater will be the obstruction to normal aortic blood flow and the larger will be the pressure gradient across the obstructive coarctation. The situation is pathophysiologically analogous to aortic stenosis; however, the stenotic lesion (and hence the pressure gradient) is present in the distal aorta rather than at the aortic valve.

The obstructive coarctation produces systemic arterial *hypertension* proximal to the narrowed region of the aorta. Arterial *hypotension* is present distal to the coarctation (Fig. 7-6). Blood flow to the arterial system distal to the coarctation is maintained by numerous collateral blood vessels that carry blood around the coarctation to the distal aorta (Fig. 7-7). The examining physician obtains a hypertensive blood pressure reading from determinations made on the arm; pulse volume and blood pressure measurements obtained on the leg are much lower than those noted in the upper extremities. The hypertensive response in the upper part of the body may be the result of more than just the aortic constriction. Elevated systemic renin and angiotensin levels may be present secondary to renin secretion in response

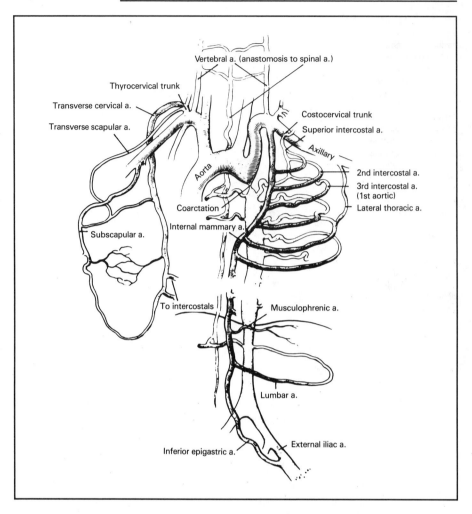

Fig. 7-7 : The extensive collateral circulation existing in patients with coarctation of the aorta. Note the remarkable increase in size of the intercostal arteries, the internal mammary artery, and the scapular arteries. (From Edwards J, in Fowler NO [ed]: *Cardiac Diagnosis and Treatment.* **New York, Harper & Row, 1980, with permission of the author and publisher.)**

to low renal artery blood pressure. Remember that the renal vascular bed is distal to the coarctation.

Coarctation imposes a pressure overload on the left ventricle. Left ventricular hypertrophy and eventually left ventricular failure develop with resultant pulmonary venous and arterial hypertension. Chronic left ventricular failure can lead to right ventricular failure in occasional individuals. Patients with coarctation may complain of intermittent claudication (crampy aching in the muscles of the calves and thighs secondary to inadequate blood flow during exercise). This symptom is due to the decreased quantity of blood reaching the distal aorta.

Longstanding coarctation can lead to aneurysmal dilatation of the ascending aorta. Complications related to such ascending aortic aneurysms include rupture and dissection of the aorta (see Chap. 15). One other complication deserves mention: bicuspid aortic valve. The majority of patients with coarctation of the aorta have this associated defect. In many of these individuals, the bicuspid aortic valve is incompetent and aortic valvular regurgitation is present. Ascending aortic hypertension increases the diastolic pressure gradient (driving pressure) across the bicuspid aortic valve and hence increases the severity of aortic regurgitation. In such patients, the left ventricle is subjected to both pressure and volume overload.

Eisenmenger Syndrome

This condition has already been discussed briefly in connection with the three congenital cardiac defects that lead to left-to-right shunts: ASD, VSD, and PDA. Eisenmenger syndrome is the result of progressive hypertrophy and fibrosis of the medial and endothelial layers of the pulmonary arterioles (Fig. 7-2). Such pathologic changes are known as "pulmonary vascular disease" and they lead to increased pulmonary vascular resistance and pulmonary arterial hypertension. Pulmonary hypertension and increased pulmonary vascular resistance decrease the quantity of blood shunted left-to-right. Eventually, pulmonary vascular resistance and pressure reach and exceed levels present in the systemic arterial circuit: reversal of shunt flow (right-to-left) results. Although it is difficult to predict which patients with intracardiac shunts will develop pulmonary hypertension, pulmonary vascular disease develops at an earlier stage and to a greater degree in individuals with larger left-to-right shunts and with transmission of left-sided pressures to the right side of the circulation, e.g., through a large VSD or PDA.

The pathologic changes that develop in the pulmonary circulation in patients with pulmonary vascular disease are identical to those seen in the lungs of individuals with primary pulmonary hypertension (see Chap. 16). It is of considerable interest that individuals living at high altitude, i.e., 5,000 feet elevation or higher, have a greater chance of developing pulmonary vascular disease than persons residing at sea level. In addition, pulmonary vascular disease and the accompanying pulmonary hypertension develop at a younger age in patients with intracardiac shunts who live at high altitude. It has been suggested that hypoxemia (decreased oxygen tension in the blood) resulting from the decreased partial pressure of oxygen in ambient air at high altitude is the cause of the earlier and more prevalent occurrence of pulmonary vascular disease. Hypoxia causes pulmonary vascular vasoconstriction in normals, and this response may be accentuated in some way in patients with intracardiac shunts.

Exercise often produces severe symptoms in patients with pulmonary vascular disease by reducing systemic vascular resistance to levels lower than those present in the pulmonary circuit. The result is increased shunting of deoxygenated blood from right-to-left into the systemic arterial circuit. The resulting hypoxemia decreases exercise tolerance.

Two manifestations of Eisenmenger syndrome deserve comment: elevated red blood cell count (polycythemia) and clubbing of the fingernails and toenails. Elevated red cell count is the result of increased secretion of erythropoeitin from the kidneys. Elevated renal secretion of erythropoeitin results when the renal parenchyma is perfused with desaturated blood that in turn reaches the systemic arterial circulation via the right-to-left shunt. Desaturated arterial blood is also the cause of rounded fingernails and toenails known as clubbing. Abnormal nail growth results when hypoxemic blood perfuses the nailbeds.

Another complication that is associated with Eisenmenger syndrome is bacterial brain abscess. This complication is apparently the result of right-to-left shunting of blood that carries bacteria entering the venous circulation (often from the gut) past the pulmonary "filter" that usually removes such organisms.

Suggested Readings

Perloff JK: *The Clinical Recognition of Congenital Heart Disease*, ed 2. Philadelphia, Saunders, 1978.

Alpert JS: Congenital Heart Disease in the Adult, in Braunwald E (ed): *Heart Disease*. Philadelphia, Saunders, 1980.

Berry WB, Austen WG: Respiratory variations in the magnitude of the left to right shunt in experimental interatrial communications. *Am J Cardiol* 14:201, 1964.

Dexter L: Atrial septal defect. *Br Heart J* 18:209, 1956.

Dow JW, Dexter L: Circulatory dynamics in atrial septal defect. *J Clin Invest* 29:809, 1950.

Rowe GG et al: Atrial septal defect and the mechanism of shunt. *Am Heart J* 61:369, 1961.

Rudolph AM, Nadas AS: The pulmonary circulation and congenital heart disease. *N Engl J Med* 267:968, 1962.

Tikoff G et al: Heart failure in atrial septal defect. *Am J Med* 39:533, 1965.

Wagenvoort CA et al: The pulmonary arterial tree in atrial septal defect. A quantitative study of anatomic features in fetuses, infants, and children. *Circulation* 23:733, 1961.

Wood P: The Eisenmenger syndrome or pulmonary hypertension with reversed central shunt. *Br Med J* 2:701, 755, 1958.

Bonow RO et al: Left ventricular functional reserve in adult patients with atrial septal defect: Pre- and post-operative studies. *Circulation* 63:1315, 1981.

Liberthson RR et al: Right ventricular function in adult atrial septal defect: Pre- and post-operative study by radionuclide ventriculography in adults. *Circulation* 63:142, 1981.

Arcilla RA et al: Further observations on the natural history of isolated ventricular septal defects in infancy and children. Serial cardiac catheterization studies in 75 patients. *Circulation* 28:560, 1963.

Blount SG Jr, Mueller H, McCord MC: Ventricular septal defect. Clinical and hemodynamic patterns. *Am J Med* 18:871, 1955.

Dammann JF Jr et al: Anatomy, physiology and natural history of simple ventricular septal defects. *Am J Cardiol* 5:136, 1960.

Clarkson PM et al: Prognosis for patients with ventricular septal defect and severe pulmonary vascular obstructive disease. *Circulation* 38:129, 1968.

Lucas RV Jr et al: The natural history of isolated ventricular septal defect. A serial physiologic study. *Circulation* 24:1372, 1961.

Kidd L et al: Ventricular septal defect in infancy. *Am Heart J* 69:4, 1965.

Weidman WH, DuShane JW, Kincaid OW: Observations concerning progressive pulmonary vascular obstruction in children with ventricular septal defects. *Am Heart J* 65:148, 1962.

Walker WJ et al: Interventricular septal defect: Analysis of 415 catheterized cases, 90 with serial hemodynamic studies. *Circulation* 31:54, 1965.

Tikoff G et al: Clinical and physiologic sequelae of large ventricular septal defects. *Am J Med* 42:497, 1967.

Tikoff G et al: Patent ductus arteriosus complicated by heart failure. *Am J Med* 46:43, 1969.

Espino-Vela J, Cardenas N, Cruz R: Patent ductus arteriosus. *Circulation* 38(suppl 5):45, 1968.

Berlind S, Bojs G, Korsgren M: Severe pulmonary hypertension accompanying patent ductus arteriosus. *Am Heart J* 73:460, 1967.

Moss AJ, Emmanouilides G, Duffie ER Jr: Closure of the ductus arteriosus in the newborn infant. *Pediatrics* 32:25, 1963.

Rudolph AM et al: Hemodynamic basis for clinical manifestations of patent ductus arteriosus. *Am Heart J* 68:447, 1964.

Reid JM et al: Moderate to severe pulmonary hypertension accompanying patent ductus arteriosus. *Br Heart J* 26:600, 1964.

Spach MS et al: Pulsatile aortopulmonary pressure-flow dynamics of patent ductus arteriosus in patients with various hemodynamic states. *Circulation* 61:110, 1980.

Amsterdam EA et al: Plasma renin activity in children with coarctation of the aorta. *Am J Cardiol* 23:396, 1969.

Dahlback O, Dahn I, Westling H: Hemodynamic observations in coarctation of the aorta, with special reference to the blood pressure above and below the stenosis at rest and during exercise. *Scand J Clin Lab Invest* 16:339, 1964.

Alpert BS et al: Role of renin-angiotensin-aldosterone system in hypertensive children with coarctation of the aorta. *Am J Cardiol* 43:828, 1979.

Dalen JE, Bruce RA, Cobb LA: Interaction of chronic hypoxia of moderate altitude on pulmonary hypertension complicating defect of the atrial septum. *N Engl J Med* 266:272, 1962.

8 : Respiratory Mechanisms in Circulatory Failure

Richard S. Irwin
Carl Teplitz

The pulmonary circulation has four major functions: (1) It provides a means for effective gas exchange between air and blood (external respiration); (2) it serves as a filter for a variety of systemic venous particles; (3) it has numerous and varied metabolic activities; and, as the bridge between the two sides of the heart; and (4) it serves as a reservoir of blood for the left ventricle. This chapter will concern itself with the pulmonary circulation as a reservoir of blood.

The Normal Pulmonary Circulation

General considerations

The pulmonary circulation begins at the main pulmonary artery and ends where the four main pulmonary veins enter the left atrium. It has a pump, the right ventricle, a system of distributing arteries and arterioles, mechanisms by which it can transfer substances between air and blood (blood-air barrier), and a collecting system of veins and venules. This circulation is unique among regional circulations: it is the only one that accepts the equivalent of the entire output of the left ventricle, since right and left ventricular outputs are almost identical.

Although the pulmonary circulation accepts the same pump output as the systemic circulation, it is normally able to do so with much lower pressures (Fig. 8-1) due to the following unique structural characteristics: (1) the pulmonary arteries have more elastic tissue and less muscle than equivalent-sized arteries in the systemic circulation (Figs. 8-2A, B); (2) the precapillary arterioles (the vessels in the systemic circulation that probably determine systemic blood pressure) and small veins are almost devoid of smooth muscle (Figs. 8-3A, B); (3) veins and venules have no valves; and (4) the rich peripheral nervous system, supplying the circulation, plays a very small role in controlling resistance, flow, and pressure. For all of these reasons, the normal pulmonary circulation passively accepts large volumes of blood at relatively low pressures.

Biophysical considerations

The central function of any circulation is to supply enough blood to meet the demands of the peripheral tissues. The pulmonary circulation must do this plus return blood to the left ventricle. By applying

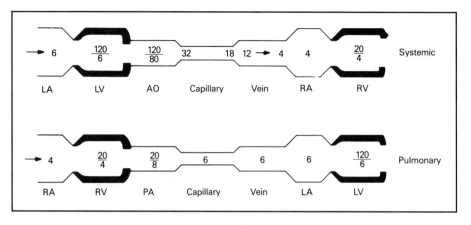

Fig. 8-1 : Comparison of pressures in mm Hg in both systemic and pulmonary circulations. LA = left atrium; LV = left ventricle; AO = aorta; RA = right atrium; RV = right ventricle. (From Robin, ED, Gaudio, R: Cor Pulmonale, in Dowling HF et al [eds]: *Disease-A-Month.* Chicago, Year Book, 1970, with permission of the authors and publisher.)

Ohm's law and the Poiseuille-Hagan formula to the pulmonary circulation, it is possible to understand its blood flow and pressure characteristics, and also appreciate its extreme distensibility.

Ohm's law (Eq. 8-1) can be applied to the study of fluids (Eq. 8-2) since current is equivalent to flow and electromotive force is equivalent to pressure.

$$\text{Current} = \frac{\text{electromotive force}}{\text{resistance}} \qquad \text{Equation 8-1}$$

$$\text{Flow (F)} = \frac{\text{pressure (P)}}{\text{resistance (R)}} \qquad \text{Equation 8-2}$$

Ohm's law can be applied to the study of the pulmonary circulation (Eq. 8-3) since flow equals the cardiac output of the right ventricle

Fig. 8-2 : The great amount of distensible elastic tissue fibers and the relatively small amount of vessel wall muscular tone due to paucity of smooth muscle fibers characterize the low resistance, low pressure pulmonary arteries as compared to systemic vasculature. A. The vessel wall media (M) of a medium-sized systemic artery (top) is composed almost entirely of smooth muscle, which morphometrically comprises 60% of the total cross-sectional vessel area, with the lumen (L) occupying only 40%. B. In a pulmonary artery of similar caliber, although the lumen occupies essentially the same percentage of total cross-sectional area (40%), the wall is morphometrically composed of both smooth muscle (sm), seen as dark fibers that comprise only 30% of total cross-sectional area (i.e., half the amount of muscle present in the systemic artery), and appreciable elastic tissue (E), the wavy light-colored fibers that also comprise 30% of the total cross-sectional vascular area. (× 340, 3μ plastic JB embedment sections, H and E stain.) (Measurements made using digital morphometer.)

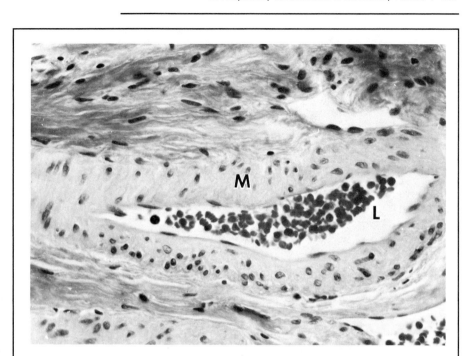

A

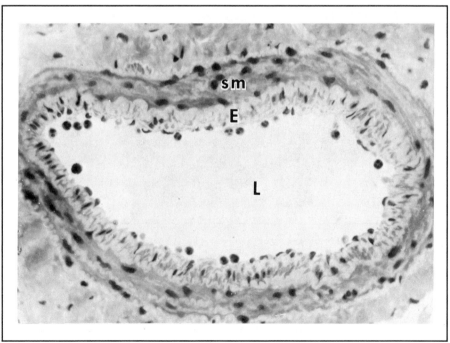

B

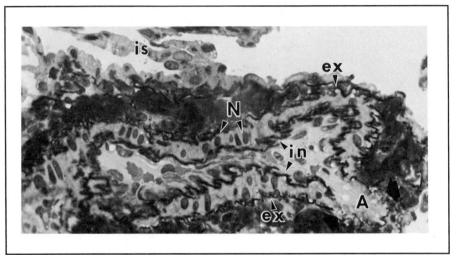

A

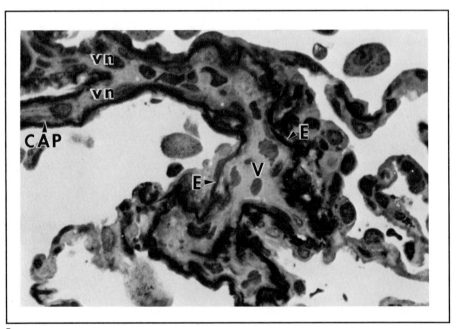

B

Fig. 8-3 : A. A small pulmonary artery has a thin media composed of a single layer of smooth muscle cells with their nuclei (N) between an internal (in) and an external (ex) elastic lamina. The two elastic laminae fuse into one thin lamina (large arrows) and the resultant prearteriole (A) has no identifiable muscle layer to contribute to pulmonary vascular resistance. Interalveolar septum (is) is seen. ($\times$ 540, 1μ epon section.) B. A small pulmonary vein (V), well delineated by an elastic tissue envelopment (E) but without light microscopically discernible smooth muscle, branches into venules (vn) that are continuous with the interalveolar septal capillaries (CAP). ($\times$ 670, 1μ epon section.)

and pressure is a pressure differential (ΔP) that drives blood from the main pulmonary artery to the left atrium.

$$F = \frac{\Delta P}{R}$$

Equation 8-3

Although this last modification of Ohm's law allows us to understand that flow to the tissues and left ventricle will be determined by a driving pressure and resistance, it does not allow us to appreciate the complexity of the resistance factor. By applying the Poiseuille-Hagan formula to the pulmonary circulation and combining it with the hydraulic extrapolation of Ohm's law, it is possible to conceive of multiple factors that might affect the resistance to blood flow. The Poiseuille-Hagan formula (Eq. 8-4) states that continuous, laminar flow through a rigid tube is influenced directly by a driving pressure $(P_A - P_B)$, a geometric factor $(\pi/8)$, and by the radius of the tube, (r^4), and inversely by a viscosity factor (n) of the fluid and the length of the tube (L).

$$F = (P_A - P_B) \times \frac{\pi}{8} \times \frac{1}{n} \times \frac{r^4}{L}$$

Equation 8-4

Since $F = (P_A - P_B)/R$, Equation 8-4 can be substituted for F and resistance can be solved for (Eq. 8-5):

$$R = \frac{8nL}{\pi r^4}$$

Equation 8-5

It follows that, theoretically, resistance in the pulmonary circulation might be affected by the viscosity of the blood and the cross-sectional diameter of the vascular bed (the length of the pulmonary circulation should not be a changing factor). Therefore, flow through the pulmonary circulation should be determined by pressure, viscosity, and cross-sectional diameter of the vascular bed.

The preceding biophysical considerations are useful in understanding what controls the overall behavior of the pulmonary circulation. However, they cannot be applied directly to predict accurately or reliably function in health or disease since blood is not a perfect fluid, the pulmonary circulation is not a rigid tube, and flow is not necessarily laminar or continuous. This point can be emphasized in normal adults by increasing cardiac output and measuring pulmonary arterial pressure (Fig. 8-4); until cardiac output increases more than two and one-half-fold in normals, the pulmonary arterial pressure will remain unchanged and resistance will decrease. Pressure remains unchanged due to the passive distention or dilatation of the pulmonary vascular bed and perhaps to the additional recruitment of previously closed vessels. Only when the pulmonary vascular bed has

Fig. 8-4 : The relationship between cardiac output (pulmonary blood flow) and mean pulmonary artery pressure. (From Robin ED, Gaudio R: Cor Pulmonale, in Dowling HF et al [eds]: *Disease-A-Month.* Chicago, Year Book, 1970, with permission of the authors and publisher.)

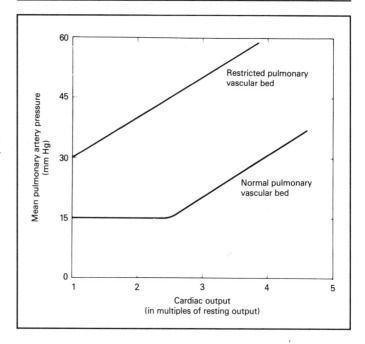

already been restricted, as in a patient with a pneumonectomy, will pulmonary artery pressure rise *acutely* secondary to an increase in blood flow (Fig. 8-4). On the other hand, *chronic* increases in pulmonary blood flow (see discussion of congenital heart disease under Active Pulmonary Hypertension) can lead to pulmonary hypertension.

Determinants of pulmonary vascular pressures

By performing cardiac catheterization and knowing the anatomy of the pulmonary circulation, it is possible to measure and understand what determines pulmonary vascular pressures. The following discussion will consider only the overall behavior of the pulmonary circulation for clear exposition. It is not meant to imply that the entire pulmonary vasculature participates homogeneously. Regional regulatory factors will be discussed later.

Pulmonary artery end-diastolic (PA_{ed}) pressure measured in the main pulmonary artery has been shown to be equal to left atrial and left ventricular end-diastolic pressures, as long as the diastolic pressure in the left ventricle is $\geq$ 5 mm Hg. When the left ventricular end-diastolic pressure is < 5 mm Hg, pulmonary arterial diastolic pressure exceeds left ventricular end-diastolic pressure by a few millimeters of mercury. Studies have suggested that this gradient represents the critical closing pressure of the pulmonary vasculature since it can be abolished by increasing left atrial pressure. Presumably, the increase in pulmonary blood volume associated with the increase in left atrial pressure increases the cross-sectional area of the pulmonary vascular bed by dilating existing vessels or opening previously closed ones. It is not surprising that PA_{ed} pressure is equal to left ventricular end-diastolic pressure for the following reasons: (1) pulmonary blood flow is not appreciable at the end of diastole and (2) no structure(s) interrupt the stream of blood between the pulmonary artery and left ventricle during end-diastole (the mitral valve is open; there are no valves in the pulmonary veins or venules; there is no smooth muscle in the precapillary arterioles; and there is little, if any, neural control over the circulation). Consequently, PA_{ed} pressure is determined by the volume of blood that distends the pulmonary vascular bed; this volume is determined by the function of the right and left ventricles.

The pressure recorded from a catheter tip wedged in a distal pulmonary artery (pulmonary capillary wedge [PCW] pressure), is also equal to left atrial and left ventricular end-diastolic pressures because it does not allow any additional blood to flow into the wedged vessel that is still part of the continuous stream. Since the PCW pressure accurately reflects pulmonary venous pressure, it is possible to evaluate right- and left-sided pressure events by passing a catheter through the systemic veins into the right heart.

Pulmonary systolic and mean pressures are determined by the stroke volume of the right ventricle and the volume of blood already distending the elastic pulmonary arteries at the end of diastole. This has been demonstrated by predicting mathematically what the systolic and mean pressures should be for given stroke volumes and diastolic pressures and then measuring by cardiac catheterization almost identical values.

The resistance to blood flow across the normal pulmonary circulation is very low; it can be appreciated in two ways. Traditionally calculated, pulmonary vascular resistance is approximately one-tenth of the resistance across the systemic vascular bed. Since mean pulmonary arterial pressure is approximately 15 mm Hg and mean left atrial pressure or PCW pressure is approximately 5 mm Hg, the pressure gradient across the normal pulmonary circulation is only about 10 mm Hg. Thus, a normal cardiac output of approximately 6 liters/minute flows from the right ventricle to the left atrium with a pressure drop of only 10 mm Hg, as opposed to a pressure drop in the systemic circulation, between the left ventricle and the right atrium of approximately 100 mm Hg. In numbers, the pulmonary vascular resistance = $(15 - 5)/6$ or about 1.7 mm Hg/liters/minute. Expressed in units of dynes/sec/cm^{-5}, this is approximately equal to 100 such units. Since pulmonary arterial mean pressure measurements reflect stroke volume, a ventricular function, it may not be the most sensitive indicator of intrinsic pulmonary vascular disease. The PA_{ed} pressure to mean atrial or PCW pressure gradient is another, perhaps more accurate, way of looking at pulmonary vascular resistance to flow. In normals, as long as left atrial pressure is 5 mm Hg, there will be no gradient. If there is intrinsic pulmonary

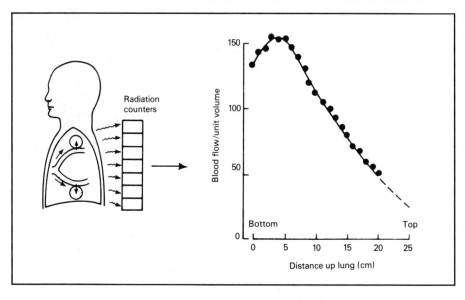

Fig. 8-5 : Measurement of the distribution of blood flow in the upright human lung using radioactive xenon. The dissolved xenon passes into alveolar gas in the pulmonary capillaries. The units of blood flow are such that if flow were uniform, all values would be 100. Blood flow is greatest at the bottom of the lung and smallest at the top. (From West JD: *Respiratory Physiology—The Essentials.* Baltimore, Williams & Wilkins, 1974, with permission of the author and publisher.)

vascular disease (e.g., pulmonary embolism), there will be a gradient with PA_{ed} pressure being greater than PCW pressure. If pulmonary hypertension is caused by passive congestion from left ventricular failure, PA_{ed} pressure and PCW pressure will both be elevated but there will not be a gradient.

Regional distribution of pulmonary blood flow

There is considerable inequality of blood flow in the lung. In the upright position, blood flow decreases almost linearly from the bottom to the top (Fig. 8-5); this uneven distribution is explained by the effect of gravity on the hydrostatic pressure differences in the blood vessels. Therefore, it is not surprising that measurements repeated in men suspended upside-down are reversed and, in the supine position, distribution of blood flow from apex to base becomes almost uniform, while blood flow in the posterior regions of the lung exceeds that in anterior regions.

The uneven distribution of blood flow in the upright posture can be explained by reviewing the pressures affecting the capillaries (Fig. 8-6). At the top of the normal lung, pulmonary arterial pressure is just enough to raise blood to the top. If alveolar pressure is raised (during positive pressure ventilation) and/or arterial pressure is reduced (during severe hemorrhage), capillaries at the top of the lung will be compressed and flow will stop. Under these conditions, blood flow is

Fig. 8-6 : The un-
even distribution of
blood flow in the lung
based on the pres-
sures affecting the
capillaries are de-
picted in this model.
See text for further
explanation. (From
West JB: *Respiratory
Physiology—The Es-
sentials.* Baltimore,
Williams & Wilkins,
1974, with permis-
sion of the author and
publisher.)

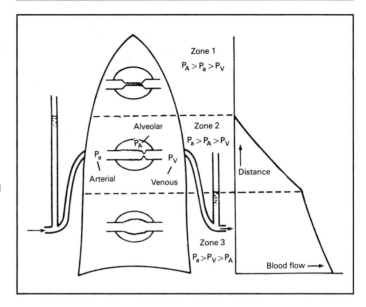

determined by the difference between alveolar and arterial pressures
(so-called zone 1 conditions). Further down the lung, pulmonary arterial pressure increases because of gravity and exceeds alveolar
pressure; both exceed venous pressure. Under these conditions,
blood flow is determined by the difference between arterial and alveolar pressures, not the usual arteriovenous pressure differences
(zone 2 conditions). Under zone 3 conditions, both pulmonary arterial and venous pressures exceed alveolar pressure and blood flow is
determined by the arteriovenous pressure difference. The increase in
pulmonary artery and venous pressures from the hydrostatic effect of
gravity distends the capillaries and increases blood flow in this zone.

The clinical relevance of this discussion will become apparent in later
sections when the knowledge of what determines regional distribution of pulmonary blood flow will help (1) interpret intravascular
pressures in patients on ventilators and (2) predict intravascular pressures by chest roentgenograms.

Pulmonary Hypertension: An Abnormality of the Pulmonary Circulation

General considerations

Pulmonary hypertension is present when systolic pressure is > 35
mm Hg, diastolic pressure is > 15 mm Hg, and mean pressure is
> 20 mm Hg. The origins of pulmonary hypertension may be (1)
totally "passive" due to increased postpulmonary capillary pressure
elevations; (2) "active" due to the active participation of capillary
and precapillary vessels in increasing the resistance to flow; and (3)

pulmonary vascular bed is obstructed. Although patients with pulmonary hypertension from thromboemboli may present with syncope, collapse, or frank shock, shortness of breath is the commonest presenting symptom, followed by easy fatigability. There may or may not be a clearcut history of embolic episodes or of phlebitis. Respiratory rates between 20 and 30 per minute are the rule. Ventilation-perfusion lung scans and, on occasion, pulmonary angiography are necessary to make the diagnosis.

In primary pulmonary hypertension, pulmonary vascular resistance increases initially from an unknown vasospastic or vasoconstrictive tendency and subsequently from primary vascular changes in the pulmonary arterioles that range from intimal thickening and fibrosis, smooth muscle hypertrophy, to arteritis with necrosis. Since the cause of primary pulmonary hypertension is unknown, the diagnosis is one of exclusion. All of the causes of pulmonary hypertension must be ruled out with chest roentgenograms, pulmonary function tests, arterial blood gases, echocardiography, ventilation/perfusion lung scans, and, on occasion, pulmonary angiography and even left heart catheterization.

In patients with VSD, PDA, and ASD, pulmonary vascular resistance increases due to intimal thickening, fibrosis, and smooth muscle hypertrophy in pulmonary arterioles that presumably occurs in response to *chronic* increases in pulmonary blood flow from the left-to-right shunt. The clinical findings and/or symptoms of VSD and PDA usually lead to their detection in childhood. However, the clinical manifestations of ASD are subtle and, therefore, this lesion may go undetected until adult life.

Diseases that may cause capillary restriction of the pulmonary vascular bed are those that replace, destroy, or compress vessels by interstitial fibrosis and include idiopathic pulmonary fibrosis, silicosis, asbestosis, and sarcoidosis. Patients with diffuse interstitial lung disease will probably only complain of dyspnea. The history of significant dust exposure will suggest the possibility of asbestosis or silicosis. Physical findings will usually be limited to crackles on auscultation of the lungs and clubbing of the fingers. Invariably, by the time pulmonary hypertension has developed, chest roentgenograms will reveal diffuse pulmonary infiltrates and pulmonary function tests decreased lung volumes (restrictive ventilatory abnormality). Lung biopsy may be necessary to make a specific diagnosis.

Whether or not increased intrapulmonary (alveolar) or intrathoracic pressures (pleural), by themselves, can cause pulmonary hypertension by compressing the pulmonary vascular bed is not known. Such pressure changes probably will not produce pulmonary hypertension since the behavior of the capillaries and the larger blood vessels is entirely different. At the same time the intraparenchymal capillaries, small arterioles and venules (alveolar vessels) may be compressed by increased alveolar pressure, all the larger arteries and veins coursing through the lung parenchyma (extraalveolar vessels) are being pulled open by the tension of the elastic tissue of the expanding lung. The large vessels near the hilum are not in the lung parenchyma and are exposed to intrathoracic (pleural) pressure that is negative in spontaneously breathing patients and less negative or slightly positive in mechanically ventilated patients. In other words, the different effects on alveolar and extraalveolar vessels most likely will cancel each other out.

"Reactive" pulmonary hypertension

Pulmonary hypertension in these individuals is due to a combination of passive and active mechanisms. Although initially due to passive congestion, pulmonary artery pressures subsequently rise out of proportion to postcapillary pressures as passive congestion becomes *chronic*. In "reactive" pulmonary hypertension, the $(PA_{ed} - PCW)$ pressure gradient is ≥ 5 mm Hg and the PCW pressure is greater than normal. This reaction most commonly occurs in patients with mitral valvular disease, particularly mitral stenosis. It is quite uncommon in patients with ventricular failure secondary to aortic valve disease, coronary heart disease, or systemic hypertension.

Chest Roentgenogram

The routine chest roentgenogram consisting of posterioanterior (PA) and lateral projections is a useful test to screen for abnormalities of the pulmonary circulation. The normal pulmonary circulation is seen in Fig. 8-7A.

Active pulmonary hypertension

Certain characteristic roentgenographic changes may be observed in the pulmonary vascular pattern of the lungs and in the size of the heart. Although these changes are similar in all forms of pulmonary hypertension (congenital and acquired) they are most easily appreciated in patients with precapillary pulmonary hypertension (Fig. 8-7B) and include marked enlargement of the main pulmonary artery segment, dilatation of the central hilar pulmonary artery branches down to the origin of the segmental vessels, and constriction of the segmental arteries. This correlates with the decreased cross-sectional area of the pulmonary vascular bed. The pulmonary veins will not be enlarged. The following measurements on routine inspiratory upright PA films suggest the presence of active pulmonary hypertension: (1) protrusion of the main pulmonary artery segment from the midline is greater than 33% of half of the internal diameter of the thorax, and (2) dilatation of the central pulmonary artery is present when the width of the descending branch of the right pulmonary artery is greater than 16 mm. Although slight elevations of pulmonary arterial pressures may not produce any abnormal clinical or roentgenographic signs, some or all of the changes described above will usu-

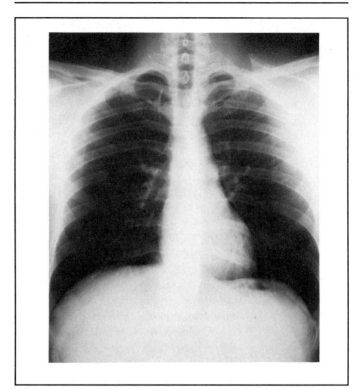

A

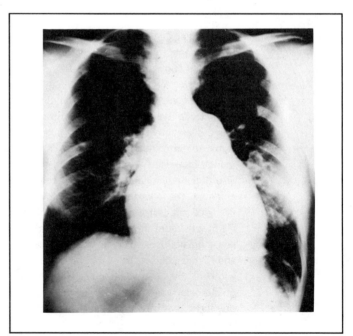

B

ally be present in active hypertensive states when the pressures reach the range of 55/25 mm Hg.

Passive pulmonary hypertension

The characteristic roentgenographic signs of passive pulmonary hypertension are the signs of pulmonary venous hypertension (Fig. 8-8A). The following sign on routine, inspiratory, upright PA films suggests the presence of pulmonary venous hypertension: prominence of upper lobe vessels (veins) over lower lobe vessels due to redistribution of pulmonary blood flow. The presence of interstitial edema (Figs. 8-8B, C, D) and alveolar edema (Fig. 8-8E) are indicative of edema accumulation; they are not specific for pulmonary venous hypertension. The clinical and roentgenographic signs of "passive" pulmonary hypertension will usually be present when PCW pressures are $\geq$ 18 mm Hg. The size and shape of the left ventricle and left atrium will depend on the cause(s) of the passive pulmonary hypertension (see Chaps. 3, 5).

Normal Liquid and Solute Transport in the Lung

Overview

The lung is not a "dry" organ. Normally, it has one of the highest water contents of any organ. The blood-free lung weighs approximately 500 mg— 80% of it is water.

A small amount of liquid leaks chiefly through the walls of pulmonary capillaries and perhaps from arterioles and venules into the interstitial tissues; but it does not accumulate and cause gas-exchange problems since it is efficiently removed by lymphatics. The anatomy of the lung is ideally suited for simultaneous transport of liquids and solutes as well as for providing a means for effective gas exchange between air and blood.

Structural considerations

The unique structure that effectively handles both functions is the interalveolar septum (Fig. 8-9). This septum, lined on its outside surface by alveolar epithelium, contains numerous pulmonary capillaries that are surrounded by an interstitial space that is thin on one side and thick on the other. Each capillary is lined by a continuous layer of endothelial cells. The basement membranes of the endothelium and epithelium fuse over approximately one-half of the capillary perimeter to form the so-called *thin* portion of the air-blood barrier

Fig. 8-7 : A. Normal chest roentgenogram. Along the left side of the mediastinum, there are three normal convexities. The first is the aorta at the level of the carina; the second is the main pulmonary artery just above the left mainstem bronchus; the third is the left ventricle just above the left hemidiaphragm. B. Chest roentgenogram of a patient with primary pulmonary hypertension. The main pulmonary artery is enlarged; the right main pulmonary artery is quite prominent and it tapers rapidly.

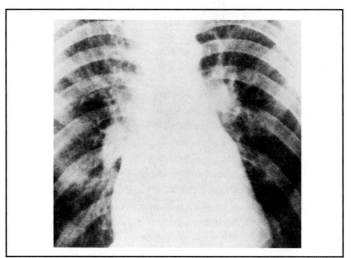

A

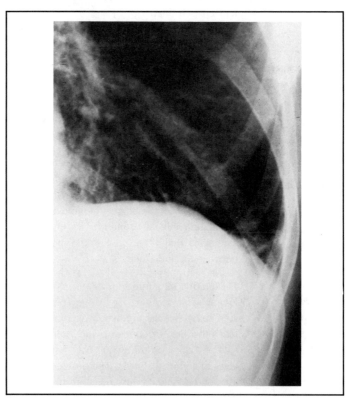

B

Fig. 8-8 : A. Pulmonary venous hypertension. The diameter of the blood vessels in the upper lung zones is greater than the diameter of the vessels in the lower lung zones. B. Kerley B lines can be seen in the cardiophrenic angle; they are no more than 1 mm in diameter thick and usually no more than 1–2 cm long. C. Kerley C lines appear as a diffuse spiderweb-like pattern. D. Kerley A lines (*arrow*) are long, sometimes sharply angulated lines that appear to arise from hilar shadows. E. Alveolar edema appearing as characteristic bat-wing alveolar filling pattern.

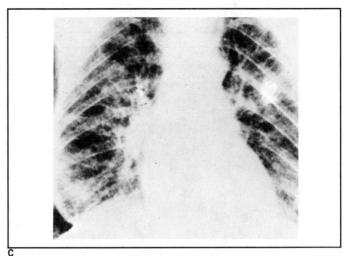

C

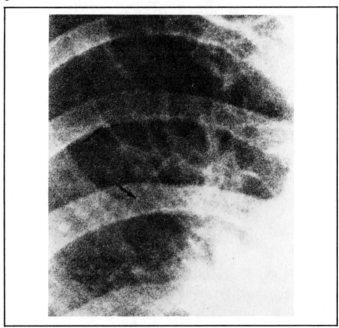

D

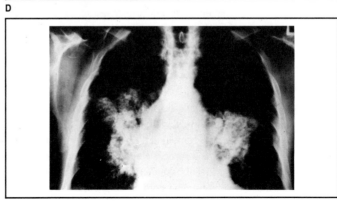

E

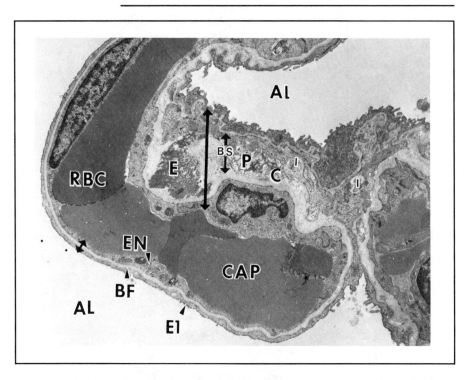

Fig. 8-9 : Electron micrograph of interalveolar septum containing pulmonary capillary (CAP). Blood-air barrier (*short double arrow*) is composed of an endothelial cell (EN), fused basement membrane (BF), and Type I alveolar epithelial lining cell (E1). The broad or thick portion of the interstitial space (*long double arrow*) is circumscribed by split basement membranes (BS) and contains elastic tissue fibers (E), collagen fibers (C), proteoglycan ground substance (P), and interstitial cells (I). The capillary is filled with red blood cells (RBC). Alveolar spaces (AL) are identified. ($\times$ 10,000.)

(presumed to be the preferential location for the diffusion of gases); the other half of the capillary perimeter, where the two basement membranes are separated by interstitium that contains chiefly connective tissue elements, is the so-called thick portion of the alveolar-capillary septum (presumed to be the site of initial fluid accumulation).

While the incompletely fused, "loose" junctions between endothelial cells allow liquid and solutes to move continuously across the endothelium into the interstitial space, the "tight" junctions of alveolar epithelial cells provide a more impenetrable barrier against liquid and solute movement into alveolar spaces (Fig. 8-10). Interstitial cells, which contain actin filaments and smooth muscle cytoplasmic membrane insertion plaques for these myofilaments, attach to alveolar epithelial basement membranes, and possibly control interstitial volume by their contractile properties (Fig. 8-10).

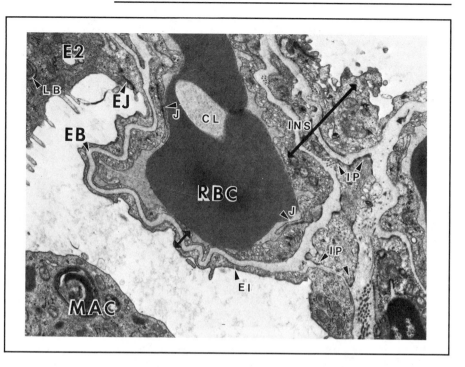

Fig. 8-10 : Electron micrography of interalveolar septum showing relatively open endothelial junctions (J) that allow fluid to pass from capillary lumen (CL) to thick portion of interstitial space (INS). The Type I alveolar epithelial cells (E1) make watertight junctions (EJ) between adjacent alveolar epithelial cells. Thin blood-air barrier (*double arrow*) and red blood cell (RBC) are identified. An interstitial cell containing actin filaments attaching to dense cytoplasmic insertion plaques (IP) crosses the thick portion of interstitium and attaches to alveolar epithelial basement (EB) membranes. This cell may regulate the interstitial compartment's volume by its contractile properties. Alveolar macrophage (MAC) and Type II alveolar epithelial cell (E2) with surfactant lamellar bodies (LB) are present. ($\times$ 22,000.)

The lung has an extensive network of lymphatic vessels that end in interstitial spaces surrounding small blood vessels and terminal bronchioles. Although lymphatic vessels have, to date, never been seen within alveolar walls, they lie, nevertheless, in close proximity to alveoli (Figs. 8-11A, B). Normally, liquid and solute drain, because of physical forces to be described, from the thick portion of the interalveolar septum into the interstitial space containing lymphatics. This liquid and solute has easy access to lymphatic channels through loose endothelial junctions of lymphatic vessels.

Physiologic considerations

In the normal lung, there is a balance between the rate of liquid movement into the interstitial space and the rate of its removal.

Net liquid flow ($\dot{Q}_f$) across an endothelial barrier can be described by the Starling equation:

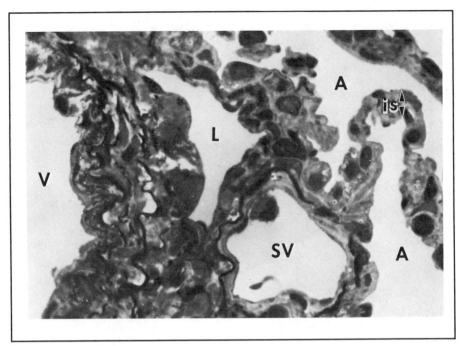

A

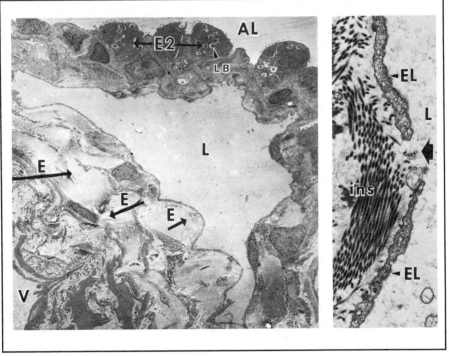

B

$$\dot{Q}_f = K\,(P_c - P_{is}) - K\,\delta\,(\pi_c - \pi_{is})$$

where

    K = capillary filtration coefficient (the ease with which fluid flows across the endothelial barrier)

    P_c and P_{is} = hydrostatic pressures in the capillary and interstitial space

    π_c and π_{is} = colloid osmotic (oncotic) pressures in the capillary and interstitial space

    δ = reflection coefficient

The reflection coefficient, which indicates the effectiveness of the membrane in preventing the flow of solute compared to water is reduced in disorders causing cells to be more permeable. Although capillary oncotic pressure is the only pressure that is known (approximately 25 mm Hg) and the reflection coefficient is assumed to be 1.0 (i.e., the endothelial membrane allows no protein to pass through it, a supposition that is not entirely true), recent data allow one to use the Starling equation to estimate reasonably the factors that contribute to liquid extravasation and how they operate (Fig. 8-12). Thus, in the normal lung, there is filtration of fluid across the endothelial membrane; it is due to the sum of four pressures (a hydrostatic pair and an osmotic pair) called "Starling's forces" and K, the ease with which fluid flows across the capillary endothelial membrane (this term refers to the permeability characteristics of the membrane). It is important to remember that oncotic pressure always opposes hydrostatic pressure.

Since capillary osmotic pressure is greater than capillary hydrostatic pressure, the difference is in favor of intravascular retention of fluids; this difference suggests that the lung is "dry." However, alveolar surfaces have been shown to be moist and liquid has been shown to be constantly removed from the lung by lymphatic channels. Therefore, since capillary (intravascular) pressures cannot explain, by themselves, why fluid is being filtered, interstitial pressures must help explain why there is net movement of fluid from the intravascular to the interstitial space.

Fig. 8-11 : A. Pulmonary lymphatic (L) between adventitia of large pulmonary vein (V) and alveolar spaces (A). A small vein (SV) is also seen. Interalveolar septum (is) is identified. The large vein contains prominent dark, wavy elastic tissue fibers with relatively inconspicuous, interspersed smooth muscle cells. ($\times$ 850, 1μ epon section.) B. Electron micrograph of the same lymphatic (L) and large vein (V) seen in (A). Large elastic tissue fibers (E) within vein and adjacent connective tissue next to lymphatic presumably contribute to the lymphatic pumping action when stretched. The lymphatic is separated from the alveolus (AL) by the Type II alveolar epithelial cells (E2) containing round lamellar bodies (LB) that are the precursors of surfactant. ($\times$ 2400.) Insert shows a high magnification of the endothelial lymphatic lining (EL) with a wide-open intercellular gap (arrow) allowing communication between interstitial space (ins) and lymphatic lumen (L), which contains flocculent lymph protein. ($\times$ 28,000.)

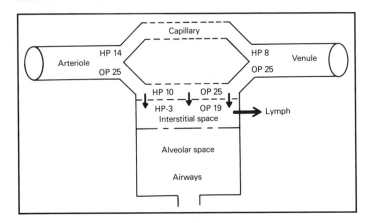

Fig. 8-12 : Normal resting hydrostatic pressure (HP) and colloid osmotic pressure (OP) relationships in the pulmonary arteriole, capillary, venule, and pericapillary interstitial space. The *arrows* indicate the direction of liquid movement. Since the difference between capillary hydrostatic and osmotic pressures is in favor of intravascular retention of liquid, the values for interstitial osmotic pressure and interstitial total pressure (liquid and solid) must be in the favor of net outward movement of liquid from the intravascular into the interstitial compartments. (From Murray JS: *The Normal Lung: The Basis for Diagnosis and Treatment of Pulmonary Disease.* Philadelphia, Saunders, 1976, with permission of the author and publisher.)

Interstitial hydrostatic pressure theoretically has to be negative around alveolar vessels due to the retractive force (surface tension) of approximately -3 to -5 cm of water created by the film of surfactant that lines alveolar walls; it also has to be negative around extraalveolar vessels since they see a pleural pressure of approximately -5 to -10 cm of water.

From data obtained in sheep, it has been estimated that interstitial oncotic pressure is less than but close to capillary oncotic pressure (i.e., 19 vs. 25 mm Hg). This information comes from lung lymph protein concentrations that have been felt to approximate closely interstitial fluid protein concentrations. Consequently, the sum of the four Starling's forces in the lung is outward (Fig. 8-12).

Liquid and solute balance in the normal lung is maintained by lymphatic drainage. Lymph capillaries provide the main disposal mechanism for water and solute. An abnormal accumulation of fluid in the extravascular spaces and tissues of the lung only occurs when the lymphatic pumping capacity is overwhelmed. While it has been estimated that steady-state lung lymph flow in a 70-kg man will normally approximate 20 ml/hour, it may be able to increase to 200 ml/hour.

Liquid that accumulates in the interstitial space of the alveolar septum moves toward the interstitial spaces that are peribronchial and contain lymphatics. The difference between alveolar and pleural pressure is the physical force that drives liquid and solute toward the lymphatics; alveolar pressure is greater (less negative) than intrathoracic (pleural) pressure. By an unknown mechanism, liquid is picked up by lymphatics and pumped toward the hilum by the smooth muscle of lymph vessels. A one-way flow of lymph is ensured by the unicuspid, funnel-shaped valves of the lymphatic vessels.

Lung Edema: An Abnormality of the Pulmonary Circulation

Overview

Since filtration of fluid across the capillary endothelium is a normal process in the lung, an abnormal accumulation of liquid (edema) is an aberration of the normal transport process. Moreover, before edema occurs, the three normal lung defenses against its formation must be overcome: (1) interstitial washdown—this first defense mechanism operates as follows: any interstitial edema that accumulates will decrease further filtration by diluting interstitial oncotic pressure; (2) low compliant interstitial space—this defense mechanism operates in the following manner: any interstitial edema that accumulates will also decrease further filtration by increasing interstitial hydrostatic pressure; and (3) lymph flow—this mechanism, perhaps the most important, has a great capacity to clear excess fluid from the lung. Lymph flow can increase tenfold over steady-state conditions.

How much edema must accumulate in the lung before it is clinically detected? Using the chest roentgenogram and arterial oxygen tension abnormalities to reflect edema accumulation, the answer is 20–30% over the amount of fluid that is normally present in the lung.

The terms *pulmonary edema* and *passive congestion* are often used, sometimes interchangeably, to refer to the state that exists when an abnormal accumulation of liquid has occurred in the lungs. However, in the interests of clinical precision, two useful distinctions should be made. *Passive congestion* is used to refer to the passive distention of the pulmonary vessels that results from elevation of pulmonary venous pressure; passive congestion occurs in those conditions that cause "passive" pulmonary hypertension. Moreover, in passive congestion, the edema fluid is solely interstitial in location. On the other hand, *pulmonary edema* should be used to refer to widespread accumulation of liquid, not only in the interstitium but also in the alveoli. While patients may have minimal symptoms with passive congestion (interstitial edema), they are almost always acutely ill with alveolar edema, complaining of severe dyspnea, even at rest, and cough. If the alveolar edema is due to passive pulmonary hypertension, these patients may cough up pink, frothy edema fluid. The pinkness is due to the presence of red blood cells.

caliber of the lower lung field vessels will be necessarily decreased as will blood flow through these vessels. In order to document the presence of increased capillary hydrostatic pressure, right heart catheterization can be performed; it will reveal elevated PCW pressures.

Since capillary permeability is preserved in this form of lung edema, little protein appears in this edema fluid. The total protein (TP) concentration of lymph edema is, on the average, only 37% of that of serum. Making the reasonable assumption that alveolar edema is similar if not identical to interstitial and lymph edema, it is clinically useful to use the total protein, alveolar edema-serum ratio (TP_e/TP_s), to distinguish increased capillary hydrostatic from increased capillary permeability lung edema. The ratio is ≤ 0.46 in the former and ≥ 0.72 in the latter.

INCREASED CAPILLARY PERMEABILITY. This occurs in a wide variety of conditions that either directly or indirectly, by some unknown mechanism, cause capillary endothelial and/or alveolar epithelial damage. Since the edema fluid contains TP concentrations that approach that of serum, this mechanism of lung edema has been called "the capillary leak syndrome" or permeability pulmonary edema. Other names for this form of lung edema are the *adult respiratory distress syndrome* (ARDS) or *noncardiogenic pulmonary edema*. ARDS can be the result of lung infection from a variety of agents, sepsis without lung infection, oxygen toxicity, aspiration of gastric juice, pancreatitis, trauma, inhalation of noxious fumes and gases, near-drowning, drug-induced damage (i.e., heroin, codeine, methadone, salicylate, propoxyphene) and fat embolism among other conditions. The initial ultrastructural finding is intracellular edema of capillary endothelial and/or alveolar type I epithelial cells. The final stage is indistinguishable from interstitial pneumonitis with hyaline membrane formation.

Clinically, a precipitating event will occur and, after a latency period during which time patients will feel and appear normal and stable, acute and often catastrophic respiratory failure will ensue. Patients will become extremely dyspneic. Roentgenographically, interstitial and alveolar edema will be obvious but there will not be any evidence of pulmonary venous hypertension. The ratio of TP_e/TP_s will be ≥ 0.72. PCW pressures will be normal. Since many of these patients will be on continuous positive pressure breathing by mechanical ventilatory support, great care must be taken in placing cardiac catheters and interpreting the results. Patients on continuous positive pressure breathing will have alveolar pressures that are much higher than atmospheric pressure, and alveolar pressure may, in different regions of the lung, be greater than capillary hydrostatic pressure. For instance, in a patient with 20 mm Hg positive end-expiratory pressure, alveolar pressure will equal 20 mm Hg. Consequently, no matter where the pulmonary artery catheter is placed, zone 1 conditions (see p. 133) will exist everywhere unless left ventricular end-diastolic pressure is 20 mm Hg and the pulmonary artery catheter tip is in the most dependent lung regions. If the left ventricular end-diastolic pressure is not > 20 mm Hg, PCW pressures will not reflect pulmonary venous pressure but rather alveolar pressure. In a patient with 10 mm Hg positive end-expiratory pressure, alveolar pressure will equal 10 mm Hg. If the pulmonary artery catheter is mistakenly passed into the uppermost part of the lung rather than being placed in the main pulmonary artery, it is also conceivable that the catheter may be measuring alveolar rather than pulmonary capillary hydrostatic pressure. Although left ventricular end-diastolic pressure may be 15 mm Hg in the most dependent lung zones, pulmonary artery pressure at the top of the lung may not be > 9 mm Hg. Consequently, zone 1 conditions regarding the distribution of perfusion in the lung may also exist in this last example.

DECREASED COLLOID ONCOTIC PRESSURE. Although this mechanism is rarely responsible for lung edema by itself, it can worsen edema caused by another mechanism such as increased capillary permeability. Hypoproteinemia from liver failure, the nephrotic syndrome, or overhydration with intravenous crystalloid fluid (i.e., saline) can decrease capillary oncotic pressure.

DECREASED INTERSTITIAL PRESSURE. Since interstitial pressure has to be negative due to surface tension and pleural pressure, lung edema theoretically might occur if interstitial pressure became acutely negative so that lymphatics become overwhelmed. The clinical situations where this occurs are acute bronchial asthma and hanging with total upper airway obstruction. In these settings, pleural pressure is extremely negative.

LYMPHATIC INSUFFICIENCY. This mechanism all by itself will lead to lung edema even if all of Starling's forces are normal. It is operative in lymphangitis carcinomatosis and silicosis in which lymphatic channels are obstructed, obliterated, and/or distorted.

UNKNOWN MECHANISM. The pathogenesis of several forms of lung edema are unknown. These include the pulmonary edema due to sojourns at high altitude and neurogenic pulmonary edema. Neither is due to any of the mechanisms mentioned above.

The mechanism of neurogenic pulmonary edema that occurs after seizures or head trauma may well be due to a combination of two mechanisms: (1) increased capillary hydrostatic pressure from acute left ventricular failure; left ventricular failure is due to systemic hypertension from the sympathetic discharge of central nervous system origin; and (2) increased capillary permeability from the very high capillary hydrostatic pressure that ruptures capillary endothelial junctions.

Clinicopathologic Correlation

In general, patients with pulmonary hypertension, no matter what the cause, will have an increased minute ventilation. This usually correlates with a respiratory rate > 16 breaths/minute (tachypnea). The increased minute ventilation is usually due to stimulation of pathologic reflexes that originate within the lung. In most situations, the pathways have not been well defined. In passive pulmonary hypertensive states, increased interstitial pressure from edema stimulates juxtapulmonary capillary (J) receptors located in the interstitium; vagal afferents, subserving this reflex, then stimulate the respiratory center in the medulla. In active pulmonary hypertensive disorders of pulmonary emboli and primary pulmonary hypertension the following pathways may be operative: the release of vasoactive substances or pulmonary hypertension by itself, in pulmonary embolic disease, is thought to somehow stimulate J receptors by increasing interstitial pressure; elevated pressures within the pulmonary arteries in primary pulmonary hypertension may stimulate stretch receptors within the walls of the arteries themselves; vagal afferents may then stimulate the respiratory center in the medulla. The exact mechanism(s) by which minute ventilation and, therefore, the work of breathing increases in all patients with pulmonary hypertension is not known. Recent studies suggest that this increased work of breathing leads to dyspnea when respiratory muscles begin to fatigue.

Dyspnea that occurs (1) when the patient assumes the recumbent position (orthopnea) or (2) after the patient has retired and been asleep for an hour or two in the recumbent position (paroxysmal nocturnal dyspnea) are helpful clues to the presence of passive pulmonary hypertension. Orthopnea and paroxysmal nocturnal dyspnea are due to the increased work of breathing secondary to accumulation of interstitial edema that, in turn, is the result of increased capillary hydrostatic pressure secondary to increased venous return to the heart in the recumbent position.

The Right Ventricle in Health

General considerations

Cardiac output of the right ventricle (RV) equals that of the left ventricle (LV) despite the fact that pressures are normally much lower in the former pump (Fig. 8-1). This fact suggests that the RV is more distensible than the LV; the following anatomic and physiologic observations of the respective, normal adult ventricles support this suspicion: (1) the outer wall of the RV (3–4 mm) is much thinner than that of the LV (8–12 mm); and (2) the pressure-volume characteristics of both ventricles demonstrate that the RV is more compliant (Fig.8-15). That is, for the same ventricular volume, chamber pressure will be greater in the LV.

Fig. 8-15 : Pressure-volume characteristics of right (RV) and left ventricles (LV).

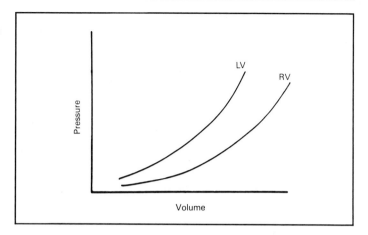

Fig. 8-16 : Right (RV) and left ventricular (LV) function curves.

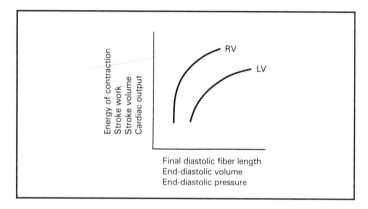

The explanation for RV and LV outputs being equal is not related to distensibility but rather to Starling's law of the heart. The RV and LV function according to the same ventricular function curve theory (Fig. 8-16). That is, cardiac output depends upon the volume of blood that is present before contraction (preload). Since the two pumps are in series and they pump according to the same principle, they will pass the same volume of blood between each other. According to Fig. 8-16, it is possible, on a beat-to-beat basis, to move up and down the corresponding ventricular function curve by varying the volume of blood that is returned to each pump. For instance, by assuming the recumbent position, venous return to the RV increases. This will increase RV preload and be responsible for increasing RV output. LV preload and output will then increase by the same amount.

Although the RV and LV function curves have essentially the same shape, the LV curve is shifted to the right because it is less compliant (i.e., for the same volume, LV end-diastolic pressure will be greater).

By briefly reviewing the anatomy of the fetal cardiovascular system, it is possible: (1) to understand why LV muscle mass is greater than RV; and (2) to appreciate that ventricular output, in addition to preload, may also be influenced by the resistance that the ventricle has to eject against (i.e., circulation peripheral to the pump). Before birth, the ductus arteriosus is patent. Since approximately 90% of RV output is pumped through the patent ductus into the same conduit (aorta) that the LV is pumping into, both ventricles are emptying into the same circulation and both ventricles are exposed to the same systemic vascular resistance. Not surprisingly, RV and LV chamber pressures and muscle masses are similar in utero. At birth, the ductus closes and the lungs become aerated; the RV pumps blood into the pulmonary circulation with a low vascular resistance to flow. Consequently, the RV no longer needs to be as strong as the LV; RV chamber pressures and muscle mass decrease.

Determinants of normal right ventricular function

Normal RV and LV cardiac outputs are determined by the same two factors: (1) stroke volume, a function of preload, myocardial contractility, and afterload, and (2) heart rate.

Preload has already been described (Fig. 8-16). It is the amount of blood that is present in the ventricle before contraction takes place.

Contractility defines the performance of the ventricular muscle. Although contractility can be described in terms of how quickly the muscle contracts, the effect of contractility on cardiac output can perhaps be best appreciated by looking at a family of RV function curves (Fig. 8-17). For the same preload, increased contractility shifts the curve upwards; decreased contractility shifts the curve downwards.

Afterload is described by the law of Laplace:

$$T = \frac{P \times r}{2 \text{ (wall thickness)}}$$

It is the tension (T) that must be developed in the ventricular muscle before the muscle fibers will shorten and eject blood. Afterload is directly proportional to the intraventricular pressure (P) (equivalent to the pressure within the circulation that the ventricle has to push against) times the radius (r) of the chamber; and it is indirectly proportional to two times the muscle wall thickness. The effect of afterload on cardiac output is a negative one. When afterload increases, cardiac output tends to decrease. For instance, before the RV will eject blood into the pulmonary circulation when pulmonary hypertension is present, a greater tension must be generated in the myocardium during contraction. Because of the extra time it takes to reach this greater tension, ejection may cease before the ventricle can empty itself entirely.

Fig. 8-17 : The effect of contractility on right ventricular function.

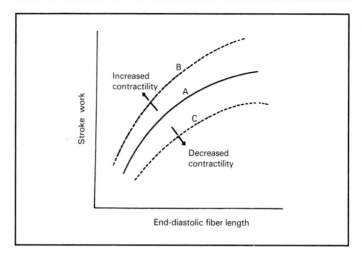

Since cardiac output is equal to stroke volume times heart rate, at any given stroke volume, cardiac output is linearly related to heart rate. Should stroke volume be reduced for any reason, a compensatory increase in heart rate can usually maintain an appropriate cardiac output.

The Right Ventricle in Disease

Pathophysiologic mechanisms in RV failure

Potentially, RV failure will be mediated functionally by disturbance(s) of contractility, heart rate, preload, and afterload.

Although primary or predominant contractility disturbances of the RV and LV may occur concomitantly in cardiomyopathies and acute myocardial infarction of the inferior wall of the LV, it is extremely unusual for RV failure to occur secondary to a primary contractility abnormality of the RV alone. Such an abnormality does occur rarely during infarction localized to the RV. RV failure due to an isolated disturbance of heart rate is also an extremely unlikely theoretical as well as clinical possibility.

By reconsidering Starling's law of the heart (Fig. 8-16), one can see that it is possible to volume underload the RV to such an extent that cardiac output would be markedly reduced. Although underloading causes concomitant LV and RV dysfunction during cardiac tamponade, decreased output from this mechanism alone is rarely seen, e.g., in patients with tricuspid stenosis.

Although it is theoretically possible to cause RV failure by overstretching the muscle fibers from volume overloading (the ventricular function curve plateaus and then descends in animal experiments), this pathophysiological mechanism is thought not to occur in most clinical situations. On the other hand, pressure overloading of the RV, caused by increasing afterload, is the most common cause of RV

Table 8-1 : Disorders that commonly lead to cor pulmonale

Neuromuscular diseases
  Primary central hypoventilation, poliomyelitis, myasthenia gravis
Chest wall deformities
  Kyphoscoliosis, thoracoplasty
Vascular diseases
  Multiple recurrent thromboemboli, schistosomiasis, sickle cell anemia,
    primary pulmonary hypertension
Restrictive lung diseases
  Idiopathic pulmonary fibrosis, sarcoidosis, scleroderma, tuberculosis,
    alveolar proteinosis, bilateral fibrothoraces
Obstructive lung diseases
  COPD, cystic fibrosis, upper airway obstruction (hypertrophied tonsils,
    tongue).

failure. It is the predominant mechanism of RV failure in all pulmonary hypertensive disorders whether they are active or passive.

Cardiac compensatory mechanisms

In order to maintain cardiac output in the face of the above functional abnormalities, the RV can compensate acutely, subacutely, and chronically. Acutely, increased sympathetic nervous system activity increases heart rate and myocardial contractility (inotropic effect). Subacutely, RV dilatation occurs due to the inability of the RV chamber to completely empty in afterload-induced heart failure. According to the law of Laplace, RV dilatation increases afterload (RV wall tension increases). However, since preload also increases, RV output increases by Starling's law of the heart. In other words, the RV will be able to eject more blood at the expense of elevating RV end-diastolic pressure and potentially causing passive congestion of the systemic venous system (RV congestive heart failure).

Chronically, RV end-diastolic pressure gradually rises, and RV hypertrophy occurs before congestive heart failure develops. According to Laplace's law, RV hypertrophy decreases afterload because of the increased muscle thickness. On the basis of the above considerations, compensated RV failure is manifested clinically by tachycardia and cardiomegaly (dilatation and/or hypertrophy).

Cor pulmonale

Cor pulmonale is a synonym for *pulmonary heart disease*. Disorders that commonly lead to cor pulmonale are listed in Table 8-1. It is defined quite specifically by the following criteria:

1. Pulmonary arterial hypertension must be present; it causes right ventricular enlargement (dilatation and/or hypertrophy).
2. Pulmonary arterial hypertension may be caused by intrinsic lung diseases of the interstitium, tracheobronchial tree, alveoli or pulmonary vascular tree; by inadequate function of the chest bellows (chest wall or muscles); or by inadequate ventilatory drive from the respiratory centers.
3. Neither congenital heart disease nor acquired disease of the left side of the heart can be implicated as the cause for the pulmonary hypertension.

Although RV failure, from a purely statistical standpoint, is most commonly due to LV failure, it is important to be able to identify RV failure from pulmonary diseases for the following reasons: (1) cor pulmonale, in random autopsy series, is a common finding, ranging between 6–40% of patients; (2) specific and successful therapies are available in the majority of cases; and (3) the prognosis for cor pulmonale is better than that for LV failure. This last point can be emphasized by comparing the five-year survival of patients with the most common causes of LV failure and cor pulmonale. The five-year survival of patients with LV failure secondary to coronary artery disease and systemic hypertension is 50% compared to 70% in cor pulmonale secondary to COPD.

ETIOLOGY OF COR PULMONALE. Among the disorders listed in Table 8-1, the neuromuscular and obstructive lung diseases cause pulmonary hypertension by vasoconstriction, chest wall deformities by anatomic restriction of the pulmonary vascular bed and vasoconstriction, and restrictive and vascular diseases by anatomic restriction.

TREATMENT OF COR PULMONALE. The treatment of compensated cor pulmonale in which passive congestion of the systemic venous system has not occurred need only concern itself with treating the cause of pulmonary hypertension. For instance, cor pulmonale usually resolves with anticoagulant therapy for pulmonary embolism, corticosteroid therapy in some cases of idiopathic interstitial fibrosis, oxygen therapy for COPD, and tracheostomy for peripheral obstructive sleep apnea (upper airway obstruction by the tongue during sleep). Since cor pulmonale does not involve a primary contractility problem of the RV, the use of digitalis preparations is not indicated.

The treatment of uncompensated cor pulmonale must concern itself with treating the cause of pulmonary hypertension plus attempts to improve the determinants of RV function. Diuretics decrease passive systemic venous congestion by decreasing RV end-diastolic pressure and thereby unloading the RV; afterload should also decrease since the radius of the ventricular chamber declines. A role for phlebotomy has only been demonstrated in patients with hematocrits above 55%. By decreasing the hematocrit below 55%, viscosity no longer contributes to pulmonary hypertension and pressure overloading. The use of digitalis in uncompensated cor pulmonale is controversial. Most recent studies do not support its use.

CAN COR PULMONALE CAUSE LV FAILURE? Since both ventricles structurally share common muscle bundles, it is not surprising that RV failure can cause LV function abnormalities. However, the abnormalities demonstrated have only been subtle ones. RV failure does not cause LV failure. If LV failure occurs in the presence of cor pulmonale, it is almost always due to primary LV disease.

Chest roentgenograms

By knowing the location of the RV in normal conventional PA and lateral roentgenograms (Fig. 8-18A, B), one can see why the detec-

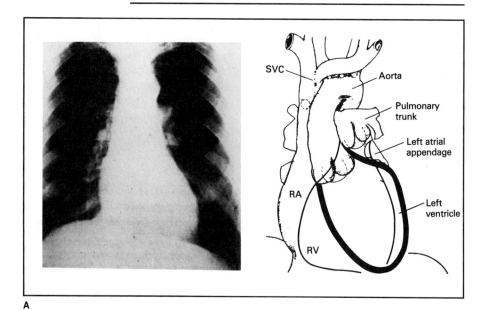

A

B

Fig. 8-18 : The normal chest roentgenogram. A. The right ventricle (RV) does not contribute to the right or left cardiac borders on the posterolateral chest roentgenogram. B. The right ventricle is the most anterior portion of the cardiac border seen on the lateral chest roentgenogram. SVC = superior vena cava; AO = aorta; PT = pulmonary trunk; RA = right atrium; LV = left ventricle; IVC = inferior vena cava.

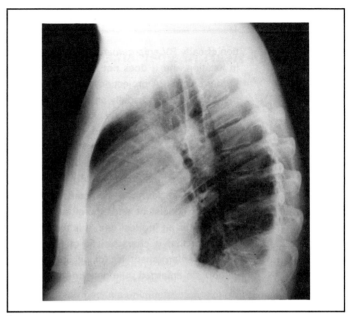

A

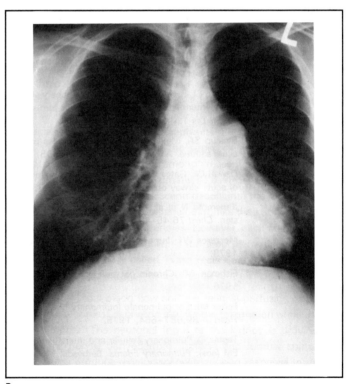

B

Fig. 8-19 : The chest roentgenogram in pulmonary hypertension and cor pulmonale. A. The right ventricle has enlarged anteriorally and obliterated the retrosternal air space in the lateral projection. B. The right ventricle is markedly enlarged; it has rotated to form all of the left cardiac border and elevated the original apex so that the left lower heart border has a characteristic rounded contour.

Fig. 9-1 : Comparison of the blood supplies of cortical and juxtamedullary nephrons. (From Pitts RF: *Physiology of the Kidney and Body Fluids*, ed 3. Chicago, Year Book, 1974, with permission of the author and publisher.)

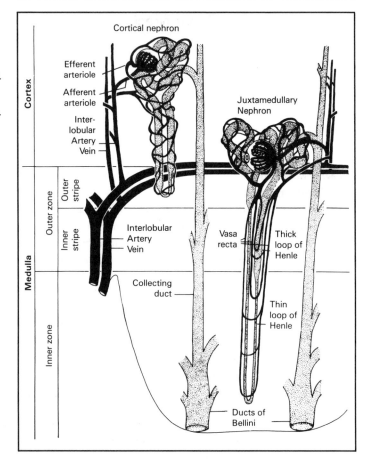

The hormonal factors that control renal perfusion are incompletely understood. However, catecholamines and angiotensin II are both known to produce renal vasoconstriction. Both circulating epinephrine and neurally released norepinephrine are renal vasoconstrictors presumably partaking in the reduction of renal blood flow that occurs with upright posture.

Increased renal sympathetic nerve traffic, circulating catecholamines, and decreased renal blood flow all stimulate renal renin release, thus initiating the renin-angiotensin-aldosterone cascade. The highly potent vasoconstrictor, angiotensin II, can reduce renal blood flow but, as we will see, it also preserves glomerular filtration rate.

When mean systemic blood pressure is varied over a wide range, between 80 and 180 mm Hg, both renal blood flow (RBF) and the glomerular filtration rate (GFR) remain relatively unaltered (Fig. 9-2). This phenomenon is referred to as "autoregulation" since the mechanisms are intrinsic to the kidney, i.e., they can be observed in the isolated organ, perfused in vitro.

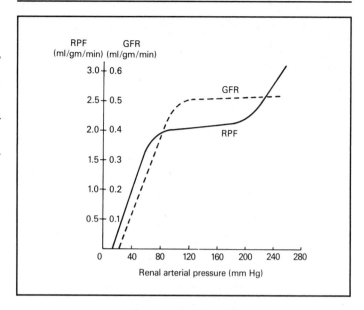

Fig. 9-2 : Autoregulation of glomerular filtration rate (GFR) and renal plasma flow (RPF) in the dog over a range of 8–180 mm Hg perfusion pressure. (From Pitts RF: *Physiology of the Kidney and Body Fluids,* ed 3. Chicago, Year Book, 1974, with permission of the author and publisher.)

The means by which the renal vasculature autoregulates RBF are incompletely understood. It appears, however, that autoregulation of RBF and GFR are independently controlled. Indeed, autoregulation of blood flow is not unique to the kidney and may be observed in many, if not all, organs. Blood flow autoregulation may be a "myogenic" process, intrinsic to vascular smooth muscle.

The first step in urine formation is the process of glomerular filtration. An ultrafiltrate, a protein-free, plasmalike solution, is formed by the combined action of several hydraulic forces across the glomerular capillary wall. The glomerular capillary is a tripartite surface: (1) the fenestrated endothelial lining, (2) the basement membrane, and (3) the epithelial cell layer that includes epithelial foot processes (podocytes) imbedded in the basement membrane. This ultrafiltration barrier permits the passage of water and other small solutes such as sodium, chloride, and inulin. Larger molecular weight substances such as albumin and other plasma proteins are largely restricted.

Filtration through glomerular capillaries is driven essentially by the same hydraulic forces that govern filtration through peripheral capillaries (Table 9-1). GFR is much greater than that of peripheral capillaries because of properties unique to glomerular capillaries:

1. The net, mean hydrostatic pressure gradient for filtration in glomerular capillaries is 13 times greater than in peripheral capillaries (Table 9-1).
2. The hydraulic permeability of glomerular capillaries to small solutes approaches 50 times that of extrarenal capillaries.

Table 9-1 : Comparison of Starling's forces in
primate muscle and glomerular capillaries*

Forces	Muscle capillary (mm Hg)	Glomerular capillary (mm Hg)
Forces favoring filtration		
Pressure in the capillary or glomerulus (P_{GC})	24	45.5
Interstitial π_{BS}	5	0
Total	29	45.5
Forces opposing filtration		
P interstitial or P_{BS}	3.5	10
π plasma or π_{GC}	25.0	29
Total	28.5	39
Net gradient for filtration (forces favoring / forces opposing)	0.5	6.5

* See text for abbreviations.

Source: Data from Landis E, Pappenheimer JR, in Hamilton WF, Dow P (eds): *Handbook of Physiology: A Critical Comprehensive Presentation of Physiologic Knowledge and Concepts.* Washington, DC, American Physiological Society, 1963, vol 2, sec 2, and Massox DA, Dean WM, Brenner BM: Dynamics of glomerular ultrafiltration. VI. Studies in the primate. *Kidney Int* 5:271, 1974. Adapted from Rose BD (ed): *Clinical Physiology of Acid-Base and Electrolyte Disorders.* New York, McGraw-Hill, 1977.

3. As seen in Figure 9-3, there are two steep pressure gradients in the renal circulation at the preglomerular and postglomerular capillary sphincters. The effective hydraulic pressure across the glomerular capillaries is nearly twice as high as in peripheral capillaries.

As is the case for peripheral capillaries, the gradient for filtration is determined by the balance of opposing hydrostatic and oncotic pressures. The GFR in a single nephron (SNGFR) can be derived simply by adding up the forces favoring and those opposing filtration and multiplying by a constant Kf, the ultrafiltration coefficient (Kf = K × S where K is the hydraulic permeability factor and S is the surface area of glomerular capillaries.)

SNGFR = Kf (forces favoring filtration) − (forces opposing filtration)
= Kf ([P_{GC} + π_{BS}] − [P_{BS} + π])

where P_{GC} = glomerular capillary hydrostatic pressure
P_{BS} = Bowman's space hydrostatic pressure
π_{GC} = glomerular capillary oncotic pressure
π_{BS} = Bowman's space oncotic pressure

or

SNGFR = Kf ($\Delta P - \Delta \pi$)

where ΔP = the transcapillary hydrostatic pressure difference, $P_{GC} - P_{BS}$
$\Delta \pi$ = the transcapillary oncotic pressure difference, $\pi_{GC} - \pi_{BS}$

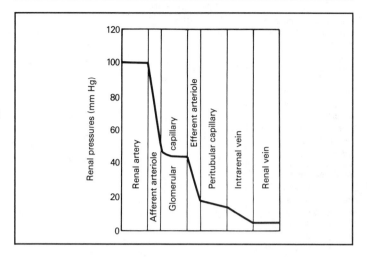

Fig. 9-3 : Pressure gradients in the renal circulation. (From Pitts RF: *Physiology of the Kidney and Body Fluids*, ed. 3. Chicago, Year Book, 1974, with permission of the author and publisher.)

The filtration fraction (FF) mathematically expresses the proportion of renal plasma flow filtered, i.e.,

$$FF = \frac{GFR}{\text{Renal plasma flow}} = \frac{GFR}{RBF\,(1-Hct)}$$

where RBF = renal blood flow
GFR = glomerular filtration rate
Hct = hematocrit

The single nephron filtration fraction (SNFF) is analogously computed, SNFF = SNGFR/GPF, where GPF is glomerular plasma flow, i.e., (glomerular blood flow) (1 − Hct).

In the postglomerular capillaries, i.e., the peritubular capillary network, the relation between ΔP and Δπ is reversed. The effect of the efferent arteriole is to reduce ΔP in the peritubular capillaries to a minimal value. On the other hand, in direct proportion to the filtration fraction, Δπ in the peritubular capillaries rises above hydrostatic pressure. Hence, the net forces in the postglomerular capillaries favor fluid and solute *uptake* and not filtration. Since solute and fluid reabsorbed by the proximal tubule are delivered to paracellular spaces in proximity to peritubular capillaries, the latter participate in the uptake of this reabsorbate.

AUTOREGULATION OF GFR. As described earlier, GFR remains near constant over wide changes in perfusion pressure. Adjustment of the relative arteriolar resistances across the glomerular capillary bed accounts for this phenomenon. In other words, as RBF (or glomerular blood flow [GBF]) is decreased, resistance at the afferent arteriole *diminishes* but efferent arteriolar resistance *increases*, thereby maintaining glomerular capillary pressure (P_{GC}). Thus, the transcapillary

Fig. 9-4 : Changes in glomerular blood flow (GBF), glomerular capillary hydrostatic pressure (P_{GC}), and afferent (R_A) and efferent (R_E) arteriolar resistances when mean arterial pressure is reduced. As shown, GBF, and to a greater extent, P_{GC} are relatively sustained over the range of pressures examined. This is accomplished by bidirectional changes in R_A and R_E. (From Buewkes R, Ichikawa J, Brenner BM: The renal circulations, in Brenner BM, Rector FC [eds]: *The Kidney,* Philadelphia, Saunders, 1981, pp 249–288, with permission of the authors and publisher.)

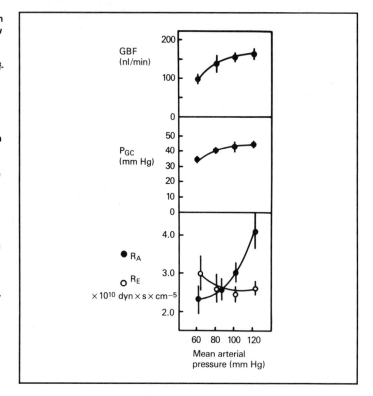

hydraulic force for ultrafiltration is preserved. These adaptations are shown in Fig. 9-4. There is considerable evidence that angiotensin II mediates filtration autoregulation and its predominant renal microcirculatory action is efferent arteriolar constriction.

Control of salt and water excretion

It is generally agreed that the acquisition or loss of sodium triggers a complex system that integrates afferent messages sensing extracellular volume and efferent signals to control renal sodium excretion restoring extracellular fluid volume (ECF) toward normal.

The afferent sensing mechanisms are incompletely understood but appear to involve both volume receptors in the intrathoracic great veins or left atrium (presumably responding to a change in wall tension) and baroreceptors in the carotid artery and the aortic arch (presumably reacting to changes in arterial blood pressure). Both of these systems activate changes in sympathetic outflow to the kidney via vagal afferent fibers that alter both renal blood flow and sodium excretion. There is evidence that both the volume receptor and baroreceptor systems play a role in the control of ECF homeostasis. Maneuvers that reduce venous return and stimulate the volume receptors such as prolonged standing or positive pressure breathing lead to reduced sodium excretion. On the other hand, augmentation of venous return such as with total body water-immersion or negative pressure respiration produces increased renal sodium excretion. Closure of an arteriovenous fistula raises mean arterial blood pressure and inhibits the baroreceptor apparatus, thereby increasing renal sodium excretion.

It should be added that both volume receptors and baroreceptors may further control extracellular fluid balance through alterations in both antidiuretic hormone (ADH) and water excretion. Both systems are stimulated by hemorrhage, for example, and via vagal afferents both can stimulate hypothalamic ADH release. This renders the collecting duct permeable to water and enhances nephronal water reabsorption and net water retention.

Tubular elements in sodium and water handling

The proximal tubule isosmotically reabsorbs roughly two-thirds of the filtered load of sodium chloride and water. This process of sodium transport is partly facilitated by entry of sodium into proximal tubular cells through a cotransport mechanism linked with glucose, bicarbonate, amino acids, and other organic substrates. However, the required "downhill gradient" for sodium entry occurs when sodium is moved outward at the peritubular side of the proximal tubular cell membrane. The energy required for this latter process is provided by Na-K-ATPase. Further along the proximal tubule, bicarbonate reabsorption is linked to hydrogen ion secretion. Here, sodium reabsorption accompanies bicarbonate reclamation. In addition, as bicarbonate is reabsorbed, a high luminal chloride concentration results in a positive electrical ("chloride diffusion") potential that further drives sodium transport.

In the loop of Henle, sodium chloride reabsorption occurs predominantly in the thick ascending limb. This nephron segment has two distinct properties: (1) active reabsorbtion of chloride, followed by sodium, and (2) impermeability to water; thus, this segment permits "dilution" to occur by the abstraction of solute. The thick ascending limb, often referred to as the "diluting segment," has the critical function of creating dilute tubular fluid that, if unaltered by the distal nephron, results in the formation of *hypotonic urine.* The function of this segment may be impaired either by the reduced delivery of solute and fluid (such as may occur when proximal tubular reabsorption is exaggerated as in congestive heart failure) or by either the socalled loop diuretics (furosemide or ethacrynic acid) or thiazide diuretics.

The distal tubule and cortical collecting duct are usually considered together. This segment of the distal nephron is sensitive to the mineralocorticoid, aldosterone, that induces an electrogenic potential for sodium reabsorption. Hence, the net reabsorption of sodium in the distal nephron is invariably linked to net secretion (and urinary loss) of potassium and/or hydrogen ion.

Fig. 9-5 : Flow diagram of forward and backward theories of edema formation in congestive heart failure.

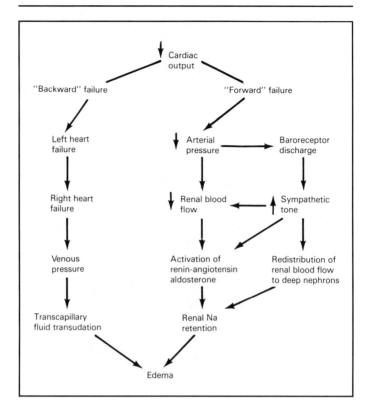

Mechanisms of Sodium Retention in Congestive Heart Failure

General theories of edema formation in CHF

Edema has been recognized as a consequence of cardiac failure since the nineteenth century. At that time it was thought that the loss of ventricular contractile force resulted in elevation of central and peripheral venous pressure. Transmitted retrograde venous hypertension thus raised capillary hydrostatic pressure, causing transcapillary exudation of fluid into the interstitial space. This "backward" hypothesis of edema formation of heart failure advanced further when it was recognized that the resultant decrease in intravascular volume leads to renal retention of salt and water thus augmenting sodium retention.

The "forward failure" (Fig. 9-5) hypothesis assumes that the primary event is diminished renal perfusion that follows as a consequence of reduced cardiac output with resultant renal conservation of sodium, chloride, and water. Thus, though plasma volume may be normal or even elevated, the "effective arteriolar blood volume" (EABV) perceived by the kidneys is reduced. "High output" congestive failure can also be explained by this mechanism even though cardiac output is supranormal (anemia, thyrotoxicosis, and large arteriovenous fistulae) since peripheral vascular resistance is reduced and effective circulation to the kidney is likewise attenuated.

It is readily apparent, however, that the forward and backward hypotheses are not mutually exclusive, and it is currently acknowledged that both mechanisms may operate simultaneously.

An integrated understanding of the various renal mechanisms that result in edema formation and water retention in heart failure requires a fundamental knowledge of the *sensing pathways* that draw upon circulatory changes occurring with heart failure. These signal a variety of effector pathways which directly stimulate either sodium chloride or water transport.

Sensing elements for sodium chloride and water retention

In mammalian organisms, the cardiac atria and great veins possess low pressure "volume receptors" that respond to changes in wall tension. These volume receptors and the high pressure baroreceptors in the carotid artery and aortic arch sense changes in EABV, thereby influencing both ADH secretion, and consequent water balance, and sodium excretion.

Acute left atrial distention results in both a sodium and a water diuresis. The former is presumably (see below) mediated by a decrease in renal sympathetic nervous stimulation; the latter, by a decrease in ADH release. The opposite findings, however, occur in heart failure.

The resolution of these conflicting data lies in three lines of evidence. First, *acute* myocardial infarction, accompanied by *acute* left atrial distention, may indeed be accompanied by a high urine output and a natriuresis. However, after the first 24 hours following acute myocardial infarction this effect becomes negligible.

Secondly, *right* atrial hypertension produces renal sodium retention. Hence, although *left* atrial stretching may acutely activate increased sodium excretion, chronic right atrial distention results in sodium conservation while the effect of left atrial distention is attenuated chronically.

Thirdly, decreases in cardiac output increase sympathetic nervous outflow, presumably by stimulating high pressure baroreceptors thereby causing renal vasoconstriction and sodium and water retention. For example, partial ligation of the thoracic inferior vena cava (TIVC) produces hemodynamic changes identical to heart failure. TIVC constriction reduces cardiac output and blood pressure. Even if renal blood flow is held constant, renal sodium excretion diminishes, which suggests that renal sodium avidity may be stimulated by the sympathetic nervous system. There are, however, other pathways involved since "high-output" cardiac failure (as in beri-beri heart disease, thyrotoxicosis, anemia, and arteriovenous [AV] fistula) is likewise associated with renal sodium avidity.

Opening of an AV fistula, for example, produces abrupt renal salt conservation and surgical closure of the fistula, as mentioned previously, results in a rapid natriuresis. Since opening and closing of the fistula is associated with decreasing and increasing diastolic blood pressure, respectively, peripheral vascular resistance and EABV, and not necessarily cardiac output, appear to cause changes in sodium excretion in these studies.

The neuronal and/or hormonal pathways through which these atrial and baroreceptor reflexes operate are incompletely understood. Cervical vagotomy interrupts the atriorenal reflex, thus indicating that the afferent message travels via the vagus nerve. However, the effector limb of the reflex appears to be through sympathetic renal nerve tone since increased left atrial pressure leads to a reduction in sympathetic outflow and renal vasodilation. On the other hand, maneuvers that cause atrial collapse, such as hemorrhage, stimulate sympathetic renal nerve discharge and produce renal vasoconstriction.

In summary, the modern understanding of renal salt retention and edema formation in heart failure acknowledges both the "forward" and "backward" hypotheses. Chronic venous (and atrial) hypertension clearly activate sodium reabsorption thereby supporting the "backward" hypothesis. However, changes in the "forward" cardiac output or EABV are also critical elements in the production of the heart failure syndrome.

Effector elements in renal sodium conservation in heart failure

The effector limb of sodium retention in cardiac failure involves several elements (Fig. 9-6) that combine to increase sodium reabsorption along the length of the nephron.

GFR, RBF, AND PERITUBULAR PHYSICAL FACTORS IN SODIUM RETENTION. Since sodium reabsorption is enhanced in heart failure along the entire length of the nephron, the whole spectrum of tubular mechanisms has been implicated. We will examine how these elements can be integrated to produce the typical sodium avidity of heart failure.

To begin with, it becomes apparent that a reduction in cardiac output, if it produces a parallel decrease in GFR, should effect a similar change in sodium excretion. However, unless cardiac output is severely reduced, GFR actually remains near normal. GFR is protected from reduced cardiac output and arterial pressure by means of filtration autoregulation. This means that while RBF is generally reduced in CHF, the filtration fraction GFR/RBF $(1 - Hct)$ is increased. This phenomenon is better understood by examining the glomerular microcirculation. The FF for a single nephron (SNFF) is given by: SNGFR/GBF $(1 - Hct)$. Just as whole kidney GFR is maintained, SNGFR also remains normal. Likewise, since RBF (and renal plasma flow) are reduced, glomerular plasma flow (GPF) is also reduced. Hence, SNFF is increased in heart failure.

Fig. 9-6 : Summary of mechanisms that lead to renal sodium retention. Note that the result of volume expansion provides a negative feedback loop (*broken arrow*) by restoring cardiac output and blood pressure. RBF = renal blood flow.

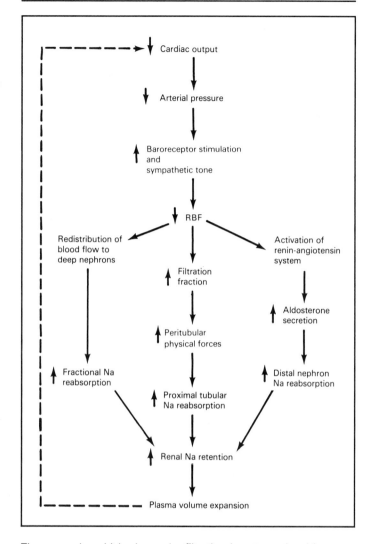

The means by which glomerular filtration is autoregulated is uncertain but appears to involve local activation of the renin-angiotensin system. Renin is released from juxtaglomerular cells along the afferent arteriole. The major controls for renin secretion include an afferent arteriolar baroreceptor that provokes renin release when renal perfusion is reduced. Juxtaglomerular cell renin release is also activated by renal sympathetic nerve stimulation and by beta-adrenergic catecholamines. There is also a tubular mechanism for renin secretion—the macula densa. This specialized group of distal tubular cells appears to respond to changes in distal nephron solute delivery by signalling the adjacent juxtaglomerular apparatus to release renin. All of the above mechanisms may be activated by reduced cardiac output with an attendant reduction in RBF, an increase in sympathetic nerve discharge, and a diminution in solute delivery to the distal nephron.

Fig. 9-8 : Pathogene-sis of water retention and hyponatremia in cardiac failure.

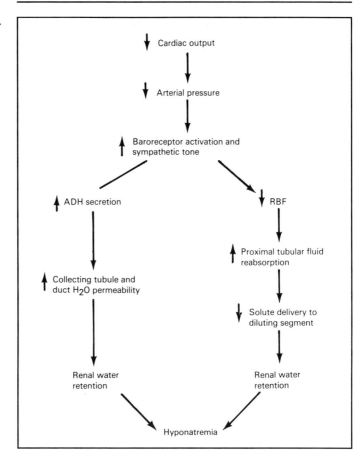

with experimental cardiac failure. However, the importance of ADH secretion in the water retention of heart failure is suggested by the finding that most patients with heart failure and hyponatremia have measurable plasma levels of ADH. Hence, despite the lack of an osmotic stimulus to ADH secretion, nonosmotic inputs are activated in heart failure. A decrease in cardiac output and blood pressure undoubtedly is registered by carotid and aortic baroreceptors that, through a decrease in vagal tone, stimulate ADH secretion. While the increased left atrial pressure of heart failure may activate vagal affer-ent fibers to shut off ADH release, this effect must be overridden by the baroreceptor mechanism. Furthermore, the left atrial volume re-ceptor is probably desensitized by chronic left atrial distention thus rendering this ADH-suppressive element less potent.

Recent studies in which ADH has been measured in heart failure patients by radioimmunoassay demonstrate that there are two groups of patients: one in which the ADH levels are persistently high despite elevations in left atrial pressure and rise no further when pulmonary capillary wedge pressure is lowered with the vasodilator, prazosin, and one in which the ADH levels are initially low and rise in response to prazosin. Furthermore, mechanical ultrafiltration to remove extracellular fluid by an artificial device appears to reduce ADH levels when cardiac output is improved by this maneuver. These studies indicate that improvement of cardiac performance reduces the baroreceptor stimulus to ADH secretion.

Homeostasis of GFR and RBF in Cardiac Failure

It is generally held by nephrologists that acute renal failure (or so-called acute tubular necrosis) is a less common clinical phenomenon in cardiogenic shock than in hemorrhagic or septic shock despite equivalent degrees of arterial hypotension. Although this clinical observation requires further documentation, there is abundant experimental data to support the notion that RBF and GFR are somewhat protected in cardiogenic shock and heart failure. In dogs, for example, an equivalent decrement in cardiac output and blood pressure produced by either cardiogenic or hemorrhagic shock is associated with only 25% reduction of RBF in the former but a 90% reduction in the latter.

The cardiorenal reflex

A reduction in RBF can be produced by increased renal sympathetic nerve traffic. This appears to be the efferent limb of a reflex activated by aortic and carotid baroreceptors and attenuated by atrial stretch receptors. Recent studies in dogs demonstrated that elevation of left atrial pressure by inflation of a balloon induced variable changes in renal nerve activity. Vagotomy (and interruption of the atrial stretch receptor pathway) followed by balloon inflation resulted in increased renal sympathetic outflow. On the other hand, when aortic and carotid baroreceptors had been denervated, the same maneuver suppressed renal nerve activity. These experiments suggest that low pressure atrial receptors and high pressure baroreceptors are both stimulated by acute left atrial distention and tend to oppose each other. Carotid and aortic denervation unmask the renal nerve inhibitory and vasodilatory effect of the atrial stretch receptor. Vagotomy unmasks the sympathetic discharge and vasoconstrictor effect of the baroreceptors. In cardiogenic shock, when both pathways are intact, these reflexes apparently balance each other with neither renal vasoconstriction or vasodilation being evident. Hemorrhagic shock, in contrast, activates only the baroreceptors and leads to profound renal vasoconstriction. Hence, RBF, and presumably GFR, are better preserved in cardiogenic than in hemorrhagic shock.

Role of prostaglandins

Prostaglandins are derived from membrane-bound phospholipids. Renal prostaglandins possess potent natriuretic and diuretic activity. They are also powerful renal vasodilators. Unlike some other humoral substances, there is no storage form of prostaglandins. They are synthesized and released immediately. Synthesis proceeds from the fatty acid arachidonate via the cyclooxygenase enzyme. Cyclooxygenase is inhibited by aspirin and nonsteroidal antiinflammatory drugs (e.g., indomethacin). The endoperoxide products of the cyclo-oxygenase step are unstable and are rapidly converted either to vaso-dilatory prostaglandins such as PGE_2 (by the kidney) and prostacyclin (by vascular endothelium) or to the vasoconstrictor prostaglandin, thromboxane (by platelets).

Since these substances are immediately synthesized and released, they are capable of producing rapid responses to hemodynamic alterations. Phospholipid release and prostaglandin synthesis can be rapidly induced by angiotensin II, a vasoconstrictor, and bradykinin, a vasodilator. It appears that renal PGE_2 is a protective vasodilator in edematous conditions such as cardiac failure.

When a state resembling heart failure is induced by balloon inflation in the thoracic vena cava of dogs, blood pressure and cardiac output fall. RBF and renal vascular resistance are not significantly changed by this maneuver despite an increase in total peripheral resistance. Plasma renin, norepinephrine, and renal venous PGE_2 are all increased by balloon inflation. When caval balloon inflation is followed by blockade of PGE_2 synthesis (with either indomethacin or meclofe-namate), renal vascular resistance is increased and RBF decreased by this maneuver with other hemodynamic parameters unchanged. Inhibition of PGE_2 synthesis in control animals has no effect on either RBF or renal vascular resistance. Thus, renal prostaglandins appear to modulate the vasoconstrictive effects of the renin-angiotensin system and renal sympathetic nerves activated in cardiac failure. Inhibition of prostaglandin synthesis unmasks the full expression of these renal vasoconstrictors.

The importance of renal prostaglandins in the maintenance of RBF and GFR in cardiac failure has been further illustrated by the observation that indomethacin has produced acute oliguric renal failure and positive sodium balance in a patient with compensated heart failure. Renal function recovered and edema abated when the prostaglandin inhibitor was stopped. Urinary prostaglandins were depressed by indomethacin during renal failure and elevated during compensated heart failure. Hence, prostaglandin synthesis inhibitors may produce either acute renal failure or aggravated sodium retention or both when given to the patient with heart failure.

Diuretics and Other Renal Considerations in the Treatment of Cardiac Failure

Diuretics

The object of therapy in cardiac failure is the improvement of organ perfusion and the alleviation of edema and vascular congestion. By restoring cardiac output and reducing the stimuli for sodium reten-

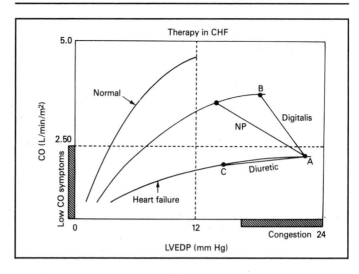

Fig. 9-9 : Relation of cardiac output (CO) to LVEDP in normal versus failing hearts. In the failing heart, a large increase in LVEDP may precipitate pulmonary edema with a persistent reduction in CO (point A). Diuretics reduce LVEDP along the same curve, out of the range of congestive symptoms, and modestly reduce CO. Inotropes such as digitalis shift the curve toward normal (Point A to point B). Vasodilators such as nitroprusside (NP) increase cardiac output by reducing afterload impedance, thus also shifting the curve upward. However, by virtue of venodilation, they also may reduce ventricular filling, thus reducing CO along the new curve. (From Grantham JJ, Chonko AM: The physiological basis and clinical use of diuretics, in Brenner BM, Stein, JH [eds]: *Sodium and Water Homeostasis.* New York, Churchill Livingstone, 1976, pp 178–211, with permission of the authors and publisher.)

tion, successful therapy for cardiac failure usually results in a diuresis. Diuretic agents work primarily by increasing renal solute and/or water excretion. As shown in Figure 9-9 diuretics lower plasma volume and left ventricular end-diastolic pressure (LVEDP), thus decreasing both pulmonary congestion and peripheral edema. Unlike vasodilators or inotropic agents, however, diuretics do not raise cardiac output, and may even lower it slightly. By doing so diuretics may compromise tissue perfusion, thus worsening azotemia (as discussed below).

Diuretics are generally classified according to their respective sites of action along the nephron. Much information regarding their mechanisms of inhibiting solute transport emanates from studies in which tubules were micropunctured in vivo or nephron segments were perfused in vitro. In the proximal nephron, where the bulk (~70%) of glomerular filtrate is reabsorbed without any alteration of total solute concentration (osmolarity), several agents are known to produce a diuresis.

MANNITOL. Mannitol is a polysaccharide, freely filtrable by the glomerulus but, unlike glucose, not reabsorbable. Its osmotic activity thus prevents fluid absorption by the proximal nephron and presents an overwhelming solute and fluid load to the distal tubules and collecting ducts. Although all diuretics increase solute excretion and therefore could be considered "osmotic," the characteristics of a mannitol diuresis are manifestations of increased fluid flow along the length of the nephron thereby producing a urine that is generally low in tonicity. Hence, mannitol induces more water than solute diuresis. It is useful, in this regard, in the treatment of hypoosmolar (hyponatremic) conditions in which the plasma volume is expanded, such as heart failure. However, since mannitol is generally given intravenously and remains confined to the extracellular space, its role in the management of congestive failure is limited, since the osmotic gradient it creates may temporarily draw more fluid into the vascular compartment, thus increasing plasma volume and vascular congestion. In patients with compromised cardiac function, particularly those with depressed glomerular filtration, worsening of congestive symptoms may result.

ACETAZOLAMIDE. Like mannitol, this agent also has its action in the proximal tubule. Unlike mannitol, this agent is *secreted* into the proximal nephron from the peritubular capillaries by a potent organic acid transport pathway. This is similar to the mechanism of secretion of thiazides and the "loop diuretics" ethacrynic acid and furosemide. Acetazolamide inactivates the enzyme carbonic anhydrase that catalyzes the conversion of carbon dioxide and water into bicarbonate. Inhibition of this enzyme results in a loss of tubular hydrogen ion secretion and consequent decrement in bicarbonate absorption. In the distal tubule, bicarbonate behaves as a nonreabsorbable anion, thus promoting a sodium and water diuresis. By reducing urinary hydrogen ion secretion, acetazolamide promotes a metabolic acidosis. It is, however, a relatively weak diuretic because metabolic acidosis reduces its efficacy. Moreover, the distal nephron can enhance solute transport, thus negating the proximal diuretic effect of this agent. In heart failure, it may be used either to correct a metabolic alkalosis or in combination with a loop diuretic for the treatment of refractory edema.

LOOP DIURETICS. As mentioned above, the thick portion of the thick ascending limb of Henle's loop is a site critical for both urinary concentration and dilution. In the *medullary* thick ascending limb, salt reabsorption is initiated by active chloride transport followed passively by sodium. In this segment, sodium chloride movement into the medullary interstitium helps to establish the osmotic gradient for urinary concentration. In the cortical thick ascending limb and early distal tubule, sodium chloride is abstracted from tubular fluid, also initiated by active reabsorption of the anion. Here, dilution of luminal fluid occurs since dilute tubular fluid remains. The entire thick ascending limb is the site of action for the potent *loop diuretics*, ethacrynic acid and furosemide. These drugs are secreted by the organic acid transport route into the proximal tubule where they may promote a weak inhibition of solute reabsorption. However, they exert their predominant effect at the luminal surface of the ascending limb. Here they apparently block chloride transport across the plasma membrane. Although 70% of glomerular filtrate sodium chloride is reabsorbed proximally, nearly 20% is absorbed by the ascending limb. Hence, complete blockade of chloride, and consequently sodium, transport in this segment will present an overwhelming solute and fluid load to the distal tubule and collecting system.

Some severely edematous patients may be refractory to the usual doses of loop diuretics (Lasix 20–40 mg PO or IV; or ethacrynic acid 25–50 mg PO or IV). This occurs either because proximal nephron reuptake is so avid that relatively little solute reaches the ascending limb, or because distal tubular and collecting system salt reabsorption compensate for the losses incurred by the ascending limb. In these instances larger doses of the agents may effect a diuresis possibly by means of moderate inhibition of proximal tubular absorption. For similar reasons, the combination of a thiazide and a loop diuretic is synergistic due to the weak proximal tubular effect of thiazides as well as their action on the distal tubule beyond the site of loop diuretic activity.

The loop diuretics appear to enhance renal prostaglandin synthesis and by doing so, increase RBF. Since PGE_2 may impair solute transport in the ascending limb, this prostaglandin has been proposed as an intermediary of the diuretic action of furosemide and ethacrynic acid. At the present time, this hypothesis requires further substantiation.

It should be noted at this juncture that the efficacy of ethacrynic acid and furosemide in reducing vascular congestion may stem partly from a nondiuretic action. These agents also increase venous capacitance. A reduction in LVEDP may be seen in the first five minutes after intravenous administration of either furosemide or ethacrynic acid and usually precedes their diuretic effect. It also can be seen in anephric patients. These observations suggest that the venodilator effect of the loop diuretics is probably responsible for their acute action in moderating pulmonary congestion.

ORGANOMERCURIAL DIURETICS. These are older, parenteral agents whose site of action has yet to be clarified but appear to work in the thick ascending limb and distal tubule. Their distal tubular site of action is suggested by the potassium sparing identified with these drugs, indicating their inhibition of distal tubular potassium secretion. Because of the necessity for parenteral administration, and the weakening of their diuretic effect in the presence of metabolic alkalosis, which is a frequent complication of diuretic therapy, these agents are seldom used.

THIAZIDE DIURETICS. The major sites of action of the thiazide diuretics has now been clearly established at the early distal tubule. These agents may also exert a modest inhibition of solute reabsorption in the proximal nephron. Compared with loop diuretics, their effect on salt and water excretion is more modest, reflecting the proportionately smaller role of the distal tubule in sodium chloride reabsorption. Nonetheless, they can raise the fraction of filtered sodium which is excreted to as much as 5%, more than a fivefold increase over normal. As with the loop diuretics, these agents also promote potassium wasting and a metabolic alkalosis. Although, like other diuretics, they are primarily secreted and not filtered into the proximal tubule, they are less effective than the loop diuretics in renal failure.

SPIRONOLACTONE, TRIAMTERENE, AND AMILORIDE. In the further reaches of the distal tubules, three drugs, spironolactone, triamterene, and amiloride, inhibit sodium reabsorption by blocking the exchange of this cation for potassium and hydrogen ion. As a consequence of these actions, they are said to be "potassium sparing" and may also induce a metabolic acidosis. Spironolactone inhibits tubular cation exchange as a competitive antagonist of aldosterone, and as such is ineffective in conditions where aldosterone is not present. Amiloride and triamterene, on the other hand, act independently of aldosterone to inhibit sodium-potassium and sodium-hydrogen exchange. All of these agents are rather weak diuretics. Both their utility and the potential hazard of their use lies in their potassium-sparing effect. In conjunction with kaliuretic agents, they permit normalization of the serum potassium, a feature which makes them useful in patients taking digitalis since the toxicity of the cardiac glycoside is enhanced by hypokalemia. They are relatively contraindicated in patients with renal insufficiency and oliguria by virtue of the hyperkalemia that may result.

Complications of diuretic use

The judicious use of diuretics for heart failure requires an understanding of their potential side effects. Some of these, such as hyperuricemia, are often mild and require no additional intervention on the part of the physician. Others, however, such as severe hyponatremia may require cessation of the offending drugs. The common adverse effects are summarized in Table 9-2.

HYPOVOLEMIA AND PRERENAL AZOTEMIA. Hypovolemia is a common complication of diuretic usage particularly in patients receiving the more potent loop diuretics or those patients with chronic renal failure and an impaired capacity to conserve sodium and thereby to compensate for diuretic-induced volume depletion. A depression in plasma volume may be obvious from clinical signs such as diminished skin turgor and postural hypotension or may be heralded by oliguria ($<$ 400 ml urine output/24 hours) and a rise in the blood urea nitrogen (BUN). This value tends to rise more rapidly than the

Table 9-2 : Summary of diuretic dose, action, and complications

Diuretic	Site of action	Type of diuresis	Frequent complications
Mannitol	Proximal tubule	Hypotonic	Hypernatremia Volume depletion
Acetazolamide	Proximal tubule	Bicarbonaturia Potassium wasting	Metabolic acidosis
Ethacrynic acid and furosemide	Thick ascending limb ($\pm$ proximal tubule)	Potassium wasting Large natriuresis Hypo- or isosmotic	Hypolkalemia Metabolic alkalosis Volume depletion (common) Azotemia
Thiazides (hydrochlorthiazide)	Distal tubules ($\pm$ proximal tubule)	Moderate natriuresis Potassium wasting	Hypokalemia Metabolic alkalosis Volume depletion
Spironolactone Triamterene Amiloride	Distal tubule Collecting tubule	Potassium sparing	Hyperkalemia Metabolic acidosis
Organomercurials (Mercurhydrin)	Ascending limb Distal tubule	Potassium sparing	Metabolic alkalosis Volume depletion

serum creatinine. Urea is filtered by the glomerulus and diffuses passively across the tubular epithelium. Passive urea diffusion increases with diminished luminal flow. In the collecting system, urea reabsorption may be facilitated by the presence of ADH. Creatinine, on the other hand, is filtered but not reabsorbed across the tubular epithelium. Hence, in heart failure, where proximal fluid uptake is enhanced and luminal flow is thereby reduced, urea clearance is more depressed than creatinine clearance. This is referred to as "prerenal" azotemia since the reduction in renal function is a result of hemodynamic factors and not intrinsic renal disease. Cardiac failure, by virtue of depressed effective renal perfusion may also be signified by prerenal azotemia.

It is important to remember that prerenal azotemia may be a complication either of severe heart failure and a profoundly reduced EABV or of diuretic therapy and absolute hypovolemia. The appropriate management of this complication depends upon identification of the underlying etiology, careful examination of the patient, and in certain instances, measurement of central venous or pulmonary capillary wedge pressure.

HYPONATREMIA. Hyponatremia, as is the case with prerenal azotemia, may either be a manifestation of severe heart failure and renal water retention, or it may be a side effect of diuretic therapy with absolute hypovolemia.

All diuretics have the capacity to induce volume depletion, as described above. With the development of hypovolemia, ADH secretion is stimulated by nonosmotic volume receptors in the left atrium and baroreceptors in the carotid artery and aortic arch. In addition, the exaggerated proximal uptake of salt and water results in a reduction of solute delivery to the diluting segment, just as may happen with severe heart failure. Furthermore, those diuretics that provoke a kaliuresis and a potassium deficit with intracellular potassium depletion may lead to translocation of sodium, the major extracellular cation, into the intracellular space.

Finally, thiazide diuretics specifically impair urinary dilution by blocking solute reabsorption in the diluting segment of the early distal tubule. The loop diuretics also impair the diluting segment, but since they act in the medullary as well as the cortical ascending limb, they inhibit urinary concentration as well. Consequently, the diuresis induced by furosemide and ethacrynic acid tends to be neither concentrated nor dilute but more nearly approximates plasma osmolarity. The loop diuretics can occasionally effect a relatively dilute urine when given in larger doses (80–200 mg IV or PO). This may occur because of "washout" of the medullary interstitial osmotic gradient which results both from the increase in RBF as well as from reduced sodium chloride delivery into the medulla. There is also evidence from isolated collecting tubule fragments that furosemide may block the action of ADH on this nephron segment.

METABOLIC ALKALOSIS. Metabolic alkalosis may ensue as a consequence of diuretic therapy because of depletion of extracellular fluid volume around a fixed amount of bicarbonate, thus raising the concentration of this anion while chloride is eliminated from the body. This phenomenon is referred to as a "contraction alkalosis." In addition, an alkalosis may reflect the increased delivery of sodium to the distal nephron secretory sites in exchange for potassium and hydrogen ions. In both instances, the alkalosis can be corrected by sodium chloride administration. Since sodium administration may not be desirable in heart failure, acetazolamide can be added to control the alkalosis.

HYPOKALEMIA. A reduced extracellular potassium concentration is seen in any form of diuretic therapy (with the exception of the potassium-sparing agents) as a result of increased distal tubular sodium delivery and resultant enhanced potassium excretion. Metabolic alkalosis as described above, often accompanies hypokalemia since a similar mechanism is involved in both the increased secretion of potassium and hydrogen. The alkalosis also causes potassium ions to enter cells in exchange for hydrogen ions. Hence, the hypokalemia may reflect both a modest total body potassium deficit as well as a transcellular shift of potassium. Since hypokalemia may promote digitalis toxic cardiac arrhythmias, this potential complication of diuretic therapy should be avoided in patients taking cardiac glycosides. This can be accomplished either with potassium chloride supplementation or by the concomitant administration of potassium-sparing diuretics.

HYPERURICEMIA. Elevated serum levels of uric acid frequently accompany diuretic therapy. This appears to reflect the enhanced proximal tubular sodium and uric acid reabsorption which ensues as a result of extracellular volume depletion. The hyperuricemia does not usually precipitate an acute gouty attack unless there is an antecedent history of gout. Furthermore, renal damage from uric acid does not occur since its excretion is reduced by diuretics. Therefore, normalization of the serum uric acid level with allopurinol is seldom required.

HYPERKALEMIA. This complication is obviously encountered only with potassium-sparing diuretics. It is particularly likely to occur in patients with renal insufficiency and oliguria. Patients with cardiac failure or hypovolemia and low urine flow are particularly at risk since potassium elimination will depend in these patients on distal tubular ionic exchange and secretion.

Renal considerations in vasodilator therapy

As discussed in greater detail elsewhere (see Chap. 13), vasodilator therapy has added a new dimension to the care of patients with refractory heart failure. These agents reduce peripheral and pulmonary edema by two mechanisms: (1) by dilating the arteriolar circuit, they reduce the impedance to ventricular ejection, thereby increasing cardiac output; (2) by dilating venules, they increase venous capacitance and reduce LVEDP (see Fig. 9-9). Pooling blood in the venous circuit, vasodilators decrease EABV in much the same way as diuretics and may reduce cardiac output. The renal effects of vasodilators reflect whether they are primarily arterial dilators such as prazosin or combined venous and arterial vasodilators such as nitroprusside. Most vasodilators promote edema formation by activating the sensing mechanisms for sodium retention such as the carotid baroreceptors and atrial volume receptors. Consequently, the simultaneous administration of a diuretic may be required to counteract this maladaptive response to therapy. Although general peripheral vascular resistance is reduced, RBF may not increase, and may in fact decrease in response to vasodilator therapy. Azotemia may result.

Recently, inhibitors of the converting enzyme for the formation of angiotensin II from angiotensin I have been added to the therapeutic modalities for severe heart failure. The oral converting enzyme inhibitor, captopril, has been shown to evoke rapid and sustained hemodynamic changes in patients with severe heart failure. These changes include a decrease in blood pressure and peripheral vascular resistance. As such, captopril acts much like other vasodilators. It has not been clearly established whether the peripheral vasodilator effect is purely on the basis of reduced angiotensin II (AII) formation or is also due to increased plasma bradykinin levels, since the converting enzyme inhibitor is also a kininase.

In addition, by blocking AII formation, captopril also attenuates aldosterone secretion and consequently decreases its effects on tubular sodium reabsorption. The usefulness of converting enzyme inhibitors

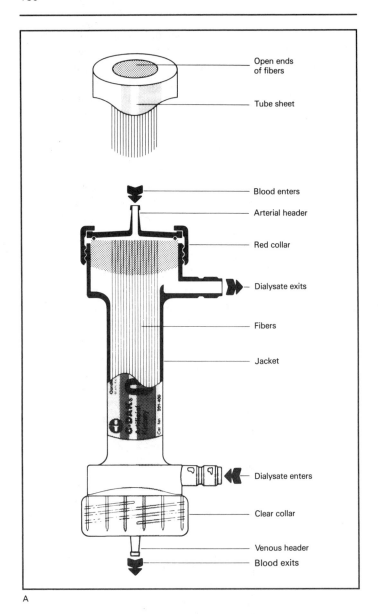

Open ends of fibers

Tube sheet

Blood enters

Arterial header

Red collar

Dialysate exits

Fibers

Jacket

Dialysate enters

Clear collar

Venous header

Blood exits

A

Fig. 9-10 : A. Hollow fiber dialyzer. Note that the tube sheet holds fibers in position and forms a gasket between blood and dialysis chambers. Both the red collar (for the arterial header) and the clear collar (for the venous header) are threaded. B. Ultrafiltration rate as a function of the hydrostatic pressure across the dialyzer. The transmembrane pressure (TMP) represents the sum of the inflow and outflow pressures. However, since only the outflow pressure varies considerably, the TMP is controlled by raising the outflow pressure usually with a clamp. (From the Cordis-Dow Corp, Miami, Fla, with permission.)

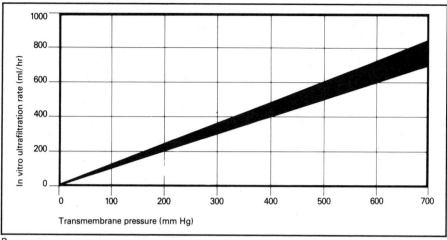

B

awaits further testing in large groups of patients with heart failure since they have potentially hazardous side effects. Since AII synthesis appears to be a major homeostatic mechanism for maintaining blood pressure in heart failure, abolished AII formation may cause profound shock. Furthermore, as detailed above, intrarenal angiotensin II formation may be the mediator of glomerular filtration autoregulation. A loss of local renal angiotensin II could result, therefore, in worsening azotemia. Furthermore, in patients with severe cardiac failure and marginal renal function, inhibition of aldosterone sometimes results in hyperkalemia.

Use of dialysis and ultrafiltration techniques in heart failure

When cardiac failure and edema are particularly refractory, and diuretic therapy is rendered useless by either parenchymal renal failure or severe prerenal azotemia, removal of excessive extracellular fluid can be accomplished with either dialysis or the technique known as "ultrafiltration."

Both hemodialysis and peritoneal dialysis may effectuate fluid removal. Peritoneal dialysis utilizes the semipermeable properties of the peritoneal membrane. The dialysate, which consists of a hypertonic solution of glucose and electrolytes, promotes fluid entry into the peritoneal space by osmotically induced bulk flow. In the cardiac patient, peritoneal dialysis may be complicated by hypokalemia and other electrolyte disturbances that may predispose to atrial and ventricular cardiac arrhythmias.

Hemodialysis utilizes an artificial cellulose membrane that is usually arranged as a bundle of tiny, hollow fibers housed in a plastic cylinder. Blood is circulated from an arteriovenous fistula or shunt to the core of the hollow fibers while dialysate enters via a side port in the cylinder and circulates in a countercurrent fashion around the fibers (see Fig. 9-10). Plasma fluid removal (ultrafiltration) is a consequence of the hydrostatic pressure gradient across the dialysis membrane. The transmembrane pressure can be raised either by increasing the resistance at the blood outflow port or by decreasing the pressure on the dialysate side of the membrane within the artificial kidney. Hemodialysis is limited in cardiac patients by its potentially adverse hemodynamic effect. Blood pressure is lowered during dialysis due to extracorporeal blood loss and fluid removal. In addition, some constituent of the hemodialysate, possibly the acetate buffer (converted in the body to bicarbonate) acts as a peripheral vasodilator and myocardial depressant, also contributing to the hypotension.

In circumstances where hemodialysis is obviated by hypotension, a bicarbonate buffer system may be substituted for acetate. Alternatively, simple ultrafiltration can be performed by removing dialysate from the system and raising transmembrane pressure.

Suggested Readings

Anderson RJ et al: Mechanism of effect of thoracic inferior vena cava constriction on renal water excretion. *J Clin Invest* 54:1473, 1974.

Auld RB, Alexander EA, Levinsky NG: Proximal tubular function in dogs with thoracic caval constriction. *J Clin Invest* 50:2150, 1971.

Cannon PJ: The kidney in heart failure. *N Engl J Med* 296:26, 1977.

Chonko AM et al: The role of renin and aldosterone in the salt retention of edema. *Am J Med* 63:881, 1977.

Davis R et al: Treatment of chronic congestive heart failure with captopril, an oral inhibitor of angiotensin-converting enzyme. *N Engl J Med* 301:117, 1979.

Gilmore JP et al: Atrial receptor modulation of renal nerve activity in the nonhuman primate. *Am J Physiol* 242:F592, 1982.

Grantham JJ, Chonko AM: The physiological basis and clinical use of diuretics, in Brenner BM, Stein JH (eds): *Sodium and Water Homeostasis.* New York, Churchill Livingstone, 1978, pp 178–211.

Hall JE et al: Control of glomerular filtration by renin-angiotensin. *Am J Physiol* 233: F366, 1977.

Humes HD, Gottlieb MN, Brenner BM: The kidney in congestive heart failure, in Brenner BM, Stein JH (eds): *Sodium and Water Homeostasis.* New York, Churchill Livingstone, 1978.

Oliver JA et al: Participation of the prostaglandins in the control of renal blood flow during acute reduction of cardiac output in the dog. *J Clin Invest* 67:229, 1981.

Paller MS, Schrier RW: Pathogenesis of sodium and water retention in edematous disorders. *Am J Kid Dis 2:241, 1982.*

Riegger GAJ, Liebau G, Kochsiek K: Antidiuretic hormone in congestive heart failure. *Am J Med* 72:49, 1982.

Rose BD: Edematous states and use of diuretics, in Rose BD (ed): *Clinical Physiology of Acid-Base and Electrolyte Disorders,* ed 2. New York, McGraw-Hill, 1983.

Silverstein ME et al: Treatment of severe fluid overload by ultrafiltration. *N Engl J Med* 291:747, 1974.

Watkins L et al: The renin-angiotensin-aldosterone system in congestive failure in conscious dogs. *J Clin Invest* 57:1606, 1976.

10 : Pathophysiology of Hypertension

Roger B. Hickler

Historical Perspective

Early investigations on the genesis of essential hypertension (EH) centered on the sympathetic nervous system (SNS). This was natural, given the primacy of the SNS in the regulation of arteriolar tone, the major determinant of mean arterial pressure in the presence of an apparently normal cardiac output. Clinical corrolaries were the widespread use of surgical sympathectomy and sympatholytic drugs in the management of the disorder. Two events shifted the focus to the kidney: (1) the classical experiment of Goldblatt (1937), who demonstrated that the production of unilateral renal ischemia in the dog produced hypertension (Fig. 10-1); (2) the demonstration by Dahl and Heine (1975) that when rats bred to develop hypertension on high dietary Na^+ intake (Dahl-S) received in transplantation (after removal of their own kidneys) a kidney from the same strain of rat that was resistant to salt-hypertension (Dahl-R), the homografted recipients showed a profound reduction in their hypertension while on the same high Na^+ diet (Fig. 10-2). The concomitant elucidation of the renal pressor system (renin-angiotensin) (Fig. 10-3) and the control by angiotensin of the adrenal secretion of the salt-retaining steroid, aldosterone, ushered in an era of prolific investigation. While this widened our understanding of fundamental blood pressure regulatory mechanisms, definition of the initiating event in essential hypertension has remained elusive. Attention to the possible primacy of sodium metabolism and the widespread use of diuretics in essential hypertension are direct consequences of these latter investigations. In the current era much of the emphasis is on (1) a study of central nervous system blood pressure control mechanisms and centers, e.g., the nucleus tractus solitariis (NTS), where lesions can produce neurogenic hypertension, and the anteroventral portion of the third ventricle (AV_3V), where lesions can prevent hypertension in several experimental models; and (2) a search for possible disorders of both active and passive ionic flux at the level of the membrane of vascular smooth muscle in hypertensive animal models (both genetic and induced) and in human blood cells. The latter approach has the merit of focusing on the "final common pathway" of practically all forms of hypertension in terms of an alteration in the contractile element of vascular smooth muscle.

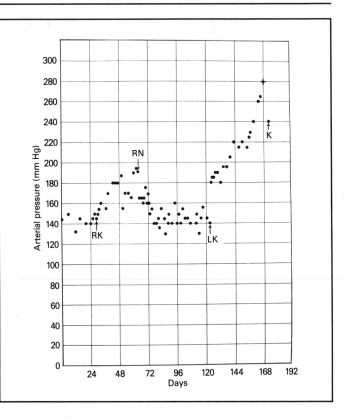

Fig. 10-1 : Experimental renal hypertension, showing rise in arterial pressure after moderate narrowing of the right renal artery (RK) in a dog, with return of pressure to normal after right nephrectomy (RN), followed by severe hypertension after severe narrowing of renal artery of remaining left kidney (LK). This demonstrated the "pressor" effect of renal ischemia and the "protective" effect of a contralateral normal kidney. (From Goldblatt H et al: The pathogenesis of experimental hypertension due to renal ischemia. *Ann Intern Med* 11:69, 1937, with permission of the authors and publisher.)

Much of the difficulty in unraveling the puzzle of EH rests with the phenomenon, both hemodynamic (Fig. 10-4) and neurohumoral (Fig. 10-5), in which a perturbation of any one of the variables produces a perturbation in many if not all of the other variables, such that it is enormously difficult to determine which came first and their comparative importance. Thus, an increased arterial pressure due to a sustained elevation in cardiac output (CO) may be transformed into a normal CO–high total peripheral resistance (TPR) state; a chronic increase in SNS activity may increase renal renin secretion, and vice versa; chronic sodium retention may increase TPR and sensitivity to catecholamines and angiotensin, and suppress renin and aldosterone secretion; increased efferent renal sympathetic nerve stimulation and activation of the intrarenal renin-angiotensin system may produce sodium retention. On the other hand, activation of intrarenal angiotensin (and bradykinin) may stimulate the intrarenal release of prostaglandin, which can produce renal vasodilation (prostacyclin [PGI$_2$]) and diuresis/natriuresis (PGE$_2$). Thus, in any given instance it is difficult to determine whether an observed change is primary or secondary, and if secondary, whether it is potentiating or antagonistic.

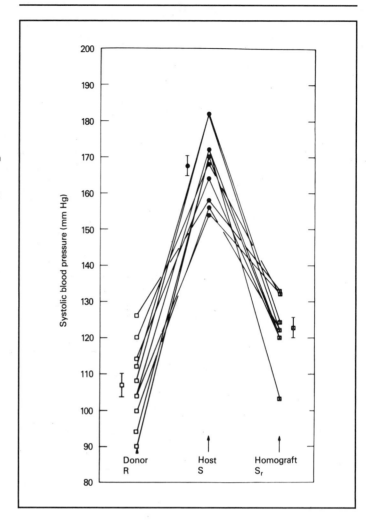

Fig. 10-2 : Effect of the genotype of the renal homograft on chronic blood pressure levels at a median time of 17 weeks after surgery. Data are for S rats with R homografts (S$_r$). The mean blood pressure is indicated for each group. (From Dahl LK, Heine M: Primary role of renal homografts in setting chronic blood pressure levels in rats. *Circ Res* 36:692, 1975, with permission of the authors and publisher.)

Etiologies of Hypertension

Blood pressure regulatory mechanisms

The *proximate* cause of mean arterial pressure (MAP) elevation indisputably is an increase in CO or TPR (or both), according to the fundamental hemodynamic relationship MAP = CO × TPR. An analysis of the major variables that determine CO and TPR are given in Figure 10-6, which includes essentially all of the known factors in blood pressure regulation. One fact emerges: in every form of clinical or experimental hypertension characterized by a diastolic pressure elevation, the key perturbation is an increase in peripheral vascular resistance due to arteriolar (resistance vessel) narrowing. This exquisitely sensitive mechanism relates to a rearrangement of the Poiseuille-Hagan formula, indicating that resistance is inversely proportional to the *fourth power* of the radius of the resistance vessels (see

Fig. 10-3 : Schema of the renin-angiotensin system.

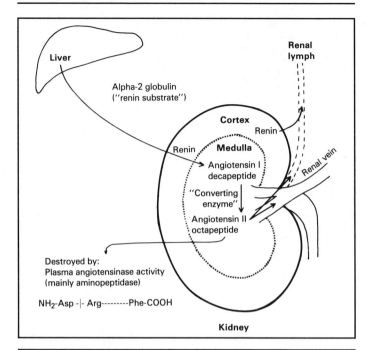

Fig. 10-4 : Schema showing the interrelationship of hemodynamic and sympathetic reflex factors in blood pressure regulation. PVR = peripheral vascular resistance; CO = cardiac output; BP = blood pressure.

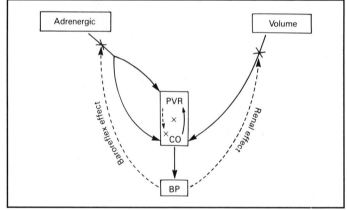

Fig. 10-5 : Schema showing the interrelationship of humoral, neurohumoral, and sodium-volume factors in blood pressure regulation.

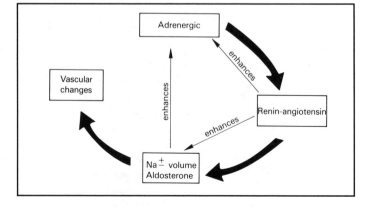

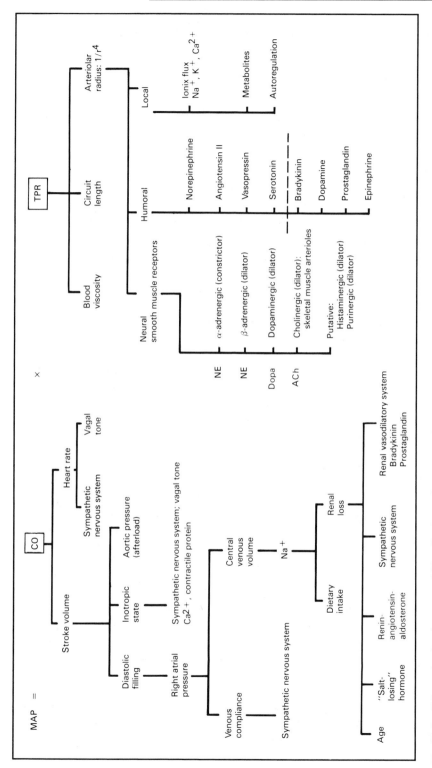

Fig. 10-6 : **Schema showing the many variables affecting cardiac output and peripheral vascular resistance in the determination of arterial pressure, essentially all of which have been under investigation to elucidate the pathophysiology of essential hypertension. MAP = mean arterial pressure; CO = cardiac output; TPR = total peripheral resistance.**

Chap. 8). The primary disturbance leading to arteriolar narrowing in any given instance of hypertension may be the result of (1) any of the factors that elevate cardiac output, which over time can be translated into an elevation of peripheral resistance through poorly understood regulatory mechanisms, or (2) of any of the factors that can decrease the cross-sectional area of the resistance vessels (blood viscosity and circuit length being comparatively minor factors). It has been hoped that an elucidation of the mechanism leading to hypertension in certain endocrine disorders, where a solitary primary secretory disturbance produces high blood pressure, would help to identify the underlying mechanism for essential hypertension.

Endocrine prototypes of hypertension

PHEOCHROMOCYTOMA. This condition is characterized by a high basal and frequently superimposed paroxysmal secretion of norepinephrine (and usually of epinephrine, as well) from a tumor of the adrenal medulla or of embryonal rests along the sympathetic ganglia. The powerful vasoconstrictor response to a high circulating level of norepinephrine accounts for the hypertension; the substantial hypotensive response to specific alpha-1 (peripheral) adrenergic blocking agents (e.g., phentolamine, phenoxybenzamine, prazosin) confirms this clear-cut relationship. The elevated plasma renin activity (PRA), found in 70% of patients with pheochromocytoma, is primarily accounted for by stimulation of renal renin secretion by elevated circulating catecholamines (norepinephrine, [NE], and epinephrine, [E]). Hypertension may also relate to renal artery stenosis produced by tumor encirclement of the renal hilum in an occasional patient with pheochromocytoma. The elevated PRA makes a comparatively minor contribution to the elevated arterial pressure, and angiotensin II (AII) blockade with saralysin is contraindicated, as it is likely to provoke a hypertensive crisis by direct tumor stimulation. A contribution by the neurogenic component of the SNS to the elevated pressure may be expected, as well, secondary to increased SNS nerve ending stores of NE, secondary to the high circulating levels. Plasma volume is contracted on average by 15% and in direct proportion to the degree of MAP elevation. Other categories of hypertension characterized by an unusually high catecholamine drive are neurogenic, as with: (1) a rapid increase in intracranial pressure (e.g., cerebral hemorrhage), and (2) peripheral neuropathy (e.g., Guillain-Barré syndrome) where the peripheral sympathetic neuronal lesion blocks the reuptake of norepinephrine, thus potentiating the vasoconstrictor effect of norepinephrine.

JUXTAGLOMERULAR CELL TUMOR. This is a condition in which the high secretory rate of renin leads to a high circulating level of angiotensin II (AII), which produces an intense, direct vasoconstriction. An additional neurogenic component of high blood pressure is contributed by the central nervous system (CNS) stimulating effect of AII on the SNS; Na$^+$ retention may make a further contribution through the stimulation of aldosterone secretion by the high level of circulating AII. Other clinical examples of hypertension directly related to a high level of renin secretion are (1) renovascular hypertension and coarctation of the aorta, (2) malignant hypertension, and (3) chronic renal failure (10–15% of instances). As with juxtaglomerular cell tumors, a neurogenic and a Na$^+$ retention factor also contribute to the hypertension in each of these clinical states of high renin secretion for the reasons just cited. In renovascular hypertension due to *unilateral* renal artery stenosis, the Na$^+$ retention may be minor, because of the intact excretory function of the contralateral kidney. The high level of renin secretion by the involved kidney will *suppress* renin secretion by the contralateral kidney, but the PRA will remain elevated in 60% of cases in the chronic state. By contrast, in renovascular hypertension associated with *bilateral* renal artery stenosis, Na$^+$ retention may predominate in the hypertensive process because of the bilateral nature of the reduction in excretory function, and PRA may not be distinctly elevated in the chronic state. It is emphasized that reduction in the renal arterial lumen must be of the order of 80% to activate the renin secretory mechanism, because renal autoregulation (dilatation to keep flow constant over a wide range of perfusion pressure) protects against stimulation of the juxtaglomerular pressure-sensitive mechanism controlling renin secretion. A number of studies indicate the importance of the renin-secretory mechanism in hypertension associated with aortic coarctation, where the reduction in renal perfusion pressure can stimulate renal renin secretion.

Malignant hypertension is the clinical example, par excellence, of the untoward effect on the vasculature of an extreme outpouring of renal renin due to the necrotizing renal arteriolitis that characterizes the disease (likened to a tiny Goldblatt clamp on each of the million glomerular afferent arterioles of each kidney). Profound secondary hyperaldosteronism with hypokalemic alkalosis is an integral part of the malignant syndrome. Chronic renal failure in 85–90% of instances relates to Na$^+$ retention and volume overload due to loss of renal excretory function; however, in 10–15% of instances hemodialysis to "dry weight" does not relieve the hypertension, and a high PRA has been implicated. The importance of secondary volume overload in sustaining the hypertension in renovascular and coarctation hypertension is indicated by the PRA, which is suppressed to normal in 40% of cases of renovascular and the majority of cases of coarctation hypertension. However, the underlying importance of renin is indicated by the supranormal rise in PRA in both conditions on Na$^+$ depletion, following which there is a markedly enhanced antihypertensive effect of angiotensin blockade with either the competitive

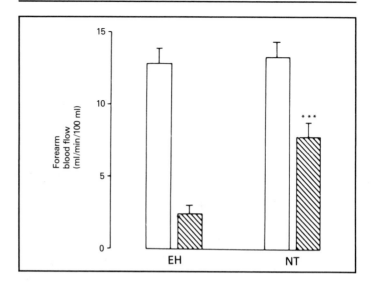

Fig. 10-7 : Forearm blood flow during nonspecific vasodilator infusion of sodium nitroprusside (0.6 µg/min/100 ml; shown as unhatched bars) and during selective postjunctional alpha-adrenoreceptor blockade with prazosin (0.5 µg/min/100 ml; shown as hatched bars) in normotensive (NT) subjects and patients with essential hypertension (EH). The greater response to prazosin in NT patients suggests enhanced alpha-adrenoreceptor-mediated vasoconstriction in essential hypertension. Mean ± SEM; *** $p < 0.001$. (From Laragh JH, Buhler FR, Seldin DW: Changing role of beta and alpha adrenoreceptor mediated cardiovascular responses in the transition from high cardiac output into a high peripheral resistance phase in essential hypertension, in Laragh JH, Buhler FR, Seldin DW [eds]: *Frontiers in Hypertension Research*. New York, Springer-Verlag, 1981, p 320, with permission of the authors and publisher.)

by the SNS to the elevated pressure in EH. As shown in Fig. 10-7, Buhler and co-workers showed a much greater increase in forearm blood flow from the brachial arterial infusion (ipsilateral) of prazosin in normotensive as compared with hypertensive subjects. Certainly, the successful application of sympatholytic agents in the management of EH resides to a great extent in the phenomenon of a major SNS contribution to elevated MAP in these individuals.

Renin-angiotensin system

The renin-angiotensin system has also been extensively surveyed in EH. When sodium balance is controlled, it is evident that some 15% of EH patients have a PRA that is *higher* than in normotensive patients. This is particularly true of *younger* hypertensive patients, and probably relates to the heightened SNS activity described above. It is well established that renal sympathetic nerve stimulation is a major factor in determining renal renin release. This SNS stimulated renal pressor mechanism may be contributing in its own right to the arterial pressure elevation and account for the reported augmented hypotensive response of such high-renin EH patients to angiotensin blocking agents (saralysin, captopril), particularly in the Na^+ depleted state. Furthermore, some 25% of EH patients have a PRA that is

Fig. 10-8 : Captopril's effect of inducing a larger increase in renal blood flow (RBF) in patients with essential hypertension than it does in normal subjects whether on a sodium restricted intake or on a liberal sodium intake. Mean arterial pressure showed a significantly larger fall in the patients with essential hypertension only when sodium intake was restricted. (From Hollenberg NK et al: Sodium intake and renal response to captopril in normal man and in essential hypertension. *Kidney Int* 20:240, 1981, with permission of the authors and publisher.)

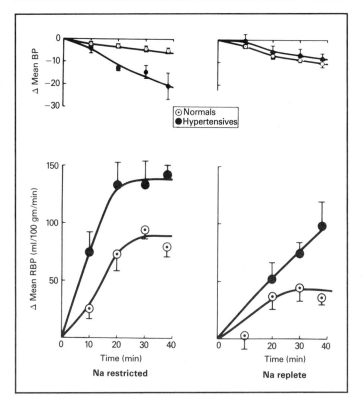

lower than in normotensive patients under conditions of controlled sodium balance. This is particularly true of *older* hypertensive patients, and of blacks. Attempts to demonstrate that this represents a "volume overload" phenomenon or is due to an unidentified circulating mineralocorticoid factor have, to date, been unsuccessful. It may well represent an age-related attrition of the renin-secretory capacity (juxtaglomerular cells) that has been *accelerated* by hypertension, as has been observed in diabetic renal disease. Despite the low PRA in such patients, aldosterone secretion remains normal, suggesting an increased sensitivity of the adrenal glomerulosa to angiotensin stimulation. Such patients have been reported to show an increased hypotensive response to diuretic (including aldosterone antagonist) agents. This is probably reflective of the fact that their PRA shows a *smaller* increase on sodium depletion, and is, therefore, less antagonistic to the hypotensive effects of volume contraction.

The *intrarenal* renin-angiotensin mechanism may be of major importance in the pathophysiology of essential hypertension. The chronically vasoconstricted state of hypertensive kidneys is probably a perturbation of fundamental significance. The degree to which this pertains and is under the control of intrarenal angiotensin was demonstrated by Hollenberg and co-workers (Fig. 10-8). After ingestion

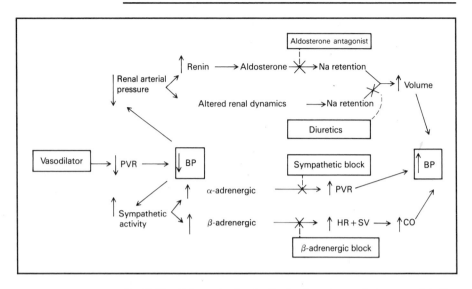

Fig. 10-10 : Schema showing details of various pharmacologic agents clinically available to oppose the possible circulatory, endocrinologic, and electrolyte compensatory adjustments to vasodilator therapy. (From Sambhi MP [ed]: *Mechanisms of Hypertension*, New York, Elsevier, 1973, p 350, with permission of the author and publisher.)

sodium load, *despite* the glomerular filtration barrier. The third is the accumulating evidence that there is a *generalized* cellular membrane defect in EH that allows a greater *passive* influx of Na^+ into cells, which, at the level of vascular smooth muscle, would permit a greater intracellular Ca^{2+} accumulation, thereby activating the contractile element (actomyosin) and render the vessel more responsive to vasoactive substances. The fourth is the evidence for a *circulating sodium transport inhibitory factor* (CSTI, the putative "salt losing hormone"), that may well emanate from osmotically sensitive neurones in the anterior hypothalamus. The latter would account for the *inhibition* of the *active* (ouabain-sensitive, Na^+/K^+ ATPase-dependent) pump observed in human blood cells of patients with EH in comparison with normotensive controls. In the study of Garay and Meyer (1981) this defect was also observed in one half of the normotensive progeny of patients with EH. The *circulating nature* of the inhibitor of the active sodium pump has been indicated in the studies of Poston and colleagues (1980), which demonstrated that the same inhibition can be produced in the red and white blood cells of normotensive individuals by cross-incubating them in the *plasma* of patients with EH. A schema demonstrating both the passive and active features of cellular ionic flux is shown in Figure 10-11.

Animal models   To complete a hypothesis it is necessary at this point to refer to a wealth of data obtained from animal models of both genetic and

Table 10-1 : Pathophysiology of essential hypertension

1. Hemodynamic mechanism: MAP (f) ↑PVR X ↔ CO
2. Fluid and electrolytes

	Young	Old (≥ 65 years)
Plasma volume	↓ in proportion to ↑MAP	↓ in proportion to ↑MAP
ECV	↔	↔
Na_E	↓ and ± α MAP	↔ and α MAP
K_E	↔ and 1/α MAP	↔ and ± 1/α MAP
Serum [Na+]	↓ and ± α DBP	α DBP
Serum [K+]	↔ and 1/α MAP	↔ and ± 1/α MAP
Serum calcium	↔ serum [Ca] but ↓ ionized serum [Ca]	↔ serum [Ca] but ↓ ionized serum [Ca]

3. Systemic neural and humoral contribution to ↑ PVR

	Young	Old (≥ 65 years)
SNS	+++	+++
Renin-angiotensin system	+	±
PRA	N to ↑	↓

4. Renal changes
   a. Intrarenal angiotensin-dependent vasoconstriction.
   b. Glomerular filtration barrier: ↑ MAP necessary to keep filtered Na+ load up.
   c. Sodium loading: Exaggerated natriuresis (unrelated to changes in colloid osmotic or hydrostatic pressure, i.e., not simply a pressure diuresis) associated with renal vascular resistance (with ↑ RBF, ↑ GFR) and tubular Fx Na+ excretion.

5. Human blood cell Na+ transport capacities[a]

	RBCs	WBCs
Passive Na+ diffusion in	↑[b]	?
Active (ouabain-inhibited) Na+ pumped out[c]	↓	↓

[a] In vascular smooth muscle such a disturbance in Na+ flux would indicate membrane instability, permitting increased intracellular $[Ca^{2+}]$, which in turn would stimulate the contractile element, actomyosin, and render the vessel hyperresponsive to vasoactive substances.
[b] Both by Na-K cotransport (furosemide inhibited) and by Na-Li countertransport.
[c] Plasma factor in HBP can transfer inhibiting effect onto blood cells from normotensive subject: putative CNS-derived, ouabain-like, circulating sodium transport inhibitor (CSTI).

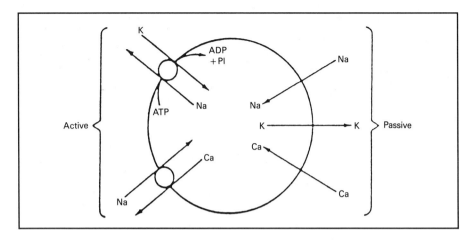

Fig. 10-11 : Vascular smooth muscle cell. Shown are postulated active and passive ion fluxes. (From Clough D, Haddy FJ: Ionic regulation of the microcirculation, in Altura BM, Davis E, Harders H (eds): *Advances in Microcirculation*. Basel, Switzerland, S. Karger, 1982, with permission of the authors and publisher.)

induced hypertension. The apparent contradiction in EH of a glomerular filtration block coexisting with an exaggerated natriuresis on salt loading has been identified in genetically hypertensive rat models *before* the development of hypertension, which suggests a *primary* (intrinsic) renal defect. This is consistent with renal transplant studies, cited above, in which the kidney of a genetically hypertensive rat imparts hypertension to a normotensive recipient rat, and vice versa. Ultrastructural studies on the kidney of young, genetically hypertensive rats *before* the development of hypertension show afferent arteriolar constriction and a reduced diameter in the glomerular endothelial fenestrae (Evan et al, 1981). During sodium loading in humans with EH there is a remarkable increase in renal blood flow and glomerular filtration rate secondary to a drop in renal vascular resistance, not observed in normotensive individuals under identical conditions; this is associated with a fractional tubular excretion of filtered sodium that is more than double that of normotensive individuals (Willassen, Ofstad, 1980). Peritubular capillary physical factors (hydrostatic and colloid osmotic pressure) remain normal, indicating that the exaggerated natriuresis is not a consequence of the elevated MAP, per se. Clearly, an intrarenal system that is nonphysical in nature is *hyperregulative* in EH under conditions of salt loading. The probable system implicated is the intrarenal renin-angiotensin mechanism, which, when activated, combines a renal arteriolar vasoconstrictive and enhanced tubular sodium reabsorptive function (Levens et al, 1981). Conversely, when inhibited, it would be *vasodilatory* and produce a *diminished* renal tubular sodium reabsorption. The exaggerated response to intrarenal captopril infusion in EH,

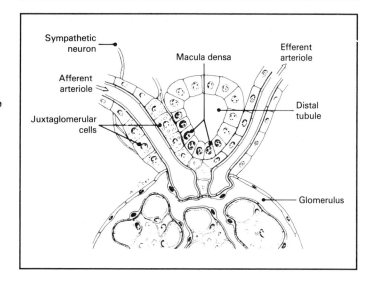

Fig. 10-12 : The renal juxtaglomerular apparatus. Note the afferent and efferent arterioles, juxtaglomerular cells, and macula densa. (From Levens NR et al: Role of the intrarenal renin-angiotensin system in the control of renin function. *Circ Res* 48:157, 1981, with permission of the authors and publisher.)

cited above, is fully consonant with this. An inhibition of renal renin secretion by the intrarenal arterial administration of ouabain, presumably by depressing the macula densa control mechanism on renal renin secretion, was demonstrated in canine studies by Churchill and co-workers (1974). Figure 10-12 shows the proximity of the macula densa of the distal nephron to the renin-secreting juxtaglomerular cells of the glomerular arterioles. According to the work of Vander (1967), when an increased sodium load is sensed by the macula densa, it inhibits renin secretion. A *supranormal* burst in the release of CSTI in EH, then, in response to a sodium load, would *maximally* depress the intrarenal secretion of renin and the generation of angiotensin. This would *maximally* release the renal vasculature from angiotensin vasoconstriction and account for the unique drop in renal vascular resistance under conditions of sodium loading in EH. Similarly, such a supranormal burst in CSTI would *maximally* depress active renal tubular sodium transport directly, which in conjunction with a maximal inhibition of angiotensin (which has a positive effect on tubular sodium transport) would account for the exaggerated increase in fractional tubular sodium excretion in EH during sodium loading. Gruber and co-workers have demonstrated increased circulating levels of an endogenous, "digoxin-like" factor in genetically hypertensive monkeys (1982). This factor was shown to have a molecular weight of less than 1,000, to have Na^+K^+-ATPase inhibitory characteristics, and to be linearly correlated with the degree of MAP elevation.

Extremely provocative with respect to these observations is the identification by Brody and associates of an AII and osmotically sensitive, hypothalamic area (anteroventral portion of the third ventricle [AV_3V]) that is essential for the full development and maintenance of experimental hypertension in the rat (1980). Lesions placed in this area retard or block the blood pressure rise in all experimental forms of induced hypertension (desoxycorticosterone acetate [DOCA]-salt, methylprednisolone, renovascular) and in genetic Dahl-S rat hypertension. Sympathetic neural connections between this area and the rat kidney have been demonstrated, and renal denervation has been shown to impede hypertension in several rat models (both induced and genetic). Further, AV_3V lesions have been shown to suppress the emergence of a humoral substance that ordinarily suppresses the active vascular Na^+ pump in rat DOCA-salt hypertension. On the strength of the available experimental data, Bohr (1981) has hypothesized that "a primary fault" in the pathophysiology of hypertension may be "a defect in calcium binding of the plasma membrane of the cells of a pressure-regulating center in the hypothalamus," which could stimulate its neural and humoral function.

Another piece in the puzzle is provided by the ingenious experiments of Campbell and associates, which establish the *requirement* of an *intact SNS innervation* for the *vascular smooth muscle* of young, spontaneously hypertensive rats (SHR) to develop an irreversibly unstable vascular smooth muscle membrane, *prior* to the emergence of hypertension (1981). The conclusion may be drawn that the fundamental genetic disorder, leading to an irreversible sodium leak in peripheral vascular smooth muscle, requires a critical interaction between the sympathetic nerve and its vascular smooth muscle membrane during the early developmental period. A comparable, primary cellular disorder (1) in the hypothalamic center responsible for the release of CSTI would provide the basis for its hyperactivity in EH, and (2) in the renal vasculature would also provide the basis for the transferability of the hypertensive state through renal transplant studies, previously cited, in genetic rat models.

At this point it may be possible to derive a theoretical construct of the fundamental pathophysiology of EH (Fig. 10-13). A genetically determined, SNS facilitated, primary cellular membrane defect leads to increased passive Na^+ intracellular flux at three critical sites: (1) hypothalamus as the putative focus of CSTI release; (2) peripheral vascular smooth muscle; (3) renal vascular smooth muscle. The increased intracellular Na^+ allows an increase in intracellular Ca^{2+} because there is a smaller Na-electrochemical gradient to drive net Ca-extrusion via Na-Ca exchange (Blaustein et al, 1981). This causes (1) peripheral vasoconstriction by activating actomyosin, leading to hypertension; (2) renal vasoconstriction (through the same mechanism), associated with structural vascular changes and a glomerular filtration barrier, which is *antinatriuretic* in effect and compensated by the rise in systemic arterial (renal perfusion) pressure; (3) enhanced secretion of CSTI from a hypothalamic, osmotically sensitive center, which is *natriuretic* in effect by inhibiting the active, renal

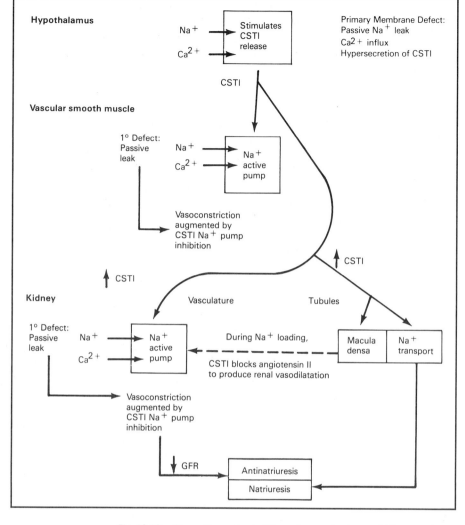

Fig. 10-13 : Theoretic construct of the pathogenesis of essential hypertension. See text for details.

tubular Na⁺ transport pump. Enhanced CSTI secretion also blocks the active (extruding) Na⁺ pump of vascular smooth muscle, allowing even *greater* intracellular Na⁺ and Ca²⁺ accumulation, which *augments* the hypertensive and renal vasoconstrictive effect of the primary passive inward Na⁺ leak. Intracellular Na⁺ and Ca²⁺ accumulation also increases the sensitivity of renal and systemic vascular smooth muscle to neural and humoral factors (e.g., NE, AII). A large sodium load will cause a supranormal increase in CSTI release, which will cause renal vasodilation through an augmented angiotensin blocking effect, as described above. The latter predominates over primary renal vasoconstriction because of the supranormal angiotensin inhibition, an effect that is augmented by the heightened sensitivity of the abnormal renal vasculature to angiotensin. This, combined with the supranormal blocking of tubular Na^+ transport accounts for the exaggerated natriuresis during Na^+ loading, which is a *transient* phenomenon.

Stages in the evaluation of essential hypertension

On the basis of these formulations, two opposing factors are operative on renal sodium excretion in the hypertensive kidney: the vaso-constriction-glomerular filtration block, which favors Na^+ retention, and the heightened CSTI effect, which favors Na^+ excretion (Fig. 10-13). It would appear that early in EH the latter effect predominates, such that Na_E is actually *diminished*, and the level of blood pressure is more strongly correlated (inversely) with K_E and serum $[K^+]$ than with Na_E. With the progression of renal vascular changes over time there would come a stage where the two opposing factors were in balance, and, finally, a stage where the glomerular filtration barrier predominated over the CSTI effect on sodium metabolism. This is consistent with the finding in *older* hypertensive patients that Na_E is no longer diminished and is positively correlated with the level of blood pressure. A point is also reached where the elevated arterial (renal perfusion) pressure cannot compensate for the renal vascular changes, and renal blood flow drops more and more below the level of normotensive individuals of the same age. The degree to which the renal vascular changes are functional (vasoconstrictive) as compared with structural is indicated by the normalization of renal blood flow in the hypertensive kidney when challenged by a sodium load (Willassen, Ofstad, 1980) and the *supra*normal increase in renal blood flow in the hypertensive kidney when intrarenal angiotensin production is blocked by the infusion of intrarenal captopril (Hollenberg, 1981).

Role of antihypertensive kidney function in EH

There is an extensive literature that documents an antihypertensive function of the kidney that is secretory (nonexcretory) in nature, and that indicates that this function resides in one or more antihypertensive lipids that are synthesized by and secreted from the interstitial cells of the renal medulla. The vasodilator prostaglandin E_2 (PGE_2) and the antihypertensive neutral renomedullary lipid (ANRL) isolated by Muirhead and co-workers (1981), have been intensively studied in this regard. PGE_2 has been shown to be depleted in the renal medulla of Dahl-S hypertensive rats, a phenomenon closely related to the reduced capacity of the genetically hypertensive rat to excrete sodium (Tobian et al, 1982). Urinary PGE_2 excretion has also been shown to be unresponsive to a low sodium intake in EH, in contrast to the rise found in normotensive subjects. Renal prostaglandin generation is stimulated by bradykinin, and urinary excretion of the bradykinin generating enzyme, kallikrein, has been reported to be low in EH in some but not all studies. However, these changes may all be *secondary* to the hypertensive state, and the fact that PGE_2 is largely degraded on one passage through the lungs would seem to make it an unlikely candidate for the *circulating* antihypertensive factor of renal origin. The molecular structure of ANRL has not yet been reported, but it may be a derivative of other potent, antihypertensive, renomedulatory lipids, the alkyl ether analogs of phosphatidylcholine; its release into the circulation has been associated with degranulation of lipid-containing renomedullary cells in experimental hypertension (Pitcock et al, 1981). Whatever their ultimate role proves to be, a *primary* (genetic) deficiency of one or more renomedullary antihypertensive lipid factors to account for the *genesis* of EH remains to be established. Renomedullary implants between ''post-salt'' hypertensive rats actually showed a significantly *greater* antihypertensive effect than implants from *normotensive* into ''post-salt'' hypertensive rats, which indicates the complexity of the subject (Tobian, 1973).

Systolic Hypertension

In certain clinical conditions there is a *disproportionate* elevation of systolic pressure. The major determinants of *systolic pressure* are: (1) left ventricular stroke volume and ejection velocity; and (2) aortic distensibility. The systolic pressure is directly proportional to the former, and inversely proportional to the latter. Clinical conditions in which a disproportionately elevated systolic pressure relates to a large stroke volume due to a *primary cardiac factor* (with or without the augmenting factor of an increased ejection velocity) are aortic regurgitation, marked bradycardia (as with complete heart block), thyrotoxicosis, and the hyperkinetic cardiac state (excessive sympathetic neural drive). Clinical conditions in which a disproportionately elevated systolic pressure relates to a large stroke volume due to a *low peripheral vascular resistance* include anemia (in association with the low blood viscosity effect), arteriovenous fistula, beriberi, and extensive Paget's disease of bone. The major condition in which a disproportionately elevated systolic pressure relates to a loss of aortic distensibility is normative aging, often accelerated by underlying, antecedent essential hypertension or diabetes mellitus.

Suggested Readings

Blaustein MP, Lang S, James-Cracke M: Cellular basis of sodium-induced hypertension, in Laragh JH, Buhler FR, Seldin DW (eds): *Frontiers in Hypertension Research.* New York, Springer-Verlag, 1981.

Bohr DF: What makes the pressure go up? *Hypertension* (II)3:160, 1981.

Brody MJ, Johnson AK: Role of the anteroventral third ventricle region in fluid and electrolyte balance, arterial pressure regulation, and hypertension, in Martini L, Ganong WF (eds): *Frontiers in Neuroendocrinology.* New York, Raven Press, 1980.

Buhler FR et al: Changing role of beta- and alpha-adrenoreceptor mediated cardiovascular responses in the transition from high-cardiac output into a high-peripheral resistance phase in essential hypertension, in Laragh JH, Buhler FR, Seldin DW (eds): *Frontiers in Hypertension Research.* New York, Springer-Verlag, 1981, p 316.

Campbell GR et al: Effect of cross-transplantation on normotensive and spontaneously hypertensive rat arterial muscle membrane. *Hypertension* 3:534, 1981.

Churchill PC, McDonald FD: Effect of ouabain on renin secretion in anaesthetized dogs. *J Physiol* 242:635, 1974.

Dahl LK, Heine M: Primary role of renal homografts in setting chronic blood pressure levels in rats. *Circ Res* 36:692, 1975.

Evan AP et al: The glomerular filtration barrier in the spontaneously hypertensive rat. *Hypertension* (I)3:154, 1981.

Garay RP, Meyer P: Erythrocyte sodium extrusion in primary hypertension, in Laragh JH, Buhler FR, Seldin DW (eds): *Frontiers in Hypertension Research.* New York, Springer-Verlag, 1981, p 81.

Goldblatt H: Studies on experimental hypertension-V. The pathogenesis of experimental hypertension due to renal ischemia. *Ann Intern Med* 11:69, 1937.

Gruber KA, Rudel LL, Bullock BC: Increased circulating levels of an endogenous digoxin-like factor in hypertensive monkeys. *Hypertension* 4:348, 1982.

Hollenberg NK et al: Sodium intake and renal response to captopril in normal man and in essential hypertension. *Kidney Int* 20:240, 1981.

Levens NR, Peach MJ, Carey RM: Role of the intrarenal renin-angiotensin system in the control of renal function. *Circ Res* 48:157, 1981.

Lever AF et al: Sodium and potassium in essential hypertension. *Br Med J* 283:463, 1981.

Pitcock JA et al: Degranulation of renomedullary interstitial cells during reversal of hypertension. *Hypertension* (II)3:75, 1981.

Poston L et al: The effect of (1) a low molecular weight natriuretic substance and (2) serum from hypertensive patients on the sodium transport of leukocytes from normal subjects, in Zumkley H, Losse H (eds): *Intracellular Electrolytes and Arterial Hypertension.* Stuttgart, Georg Thieme Verlag, 1980, p 93.

Vander AJ: Control of renin release. *Physiol Rev* 47:359, 1967.

Willassen Y, Ofstad J: Renal sodium excretion and the peritubular capillary physical factors in essential hypertension. *Hypertension* 2:771, 1980.

Muirhead EE et al: Alkyl ether analogs of phosphatidylcholine are orally active in hypertensive rabbits. *Hypertension* I-3:107, 1981.

Tobian L et al: Influence of renal prostaglandins and dietary linoleate on hypertension in Dahl-S rats. *Hypertension* (II)4:149, 1982.

Tobian L: Renal medullary interstitial cells and the antihypertensive action of normal and "hypertensive" kidneys, in Onesti G, Kim KE, Moyer, JH (eds): *Hypertension: Mechanisms and Management.* New York, Grune & Stratton, 1973, p 645.

11 : Synthesis of Pathophysiologic Mechanisms in Heart Failure

As noted in Chapters 1, 8, and 9, the clinical syndromes of heart failure represent the end-result of an entire series of reactions and counterreactions involving the heart, the central and peripheral circulations, the lung, and the kidney.

The material reviewed in this chapter is discussed in greater detail in each of these three chapters. This chapter is an attempt to describe in an integrated fashion the various mechanisms operative in heart failure.

Central to the pathophysiology of heart failure is the inability of the right and/or left ventricles to pump adequate quantities of blood to meet the metabolic requirements of the various organs of the body. A wide spectrum of diseases (see Chaps. 3, 5, 6) can result in impairment of cardiac function with resultant heart failure. A second form of heart failure occurs when peripheral demand exceeds the ability of an otherwise normal heart to pump adequate quantities of blood to the periphery. Thus, heart failure is invariably the result of an imbalance between the heart's ability to *supply* blood to the body and the body's *demand* for that blood. Heart failure can result from either inadequate function on the part of the *supplying organ*, the heart, or excessive demand on the part of the *supplied organs*. Therapy to correct the pathophysiologic mechanisms that underlie heart failure should focus on attempts to improve cardiac function or decrease peripheral demand depending on which of these two is the major instigator of cardiac decompensation. There are two major cardiac compensatory responses to impaired myocardial function or excessive peripheral demand: (1) increased sympathetic nervous stimulation of the heart, and (2) ventricular chamber dilatation and/or hypertrophy of the myocardium leading to increased myocardial mass. Dilatation and hypertrophy (and ischemia in patients with coronary artery disease) reduce myocardial compliance (increased stiffness) leading to increases in ventricular filling pressures that, in turn, increase atrial (left and/or right) and venous (pulmonary and/or systemic) pressures.

Cardiac sympathetic and parasympathetic nervous function is depressed in patients with heart failure. Myocardial norepinephrine stores are exhausted because synthesis of this neurotransmitter is inadequate to maintain cardiac stores in the face of markedly increased sympathetic nervous stimulation of the heart. The myocardium remains responsive, however, to the inotropic and chronotropic effects of circulating norepinephrine and epinephrine released by peripheral nerves and the adrenal medulla. Blood levels of norepinephrine and epinephrine rise dramatically in patients with heart failure.

Cardiac pumping ability (cardiac output) is depressed at rest only in patients with advanced heart failure. Initially, cardiac output is normal at rest but fails to rise normally during exercise. The result is greater extraction of oxygen and nutrients from the blood by peripheral tissues. Thus, the systemic arteriovenous oxygen (AVO) difference is abnormally increased during exercise in patients with heart failure. Inadequate rise in cardiac output during exercise leads to the sensation of easy fatigability. In patients with advanced heart failure, cardiac output is depressed and AVO difference is increased even at rest.

Peripheral vasculature maintains its norepinephrine stores and responds to decreased cardiac output with vasoconstriction. This vasoconstrictor response is the result of a sympathetic reflex activated by decreased arterial baroreceptor stimulation that, in turn, is the result of the decrease in cardiac output (Fig. 11-1). Constriction of arterioles and veins results in decreases in perfusion to a variety of organs (splanchnic organs, skin, kidney). Blood flow to brain and heart are maintained until cardiac output is reduced to dangerously low levels.

As noted in Figure 11-1, arteriolar vasoconstriction increases total peripheral resistance and helps to maintain blood pressure in the face of reduced cardiac output (blood pressure = cardiac output × total peripheral resistance). Increased sympathetic nervous stimulation results in a number of alterations in renal function. Constriction of the renal afferent arterioles decreases the glomerular filtration rate (GFR) leading to increased reabsorption of sodium from the tubular filtrate. Moreover, increased reabsorption of sodium results from other mechanisms including the renin-angiotensin-aldosterone axis (increased renin release) and peritubular physical forces. Release of antidiuretic hormone (ADH) by the pituitary hypothalamic axis increases water reabsorption in the collecting ducts of the kidney (Fig. 11-1). Other substances, e.g., prostaglandins, may play a role in the increased renal sodium and water retention noted in patients with heart failure.

Increased salt and water reabsorption by the kidney increases circulating blood volume thereby increasing ventricular volume (dilatation) and moving the ventricle to the right along the Starling curve (Chap. 1, Fig. 1-2). However, such further increases in ventricular volume produce increases in ventricular filling pressures that are

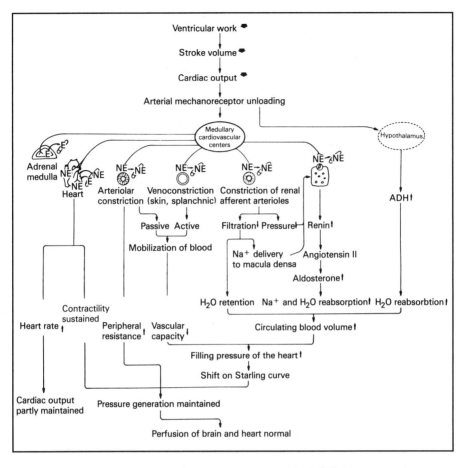

Fig. 11-1 : Reflex adjustments that occur in the body in response to heart failure. ADH = antidiuretic hormone, β = beta-adrenergic receptor; NE = norepinephrine; E = epinephrine; ↑ = augmentation; ↓ = depression. (From Shepherd JT, Van Houtte PM: *The Human Vascular System: Facts and Concepts.* New York, Raven Press, 1979, with permission of the authors and publisher.)

eventually transmitted to the capillaries of the lung in the case of the left ventricle and the systemic capillaries in the case of the right ventricle (Fig. 11-2). Systemic capillary hypertension leads to fluid transudation with resultant edema of peripheral tissues. Increased flow of lymph results; edema forms only when more fluid enters the interstitial space than can be effectively cleared by the lymphatic drainage. Capillary hypertension in the splanchnic circulation leads to ascites and impaired hepatic function. A vicious spiral can result since disturbance of hepatic function decreases the synthesis of serum proteins thereby depressing plasma oncotic pressure that, in turn, increases the tendency for extravasation of fluid from the capillaries and into the interstitial space. Edema formation is thereby increased.

12 : Clinical Demonstration of Heart Failure and Myocardial Ischemia: Relation to Pathophysiologic Mechanisms

A good physician thinks about a patient's illness in terms of the pathophysiology of that disease. Symptoms and signs are interpreted in light of the pathophysiology of the illness, and therapeutic strategies attempt to reverse the pathophysiologic sequence of the disease. Clinical and laboratory findings of heart failure and myocardial ischemia are reviewed below with reference to the pathophysiology of these two entities.

Heart Failure

History

As noted in Chapter 8, increased left atrial pressure is transmitted to the pulmonary capillaries with resultant transudation of fluid into the pulmonary interstitium. Changes in pulmonary compliance and blood gas exchange result (see Chap. 8); patients initially note dyspnea on exertion followed by dyspnea at rest as the quantity of pulmonary interstitial fluid increases. Thus, patients with left ventricular failure or mitral stenosis first complain of dyspnea on exertion that gradually worsens. Orthopnea, paroxysmal nocturnal dyspnea, and finally pulmonary edema with unrelenting dyspnea at rest follow as pulmonary interstitial fluid volume increases.

Right ventricular failure or tricuspid stenosis produce elevated right atrial pressure with resultant increased systemic capillary pressure. Interstitial edema develops in a variety of tissues, for example, liver, gut, muscle, and skin. Patients with right ventricular failure, therefore, commonly complain of ankle swelling secondary to skin edema of the lower extremities and anorexia secondary to edema of the gut wall. Edema of the lower extremities is usually noted first since increased capillary hydrostatic pressure resulting from standing or sitting combines with increased capillary pressure secondary to right ventricular failure to produce obvious edema of the skin of the lower extremities. Further increases in right atrial pressure, resulting from worsening right ventricular failure, augment the severity and extent of edema of the lower extremities. Moreover, edema of the liver and gut produce anorexia and occasionally malabsorption with associated diarrhea. Fatigue is commonly noted in patients with right ventricular failure. This symptom results from decreased cardiac output, a common finding in patients with right ventricular decompensation.

217

Pulmonary congestion secondary to left ventricular failure and the associated increase in pulmonary interstitial fluid produce a number of well-known physical findings: rales result from intraalveolar fluid, wheezing results from edematous, narrowed airways, and dullness to percussion results from pleural effusions. Decreased compliance (increased stiffness) of left ventricular myocardium is the cause of the third (S_3) and fourth (S_4) heart sounds. Modestly decreased left ventricular compliance is associated with an S_4; markedly decreased compliance leads to an S_3. Occasional patients with very severe left ventricular failure have pulsus alternans (alternating stronger and weaker beats in the peripheral pulse). Pulsus alternans is the result of beat-to-beat variation in left ventricular filling with resultant beat-to-beat variation in stroke volume and hence pulse volume.

Patients with right ventricular failure may demonstrate a number of physical findings that can be directly related to the pathophysiology of this entity. Jugular venous distension is a reflection of increased right atrial pressure transmitted to the jugular veins. Hepatomegaly results from congestion of the liver with blood secondary to increased systemic venous pressure. Similarly, peripheral edema is the result of increased systemic venous and capillary pressure. Individuals with long-standing right ventricular failure often have severe, widespread peripheral edema that may even reach the groin and lower abdominal wall. Such patients may also develop ascites as a result of increased hepatic and mesenteric venous pressure. Individuals with either left or right ventricular failure (or both) may have reduced cardiac output that may be suspected during the physical examination because of a small peripheral pulse volume. In addition, compensatory mechanisms set in motion by reduced cardiac output often increase the heart rate in patients with failure of either ventricle.

Confirmation of the presence of heart failure or clues to its etiology are frequently obtained from laboratory studies. Thus, the electrocardiogram may confirm the presence of a rapid heart rate; patterns of myocardial infarction or ventricular hypertrophy may suggest the etiology of heart failure. Persistent cardiac arrhythmias can lead to heart failure; the electrocardiogram may be helpful in this regard by demonstrating the offending arrhythmia.

Pulmonary vascular congestion and abnormally increased pulmonary interstitial fluid are evident on the chest x-ray of a patient with left ventricular failure or mitral stenosis. A semiquantitative estimate of the pulmonary capillary wedge pressure can often be obtained by closely examining the chest x-ray of a patient with left ventricular failure or mitral stenosis (Table 12-1). Compensatory ventricular dilatation (Starling mechanism) can be inferred from the chest x-ray when cardiomegaly (enlargement of the transverse cardiac diameter

Table 12-1 : Radiologic signs of pulmonary capillary hypertension

X-ray findings	Pulmonary capillary pressure (mm Hg)
Vessels in lower lobes larger than vessels in upper lobes = normal	<13
Equalization of vessel size in upper and lower lobes	13–17
Vessels in upper lobes larger than vessels in lower lobes = pulmonary vascular redistribution	18–23
Interstitial pulmonary edema = Kerley B lines, perivascular cuffing, pleural effusion (small)	20–25
Alveolar pulmonary edema	>25

to greater than 50% of the overall transthoracic diameter) is observed. Careful examination of the chest-film will also disclose specific cardiac chamber enlargement and valvular calcification; both can be used as clues concerning the etiology of pulmonary capillary hypertension.

Echocardiography employs ultrasound to examine cardiac chamber size, regional ventricular wall motion and contractility, valvular function, and the presence of pericardial effusion. Left ventricular volumes (end-diastolic and end-systolic) and a variety of contractility parameters (ejection fraction, velocity of circumferential fiber shortening [V_{cf}], posterior wall velocity, percentage of minor axis shortening [%ΔD], velocity of posterior and septal wall thickening) can be derived from echocardiographic examination of the heart. Table 12-2 lists a number of cardiac conditions that can be definitively diag-

Table 12-2 : Cardiac conditions that can be defined by echocardiography

Mitral valve disease
  Mitral stenosis
  Mitral valve prolapse
  Ruptured chordae tendineae
Aortic valve disease
  Aortic stenosis
  Aortic regurgitation
Tricuspid valve disease
  Tricuspid stenosis
  Ebstein's anomaly of the tricuspid valve
Pulmonic valve disease
  Pulmonic stenosis
Cardiomyopathy
  Congestive cardiomyopathy
  Hypertrophic cardiomyopathy
Cardiac tumors
Pericardial effusion
Infectious endocarditis
Various forms of congenital heart disease

Table 12-3 : Systolic time intervals

Interval	Significance
Preejection period (PEP)	Reflects overall left ventricular contractility
Ejection time (ET)	Reflects stroke volume
PEP/ET ratio	Correlates with left ventricular ejection fraction
Carotid pulse upstroke time	Reflects aortic valve function

nosed or inferred by echocardiography. Two forms of echocardiography are in common use: M-mode (small sample or "ice-pick view") and B-mode (cross-sectional or large sample). Patients with heart failure usually demonstrate increased ventricular volumes (dilatation secondary to the Starling mechanism) and depressed indices of myocardial and ventricular contractility.

Quantitative estimates of left ventricular and aortic valve function can be obtained from simultaneous recordings of the electrocardiogram, the first and second heart sounds, and a tracing of the carotid pulse contour. Measurements made from these recordings are translated into a variety of derived variables known collectively as "systolic time intervals" (Table 12-3). Overall left ventricular function and the presence of aortic stenosis can be inferred from such measurements—abnormal systolic intervals are commonly found in patients with heart failure and/or severe aortic stenosis.

Radioisotopes can be employed to quantitate left and right ventricular function, valvular regurgitation, and shunt flow associated with congenital cardiac defects. Small quantities of technetium 99m are bound to either serum albumin or red blood cells and injected intravenously. A scintillation detector is placed over the heart and measurements are obtained of the amount of radioactivity present during systole and diastole. From such determinations, it is possible to derive the following variables: left and right ventricular ejection fraction, the volume of aortic or mitral valvular regurgitation, and the volume of blood flowing through an intracardiac shunt, e.g., atrial or ventricular septal defect. Ventricular volumes are commonly increased in patients with heart failure (ventricular dilatation); contractility indices such as ejection fraction are usually depressed in these individuals.

Cardiac catheterization is an invasive procedure whereby a variety of catheters are advanced from peripheral arteries and/or veins into various cardiac chambers. Measurements of intracardiac pressures, blood flow and "contractility" parameters can be obtained with the aid of such catheters. Moreover, liquid contrast medium can be injected through the catheters enabling the physician to see and record on film pictures of various cardiac chambers. From such angiographic studies, a variety of measurements can be made reflecting

Table 12-4 : Variables that can be measured during cardiac catheterization and angiography

1. Pressures in all four cardiac chambers, the aorta, and the pulmonary artery
2. Cardiac output and stroke volume
3. Valve area of a stenotic valve
4. Volume of intracardiac shunt flow (severity of shunt)
5. Volume of regurgitant valvular flow (severity of regurgitation)
6. Left ventricular "contractility" indices
   a. Isovolumic phase indices—derived from the upstroke of the left ventricular pressure tracing
      (1) dp/dt = velocity of the upstroke
      (2) V_{max} = maximum velocity of the upstroke
      (3) V_{ce} = velocity of the contractile elements
   b. Ejection phase indices—derived from cineangiography of the left ventricle
      (1) V_{cf} = velocity of circumferential fiber shortening
      (2) MNSER = mean normalized systolic ejection rate
      (3) Systolic wall tension
      (4) End-systolic pressure–volume ratio
7. Left ventricular "relaxation" (compliance) indices
      (1) $-dp/dt$ = velocity of the downstroke of the left ventricular pressure tracing
      (2) End-diastolic pressure–volume ratio
      (3) dp/dv = rate of change of pressure to volume ratio during diastole
      (4) K_p = modulus of left ventricular chamber stiffness
8. Vascular resistance in systemic and pulmonary circuits
9. Regional wall motion of segments of the left ventricle
10. Anatomic alterations in cardiac chambers and/or great vessels
11. Coronary arerial anatomy
12. Electrophysiologic properties of the cardiac conduction system and myocardium

cardiac function, valvular regurgitation, and intracardiac shunt flow. Table 12-4 lists some (but not all) of the variables that can be measured during cardiac catheterization and angiography. Many of the variables listed in Table 12-4 can be estimated noninvasively by techniques already mentioned (echocardiography, radioisotopic studies, and systolic time intervals). The accuracy of noninvasive techniques in determining such variables is usually less than that obtained with invasive techniques.

Patients with heart failure commonly demonstrate elevated ventricular filling pressures, depressed cardiac output, and reduced ventricular contractility and relaxation indices. Abnormalities of ventricular wall motion and valvular function may be observed depending on the etiology of heart failure.

Myocardial Ischemia

History

The overwhelming majority of patients with atherosclerotic coronary artery disease and myocardial ischemia clearly describe episodic attacks of chest discomfort (angina pectoris) associated with effort, heavy meals, or emotional situations. There may be a history of the more intense and prolonged discomfort associated with myocardial infarction. Individuals with effort-induced angina probably develop myocardial ischemia as a result of the increased heart rate and blood pressure associated with effort. In such patients, increased myocardial metabolic demand (MVO_2) outstrips reduced myocardial blood flow that results from coronary arterial obstruction (demand angina pectoris). Individuals with angina at rest (so-called unstable angina) apparently develop myocardial ischemia as a result of decreased myocardial blood flow secondary to coronary arterial obstruction and spasm (supply angina pectoris). In such individuals, heart rate and blood pressure, and hence myocardial metabolic demand, remain unchanged before the attack of angina. Exactly how myocardial ischemia causes the discomfort of angina pectoris is unclear. Presumably, ischemia irritates nerve endings in the myocardium.

Episodes of myocardial ischemia or infarction are associated with decreased myocardial compliance (increased stiffness). Depressed myocardial compliance, in turn, leads to elevated ventricular filling pressure, which is eventually transmitted to the pulmonary capillaries. Increased pulmonary capillary pressure leads to increased pulmonary interstitial fluid with resultant dyspnea. Consequently, patients may complain of dyspnea during angina pectoris or acute myocardial infarction. Lasting symptoms of left ventricular failure (e.g., dyspnea, paroxysmal nocturnal dyspnea [PND]) may develop in patients with extensive destruction of left ventricular myocardium secondary to myocardial infarction. Similarly, patients with extensive right ventricular infarction may complain of fatigue, anorexia, and ankle swelling as a result of right ventricular failure (see above).

Complications of myocardial infarction may cause symptoms. Patients with postmyocardial infarction pericarditis (Dressler syndrome) may complain of severe pleuritic chest discomfort that lessens when the individual sits upright and leans forward. This discomfort is the result of irritation of pericardial nerve endings. The pleuritic nature of the discomfort is presumably the result of stretching of the pleura and pericardium during inspiration. The upright position may alleviate pericardial discomfort by allowing the heart to be suspended within the pericardial sac thereby minimizing contact between the moving heart and the surrounding inflamed pleura and pericardium.

Patients with ruptured ventricular septum or papillary muscle infarction may develop very severe mitral regurgitation and left ventricular dysfunction. Such patients may complain of severe dyspnea and fatigue. Many of these individuals develop cardiogenic shock and thus become somnolent or confused. These latter patients often have minimal or no complaints because of the resultant obtundation.

Two other symptom complexes associated with acute myocardial infarction deserve to be mentioned. Patients with inferior wall myocardial infarction often complain of anorexia, nausea, vomiting, or diarrhea. These symptoms are probably the result of stimulation of vagal ganglia lying near the inferior wall of the left ventricle. Vagal stimulation leads to the observed gastrointestinal symptoms. Many patients report a cold sweat and a sense of impending doom soon after the onset of acute myocardial infarction. These symptoms apparently result from reflex-mediated release of circulating catecholamines.

Physical examination

Myocardial ischemia and infarction impair regional left ventricular systolic and diastolic function. As discussed in Chapter 3, depressed myocardial contractile function and increased myocardial stiffness both lead to increased left ventricular filling pressures with resultant increases in pulmonary interstitial fluid. Thus, the physical examination in such patients often discloses pulmonary rales and occasionally expiratory wheezes. Decreased left ventricular contractile function depresses stroke volume with resultant diminution in pulse amplitude and vigor. Tachycardia may be present as compensatory mechanisms in the form of increased sympathetic nervous stimulation attempt to compensate for the decrease in stroke volume. Remember that cardiac output $=$ heart rate $\times$ stroke volume, and cardiac output may remain unchanged if a decrease in stroke volume is accompanied by an increase in heart rate of compensating magnitude. Right ventricular infarction is often associated with visibly elevated jugular venous pressure secondary to increased right ventricular filling pressure.

Ischemic or infarcted myocardium often bulges passively during left ventricular systole. This passive bulge can produce an abnormal, systolic impulse (the so-called dyskinetic or abnormal movement impulse) that is palpable alongside the normal apex impulse.

The heart sounds are quite soft and muffled in patients with myocardial ischemia or infarction. This finding is caused by depressed ventricular function with a resultant decrease in velocity and amplitude of valvular closure. A murmur of mitral regurgitation may also be heard in these patients. Mitral regurgitation is the result of ischemia or infarction of a mitral valvular papillary muscle. Similarly, the systolic murmur of a ventricular septal defect is heard in patients with post-infarction ventricular septal rupture. Decreased ventricular diastolic compliance (increased stiffness) is the cause of third (S_3) or fourth (S_4) heart sounds that are often present in patients with myocardial ischemia or infarction. These sounds result when there is rapid inflow of blood into the stiff left ventricle. Rapid inflow of blood occurs during two phases of ventricular diastole: (1) a rapid filling phase occurs during the first third of diastole; S_3 correlates with this phase of ventricular diastolic filling; and (2) a second phase of rapid ventricular filling occurs during atrial systole near the end of diastole; S_4 correlates with this phase of ventricular diastolic filling. A pericardial rub may be audible in patients with post-myocardial infarction pericarditis. This sound results from friction between the two inflamed layers of the pericardium.

Physical findings associated with myocardial ischemia and infarction are often transient since the pathophysiologic process is dynamic. Thus, a murmur of mitral regurgitation secondary to papillary muscle ischemia may be audible during but not after an attack of angina pectoris.

Laboratory data

A number of laboratory examinations are employed in order to confirm the clinical diagnosis of ischemic heart disease. The accuracy of these tests usually depends on their ability to identify ischemic or necrotic regions of left ventricular myocardium.

The electrocardiogram reflects summated electrical potentials from the entire myocardial mass. Necrotic or fibrotic zones of myocardium such as those that occur in patients with myocardial infarction are electrically dead; these regions appear on the electrocardiogram as electrically silent areas or "bites" taken out of the normal electrocardiographic tracing. Ischemic myocardial cells have abnormal mechanical and electrical function (see Chap. 14). Ischemia without infarction can result in partial depolarization of myocardial fibers, shortening or lengthening of the myocardial action potential, and even complete loss of electrical potential (see Chap. 14). These changes in electrical activity may lead to nonuniform repolarization of the various myocardial layers (subendocardium to subepicardium) with resultant electrocardiographic abnormalities such as depressed S-T segments and inverted T waves. Patients with "demand" angina may develop myocardial ischemia only during periods of increased myocardial metabolic demand, for example, during exercise. Such individuals may have a normal electrocardiogram at rest but develop markedly abnormal S-T segments and T waves during exercise. This phenomenon is the basis for the widespread use of the electrocardiographic exercise (or stress) test.

Chest radiography is usually normal in patients with atherosclerotic coronary artery disease without myocardial infarction. Resting cardiac function is usually normal in such patients and hence cardiac size and pulmonary interstitial markings are unremarkable. Compensatory ventricular dilatation is common following myocardial infarction. In addition, ventricular compliance is commonly reduced in these individuals. The roentgenographic result of these two pathophysiologic changes is cardiomegaly and the pulmonary vascular alterations observed with increased pulmonary capillary pressure secondary to left ventricular failure. A fluoroscopic examination of the

Table 12-5 : Cardiovascular nuclear medical techniques in ischemic heart disease

Technique	Variables measured	Indication	Comments
Radioisotopic ventriculography (MUGA scan, blood pool or first pass RVG)	Left and right ventricular ejection fraction and volumes, regional wall motion	Quantitate left and right ventricular function; diagnosis of ischemic heart disease	Can be done at rest or with exercise
Thallium 201 exercise test	Uniformity of left ventricular perfusion	Diagnosis of ischemic heart disease	Usually done during and following exercise
Technetium 99m pyrophosphate	Identify areas of myocardial necrosis	Diagnosis of acute myocardial infarction	Done only at rest; test only useful during first 7–14 days after infarction

heart in patients with coronary atherosclerosis often discloses areas of coronary arterial calcification.

Echocardiography may reveal areas of myocardium that contract weakly or not at all in patients with ischemic heart disease. In some of these patients abnormal myocardial contractility is the result of ischemia and in others it is secondary to myocardial necrosis. In most of these individuals, areas of abnormal ventricular wall motion are the result of myocardial infarction since ischemia alone usually develops during exercise rather than at rest. Compensatory ventricular dilatation following myocardial infarction can also be documented by echocardiographic examination. Finally, severe coronary arterial stenoses in the initial 1–2 cm of the left main coronary artery can be visualized by cross-sectional (B-mode) echocardiography. Unfortunately, the rest of the coronary arterial tree cannot be examined by echocardiography.

Systolic time intervals reflect overall left ventricular function. Patients with acute ischemia and/or myocardial infarction may have abnormal left ventricular function that can be detected by measuring systolic time intervals. However, these determinations are not commonly performed during the diagnostic evaluation of a patient with suspected ischemic heart disease.

Radioisotopic techniques have recently become very popular in the diagnostic evaluation of patients with known or suspected ischemic heart disease. Three nuclear medical examinations are commonly performed in such individuals (Table 12-5). Radioisotopic ventriculography (RVG) is an accurate technique for determining left and right ventricular ejection fraction and volumes. The technique is employed both at rest and during exercise. A small amount of technetium 99m is bound to serum albumin or the patient's red blood cells and injected intravenously. A scintillation detector is placed over the

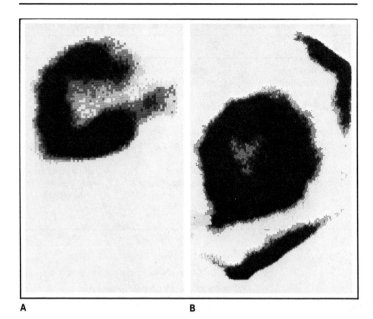

A   B

Fig. 12-1 : Positive thallium-201 exercise test result in a patient with coronary artery disease. Note that in panel A, there is a defect in the thallium-201 image (at 2–3 o'clock). This represents an ischemic area occurring during exercise. In panel B, the ischemic area has resolved during the ensuing 4-hour rest period. It is important to remember that thallium 201 distributes in the myocardium with myocardial blood flow. Thus, during exercise when ischemia develops, a defect is seen in the thallium-201 image. When ischemia is relieved by rest, the defect in the thallium-201 image resolves. (Courtesy of Dr. J. Bianco.)

chest and records radioactivity in the heart during the various phases of the cardiac cycle. Resting RVG is most useful in confirming clinical impressions concerning the adequacy of left ventricular function. Exercise RVG is useful in the diagnosis of ischemic heart disease: normal individuals demonstrate increasing left ventricular ejection fraction during exercise, while patients with coronary artery disease demonstrate unchanged or decreasing ejection fraction during exercise.

Thallium 201 exercise testing is a technique employed for measuring myocardial perfusion during rest and exercise periods. Patients exercise to peak capacity; at this point, radioactive thallium 201 is injected intravenously. This isotope is an analogue of potassium and is therefore avidly taken up by myocardial cells if they are adequately perfused. Patients who have ischemia during exercise demonstrate areas of the left ventricle that fail to take up the radioisotope ("cold spots," Fig. 12-1). On the resting image obtained several hours later, these regions of deficient blood flow disappear. Infarcted zones of myocardium demonstrate decreased perfusion both at rest and during exercise since necrotic myocardium and/or fibrous tissue receives less blood flow than normal myocardium.

Fig. 12-2 : Protocol for diagnostic evaluation of patients with suspected ischemic heart disease. Procedures almost always performed are represented by solid arrows; those performed on selected patients are represented by broken arrows.

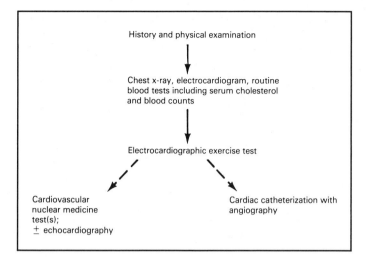

The third cardiac nuclear examination is the technetium 99m pyrophosphate ("hot spot") scan. Intravenously injected technetium 99m pyrophosphate accumulates in recently necrotic myocardium. If a scintillation detector is placed over the chest, a zone of increased radioactivity (hot spot) can be recorded if infarction has occurred during the last 7–14 days.

Cardiac catheterization and angiography yield very accurate anatomic and physiologic information concerning the severity of the pathologic process in patients with ischemic heart disease. Of course, these procedures are invasive and entail some small but definite risk for the patient. Therefore, cardiac catheterization is not performed routinely in all patients with suspected coronary artery disease. These examinations are reserved for patients in whom specific anatomic or diagnostic information is required (Fig. 12-2).

Hemodynamic evaluation (as described above) defines the level of cardiac function and demonstrates if heart failure is present. Angiography reveals regions of the left ventricle that contract abnormally (Table 12-6) and the location and severity of coronary arterial obstruction.

Information can also be obtained during catheterization concerning the state of myocardial metabolism: a catheter is placed in the coro-

Table 12-6 : Types of ventricular wall motion in patients with ischemic heart disease

1. Normal wall motion
2. Hypokinesis—decreased vigor of contraction
3. Akinesis—absence of contraction
4. Dyskinesis—passive bulging of a region of myocardium during ventricular systole
5. Hyperkinesis—compensatory increased vigor of contraction

nary sinus to collect samples of myocardial venous blood and to measure total coronary sinus blood flow by the thermodilution technique. Patients exercise or have the heart electrically paced in order to induce myocardial ischemia. Lactate levels are measured in the samples of myocardial venous blood. Under normal conditions, the myocardium, like the liver, consumes lactate both at rest and during exercise. The myocardium of patients with ischemic heart disease usually consumes lactate at rest but *produces* this metabolite during periods of exercise or pacing-induced ischemia. The myocardial blood flow response to exercise or pacing may also be abnormal in patients with coronary artery disease.

Suggested Readings

Cohn PF (ed): *Diagnosis and Therapy of Coronary Artery Disease.* Boston, Little, Brown, 1979.
Of particular interest are Chapters 2, 4, 5, 6, 7, and 8.

Braunwald E, Ross J Jr, Sonnenblick EH: *Mechanisms of Contraction of the Normal and Failing Heart,* ed 2. Boston, Little, Brown, 1976, chaps 11, 12.

Shepherd JT, Van Houtte PM: *The Human Cardiovascular System: Facts and Concepts.* New York, Raven Press, 1979, chap 12.

13 : Therapy of Heart Failure and Myocardial Ischemia: Relation to Pathophysiologic Principles

The best therapeutic approach to any disease is based on a sound understanding of the pathophysiology of the condition under treatment. Medical or surgical therapy seeks to interrupt or reverse the pathophysiologic sequence of the illness. A simple example follows: multiplication of staphylococci with production of a variety of toxins plays a central role in the pathophysiology of a staphylococcal skin abscess. An understanding of the pathophysiology of this entity enables one to select an antistaphylococcal antibiotic to treat this condition, thereby eradicating the central factor in the pathophysiologic sequence of staphylococcal skin abscess. In a similar manner, an understanding of the pathophysiology of heart failure or myocardial ischemia enables the physician to select medical or surgical therapeutic interventions that interrupt or reverse the pathophysiologic sequence.

Heart Failure

As noted in earlier chapters, heart failure with its attendant signs and symptoms is the result of inadequate cardiac output with respect to the demand of the peripheral tissues for blood flow. A variety of compensatory mechanisms are set into motion (autonomic nervous system, renal, and pulmonary) in an attempt to correct the decrease in tissue perfusion that results from the depressed cardiac function. A variety of medical and surgical interventions attempt to correct these abnormal physiologic events in patients with heart failure.

Positive inotropic agents

Decreased cardiac function is the hallmark of heart failure. Therefore, one logical approach to reverse the pathophysiologic sequence of heart failure is an improvement in overall cardiac function. A number of pharmacologic agents have been shown to possess positive inotropic action on the myocardium, that is, they increase the vigor of myocardial contraction and thereby augment cardiac output (Fig. 13-1). Digitalis glycosides seem to increase myocardial contractility by inhibiting the function of membrane-bound Na^+/K^+ ATPase. This results in a net increase in intracellular Na^+ and Ca^{2+}. Increased Ca^{2+} availability in the intracellular environment apparently leads to augmented actin-myosin interaction with a resultant increase in myocardial contractility. Increased myocardial contractile state leads to improved overall cardiac function: cardiac output rises, peripheral

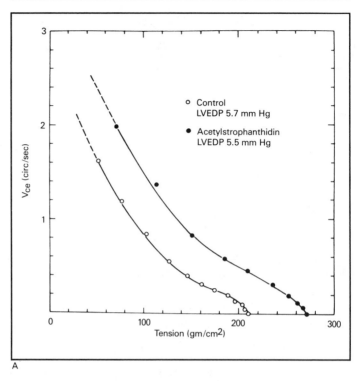

A

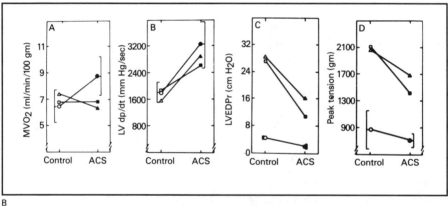

B

Fig. 13-1 : A. Myocardial contractility (as measured by velocity of contractile element shortening [V_{ce}]) in an open chested dog left ventricle during single induced isovolumetric beats before and approximately 30 mintues after intravenous administration of the digitalis preparation, acetylstrophanthidin (ACS). Left ventricular end diastolic pressure (LVEDP) was held constant. (From Taylor RR et al: A quantitative analysis of left ventricular myocardial function in the intact, sedated dog. *Circ Res* 21:99, 1967, with permission of the authors and publisher.) B. Effect of the digitalis preparation, acetylstrophanthidin, before and after acute cardiac dilatation and failure were induced in the left ventricle of an anesthetized dog. In each panel the response in a group of normal dogs is represented by circles (open circles before and closed circles after ACS). The brackets represent ± 1 standard deviation. Triangles and squares represent experiments in which acute cardiac failure was produced experimentally with marked elevation of left ventricular end-diastolic pressure and peak calculated perfusion improves, and ventricular filling pressures fall. Excess pulmonary and/or systemic interstitial fluid, generated by high capillary pressures associated with heart failure, is reabsorbed when capillary hydrostatic pressure falls. Blood volume increases activating renal compensatory mechanisms that lead to an increase in salt and water excretion. Early observers thought that digitalis was a diuretic (i.e., it increased urine flow) because they observed an increase in urine output following the administration of digitalis to patients with edema secondary to heart failure.

Increases in myocardial contractility lead to increased myocardial oxygen consumption (MVO_2) in normal myocardium. Digitalis glycosides *increase* MVO_2 in normal myocardium. As noted in Chapter 2, increased MVO_2 in the setting of restricted myocardial blood flow (coronary artery disease) can lead to myocardial ischemia. In failing myocardium, digitalis administration leads to a *decrease* in MVO_2 secondary to improved myocardial function with resultant decreased ventricular wall stress (Fig. 13-1).

Compounds that stimulate beta-adrenergic receptors in the myocardium also lead to increases in myocardial contractility. A number of catecholamines stimulate myocardial beta receptors with resultant improved overall myocardial performance (Fig. 13-2). Natural and synthetic catecholamines that possess such myocardial stimulatory properties are listed in Table 13-1.

Diuretics

Diuretic compounds increase urine flow by impairing the kidney's ability to reabsorb salt and water (see Chap. 9). Paralysis of normal renal salt and water reabsorption can be induced at a variety of sites along the nephron. For example, thiazide diuretics inhibit Na^+ reabsorption in the proximal portion of the distal convoluted tubule; furosemide, on the other hand, inhibits Na^+ reabsorption in the ascending limb of the loop of Henle.

Diuresis reduces blood volume thereby decreasing ventricular filling pressures with resultant decrements in systemic and pulmonary capillary pressures. Interstitial fluid is reabsorbed leading to a resolution of signs and symptoms of heart failure.

---

wall tension. Stroke volume, heart rate, and cardiac output were maintained constant in this experimental preparation. In normal dogs, myocardial oxygen consumption (MVO_2) was increased by the administration of ACS, myocardial contractility of the left ventricle (LV dp/dt) was increased by the administration of ACS, and there was little change in left ventricular end-diastolic pressure (LVEDPr) and peak wall tension following the administration of ACS. In contrast, in the acutely failing ventricle (triangles and squares), ACS produced no change or a slight decrease in myocardial oxygen consumption, an increase in myocardial contractility (LV dp/dt), and a substantial decrease in left ventricular end-diastolic pressure and peak wall tension. (From Covell JW et al: Studies on digitalis: XVI. Effects on myocardial oxygen consumption. *J Clin Invest* 45:1535, 1966, with permission of the authors and publisher.)

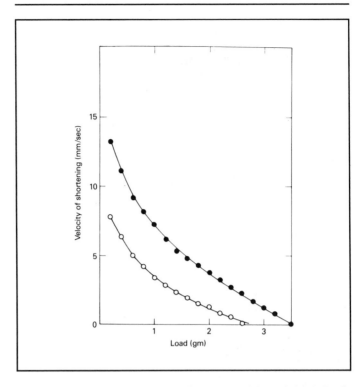

Fig. 13-2 : Effect on myocardial contractility (velocity of shortening) in isolated myocardial muscle of addition of norepinephrine (NE) to the experimental preparation. A small amount of norepinephrine induces a marked increase in the force-velocity relationship for the small piece of myocardium. In intact ventricles a similar increase in myocardial contractility results from norepinephrine induced stimulation of the myocardium. Control values are shown as open circles and values obtained following the addition of 0.05 γ/ml norepinephrine (rate 60) to the experimental preparation shown as closed circles. (From Braunwald E, Ross J Jr, Sonneblick EH: *Mechanisms of Contraction of the Normal and Failing Heart.* Boston, Little, Brown, 1976, with permission of the authors and publisher.)

Table 13-1 : Naturally occurring and synthetic catecholamines with beta₁-stimulating properties

Epinephrine
Norepinephrine
Isoproterenol
Dopamine
Dobutamine

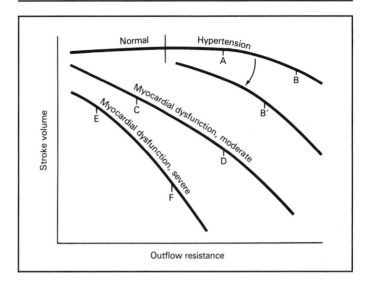

Fig. 13-3 : Relationship between left ventricular stroke volume and systemic aortic outflow resistance in normal and diseased hearts. A family of curves may be described depending on the severity of the myocardial disease. If cardiac function is reasonably normal, a rise in outflow resistance results in hypertension since cardiac output remains fairly constant. Heart failure in a hypertensive patient would occur in an individual who moves from point A to point B (high resistance with normal myocardial function) or point B′ (high resistance with slightly depressed left ventricular function). When myocardial dysfunction is more severe, minor changes in outflow resistance and blood pressure may result in marked changes in stroke volume. Thus, a patient with moderate or severe myocardial dysfunction and high outflow resistance would move from point D or F to point C and E with only modest decrease in resistance but with a rather remarkable increase in stroke volume. In a patient with normal myocardial function (the uppermost curve), reduction in outflow resistance (from point B to A) results in only a very small increase in stroke volume. (From Cohn JN, Franciosa JA: Vasodilator therapy of cardiac failure. *N Engl J Med* 297:27, 1977, with permission of the authors and publisher.)

Vasodilators

Heart failure activates the same autonomic nervous responses as hemorrhage. Decreased cardiac output is perceived by arterial baro-receptors and the renal juxtaglomerular apparatus as decreased circulating blood volume. The adrenergic nervous system and the renin-angiotensin cascade is activated with resultant arteriolar vasoconstriction and increased peripheral vascular resistance.

Left ventricular ejection into the aorta is ultimately impeded by the increased level of peripheral vascular resistance. Thus, excessive increases in peripheral vascular resistance in patients with heart failure can actually lead to increased left ventricular work (and further decreases in left ventricular function) at a time when cardiac function is already compromised and least able to tolerate such alterations (Fig. 13-3). Many patients with left ventricular failure have excessively increased peripheral vascular resistance. These individuals benefit from a reduction in peripheral vascular resistance and the associated decrease in left ventricular work. A variety of vasodilator compounds can decrease peripheral vascular resistance, thereby decreasing left ventricular work (afterload, wall tension) and improving cardiac function (Fig. 13-3). Cardiac output rises and ventricular filling pressure declines as do systemic and pulmonary capillary pressures.

Surgical interventions

A number of cardiovascular diseases that lead to left and/or right ventricular failure require surgical therapy to alleviate signs and symptoms of heart failure. For example, patients with aortic stenosis who develop left ventricular failure achieve transient amelioration from medical therapy, i.e., digitalis glycosides, diuretics, and vasodilators. Surgical relief of obstruction by valvulotomy or valve replacement is the only form of therapy that offers major and lasting improvement to patients with aortic stenosis. Other valvular lesions (stenosis, regurgitation), coarctation of the aorta, atrial and ventricular septal defects, patent ductus arteriosus, and ventricular aneurysm are some of the relatively common cardiovascular conditions that often require surgical intervention in order to relieve signs and symptoms of heart failure.

Myocardial ischemia

As noted in Chapter 2, myocardial ischemia with its attendant symptoms occurs as a result of imbalance between myocardial blood flow (supply) and myocardial oxygen consumption (demand). In patients with severe atherosclerotic coronary arterial narrowings, myocardial ischemia results from an increase in myocardial oxygen consumption (MVO_2) beyond the capacity of the pathologically altered coronary arterial network to supply the needed quantity of oxygen and nutrient containing blood. In such individuals, therapy attempts to decrease myocardial oxygen consumption. A subset of patients with atherosclerotic coronary artery disease have episodes of dynamic coronary arterial obstruction. That is, contraction of vascular smooth muscle of large epicardial coronary arteries (usually in the vicinity of atherosclerotic coronary arterial plaques) produces reversible coronary artery obstruction. In such patients, therapy focuses on relaxing vascular smooth muscle and thereby reversing the episode of dynamic arterial obstruction or coronary spasm. Many patients with coronary artery disease have a mixture of the two pathophysiologic mechanisms (excessive myocardial metabolic demand and coronary spasm) that lead to myocardial ischemia. In such patients, therapeutic endeavors focus on reversing both mechanisms that lead to myocardial ischemia.

Medical Therapy to Lower Myocardial Oxygen Consumption

Beta-adrenergic blocking agents

Beta-adrenergic blocking agents (or "beta-blockers") decrease myocardial oxygen consumption (MVO_2) in three ways (Fig. 13-4). First,

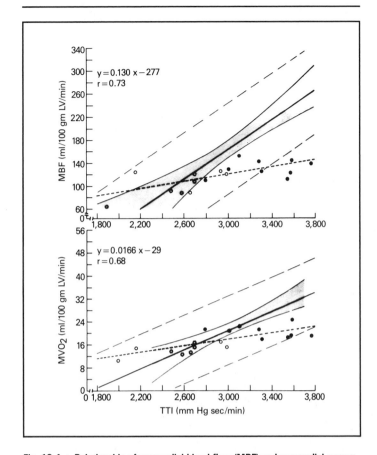

Fig. 13-4 : Relationship of myocardial blood flow (MBF) and myocardial oxygen consumption (MVO₂) to the tension time index (systolic blood pressure × heart rate) in young healthy men during upright bicycle exercise before and after the administration of a beta-adrenergic blocking agent, propranolol. The solid center line surrounded by the shaded area represents the 95% confidence limits for data obtained in the absence of propranolol. The single dotted line, along which are plotted the circles, represents the regression line for values obtained following the administration of propranolol. It is clear that the relationship of myocardial blood flow and oxygen consumption to tension time index is markedly altered by the administration of propranolol. Myocardial blood flow and myocardial oxygen consumption increase at a much slower rate following the addition of propranolol. Patients worked at relatively light workloads (open circles) and at higher workloads (solid circles). (From Jorgensen CR et al: Effect of propranolol on myocardial oxygen consumption and its hemodynamic correlates during upright exercise. *Circulation* 48:1173, 1973, with permission of the authors and publisher.)

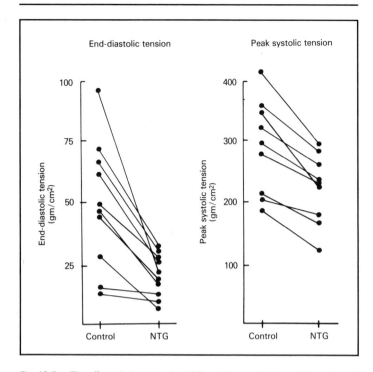

Fig. 13-5 : The effect of nitroglycerin (NTG) on left ventricular end-diastolic and peak systolic wall tension in 10 patients. End-diastolic tension and peak systolic tension are markedly and significantly reduced by the administration of nitroglycerin. End-diastolic and end-systolic wall tensions are determinants of myocardial oxygen consumption. Therefore the reduction in these two variables by nitroglycerin should result in a marked reduction in myocardial oxygen consumption as well. (From Greenberg H et al: Effects of nitroglycerin on the major determinants of myocardial oxygen consumption. An angiographic and hemodynamic assessment. *Am J Cardiol* **36:426, 1975, with permission of the authors and the publisher.)**

beta-blockers decrease adrenergic chronotropic stimulation of the heart. Resting and exercise heart rate decreases, thereby lessening MVO_2 both at rest and during exercise. Second, beta-blockers decrease arterial blood pressure thereby lessening left ventricular afterload and consequently MVO_2. Finally, beta-blockers depress myocardial contractility, another factor in the determination of MVO_2 (see Chap. 2). Taken together, these properties of beta-blocking compounds decrease MVO_2 and the tendency for an individual with coronary arterial narrowings to develop myocardial ischemia. Beta-blockers have also been employed in the therapy of early phases of acute myocardial infarction to lessen MVO_2 in the border zone between normal and critically ischemic myocardium. It is the aim of such therapy to reduce the extent of the myocardial infarct.

Nitrates   Nitrates decrease MVO_2 by two mechanisms: reduction in ventricular cavity size and reduction in arterial blood pressure (Fig. 13-5). Nitrates relax vascular smooth muscle, particularly on the venous side of the circulation. This leads to venodilatation and pooling of blood in the venous system with a resultant shift of blood volume away from the central circulation. Ventricular volume is therefore lessened, and ventricular wall tension and MVO$_2$ consequently decline. Nitrates induce a modest degree of arteriolar smooth muscle relaxation. Arteriolar vasodilatation and the shifting of blood to the venous side of the circulation combine to produce a modest decline in arterial blood pressure—left ventricular afterload and MVO$_2$ are thereby reduced. Nitrates are therapeutically employed in patients with stable ischemic heart disease as well as in patients with acute myocardial infarction. In the latter group of patients, nitrate therapy is employed in an effort to reduce myocardial infarction size.

Calcium channel blocking agents

This heterogeneous group of compounds are potent relaxors of vascular smooth muscle. Thus, they reduce MVO$_2$ in the same manner as nitrates by reducing ventricular volume and arterial blood pressure. In addition, certain calcium channel blockers depress myocardial contractility and others decrease the heart rate. Both of these latter two properties result in a decrease in MVO$_2$.

Modification of activity

Exercise leads to increases in heart rate, arterial blood pressure, and myocardial contractility with resultant augmentation of MVO$_2$. Therefore, medical regimens for patients with coronary artery disease should preclude periods of heavy, strenuous exercise with attendant marked increase in MVO$_2$. Regular, moderate exercise sessions, however, have been shown to be beneficial in these patients.

Surgical therapy to lower myocardial oxygen consumption

Certain pathologic entities produce marked increases in myocardial oxygen consumption that can lead to myocardial ischemia. For example, aortic stenosis produces increases in left ventricular myocardial mass and workload that can lead to myocardial ischemia even in the absence of coronary arterial obstruction (see Chap. 5). In such individuals, aortic valvulotomy or replacement results in a marked decrease in MVO$_2$ often with relief of signs and symptoms of myocardial ischemia. Another example of surgical therapy that decreases MVO$_2$ is found in the patient with left ventricular aneurysm. In these individuals, the aneurysm impairs normal left ventricular function leading to left ventricular dilatation with resultant increase in MVO$_2$. Removal of the aneurysm results in improved left ventricular function, and a decrease in ventricular cavity size and MVO$_2$.

Medical therapy to increase myocardial blood flow

Nitrates and calcium channel blockers are both potent relaxors of vascular smooth muscle. As such, they are both capable of producing coronary arterial vasodilatation with resultant increases in myocardial blood flow. Episodes of coronary arterial vasospasm can be lysed or prevented with these two pharmacologic agents.

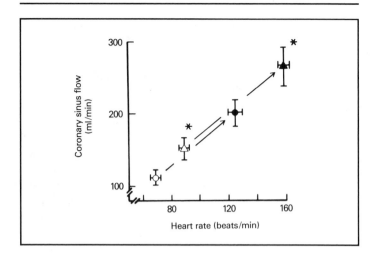

Fig. 13-6 : Coronary sinus blood flow (total heart blood flow) before and after aortocoronary artery bypass grafting in patients with coronary artery disease. The open circle represents preoperative resting value for heart blood flow; the closed circle represents the preoperative blood flow value during pacing-induced angina pectoris; the open triangle represents postoperative myocardial blood flow at rest; and the closed triangle represents postoperative myocardial blood flow at the maximum pacing rate (angina pectoris could no longer be induced by pacing). There are higher coronary sinus blood flow (myocardial blood flow) values following operation both at rest and during pacing. *p $<$ 0.01. (From Chatterjee K et al: Improved angina threshold and coronary reserve following direct myocardial revascularization. *Circulation* 51/52 (Suppl 1):I-81, 1975, with permission of the authors and publisher.)

Surgical therapy to increase myocardial blood flow

Coronary arterial bypass grafting with a reversed segment of saphenous vein is a surgical procedure commonly employed to increase myocardial blood flow in patients with critical coronary arterial obstruction (Fig. 13-6). The vein grafts are placed between the aorta and a segment of coronary artery that lies distal to the atherosclerotic obstruction. This procedure results in an unobstructed conduit between the aorta and the distal coronary arterial system. Myocardial blood flow is no longer impeded by the atherosclerotic narrowings in the proximal coronary arterial circulation. Increased MVO_2 such as that resulting from exercise is accompanied by increased myocardial blood flow in patients with patent coronary arterial bypass grafts.

14 : Pathophysiology of Cardiac Electrical Disturbances

Emil R. Smith

Each normal heart beat is the result of a series of highly complex, coordinated electrical and mechanical events that serve the sole purpose of delivering blood into the aorta. Among the more common derangements of cardiac function are the *cardiac arrhythmias*, a large number of conditions characterized by disturbances in the heart's ability to initiate and/or conduct impulses in the normal manner. As might be expected, when arrhythmias interfere with the pumping action of the heart, they can produce a spectrum of effects including palpitations, hypotension, fatigue, lightheadedness, dizziness, syncope, convulsions, coma, and death. In susceptible subjects they can also cause angina, congestive heart failure, and pulmonary edema. This chapter will first review briefly some basic cardiac electrophysiology and pathophysiology. Then after a description of the major classes of arrhythmias and the general methods available for their treatment, the most common cardiac arrhythmias and their specific treatments will be reviewed.

The Electrical Activity of the Heart

It has been known for many years that there are electrical events associated with each heart beat and that they can be recorded from metal electrodes placed on the surface of the body. Based on standardized recordings (12 leads) of these patterns of activity, electrocardiography has become a very sophisticated means of assessing the status of the heart. For dealing with cardiac arrhythmias, the *rhythm-strip* has proved of particular value. This is a long electrocardiographic recording that has clear and prominent waves allowing an accurate assessment of the site of origin and course of conduction of the individual beats. Lead II (right arm to left leg) is most often used for this purpose, although at times other leads, especially leads I (right arm to left arm) and III (left arm to left leg), may be used. For the present purposes emphasis will be placed on interpretations of cardiac rhythm based upon recordings of lead II.

The electrocardiogram

Normally, each heart beat arises from a group of specialized cells within the sinoatrial (SA) node and is conducted throughout the heart in an orderly manner (Fig. 14-1). The resultant rhythm is called "normal sinus rhythm." During such rhythm, electrical activity spreads out of the SA node and over the specialized atrial conduction

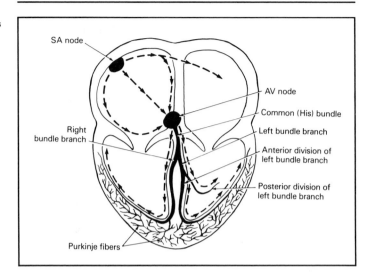

system into atrial working myocardium; the resulting atrial depolarization gives rise to the P wave of the electrocardiogram (ECG). After a delay encountered in passing along slowly conducting cells within the atrioventricular (AV) node, the activity propagates more rapidly over the specialized conduction system and the ventricle, producing the QRS complex. Repolarization of the ventricle is associated with the T wave. Under some circumstances a small U wave may follow the T wave.

Fig. 14-2 shows a short strip of normal sinus rhythm recorded via lead II and a diagram of two consecutive beats showing the universal designation for the characteristic waves (P, QRS, T, and U) and the corresponding intervals (P–R, QRS, and Q-T). By convention, standard tracings are recorded at a paper speed of 25 mm/second (five large divisions/ mV). The voltage calibration is seen below the arrow in the tracing. The R-R intervals for the beats shown are all about 20 mm (0.80 sec). The P-R, QRS and Q-T intervals are 0.14, 0.06 and 0.36 seconds, respectively. Normal ranges for P-R and QRS are 0.12–0.20 and 0.06–0.10 second, respectively. The Q-T interval is inversely related to heart rate and varies accordingly.

Normal and abnormal cardiac pacemakers

Starting with this basic knowledge of cardiac electrophysiology and electrocardiography, it is not difficult to understand arrhythmias attributable to conduction defects. However, arrhythmias due to defects in impulse formation require a greater appreciation of the potential of cardiac cells to initiate beats.

THE PACEMAKER HIERARCHY. Central to the understanding of cardiac arrhythmias is the principle that there is a hierarchy of pacemakers in the heart. There are a number of cells that, because of their inherent automaticity, possess the potential to act as the primary pacemaker

Fig. 14-2 : Normal sinus rhythm. (This tracing and those in all subsequent figures except Fig. 14-20 are reproduced and modified with permission of the California Heart Association.)

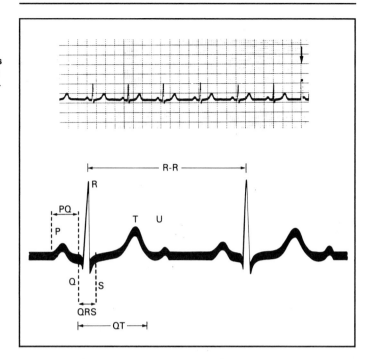

or initiator of the heart beat. Prominent among these are cells within the SA node, the AV node, and the Purkinje system. However, at any given time the cardiac rhythm is determined by the fastest beating cell(s) because each beat depolarizes all other potential pacemaker cells and interferes with their ability to initiate impulses. Since, under normal conditions, the cells in the SA node beat fastest, each normal beat is initiated within this node; i.e. as in normal sinus rhythm (Fig. 14-2).

If, for whatever reason, the activity of the SA node is disrupted, the fastest beating of the remaining functioning cells becomes the pacemaker. These secondary pacemaker cells are usually within the AV node and the resultant rhythm is called ''nodal rhythm.'' This rhythm is characterized by a slower rate than accompanies sinus rhythm (reflecting less inherent automaticity) and the absence of upright P waves in the electrocardiogram (the atria are not activated, at least in the normal manner). On the other hand, the QRS complex and T waves are generally normal because the activation of the ventricle occurs normally. Figure 14-3 shows an example of nodal rhythm; the heart rate in this case is 53 beats/minute and the morphology of the ventricular complex is relatively normal.

Under circumstances where both the SA node and the AV node fail to pace the heart, the latent automatic cells of the ventricular Purkinje system will usually assume the role of pacemaker. The resultant *idioventricular rhythm* is characterized by its slow rate, from 20 to

Fig. 14-3 : Nodal
rhythm.

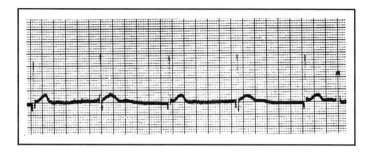

Fig. 14-4 : Idioven-
tricular rhythm.

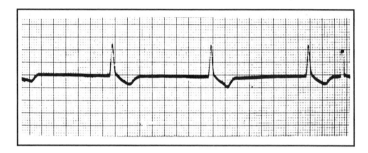

45 beats/minute; in addition, rather than exhibiting the normal con-
figurations, the ventricular complexes assume a configuration dependent upon the site of origin of the beat and the pathway of its propagation. Since the beat is not propagated over the ventricles in a
normal manner, the morphology of the beat will not be normal—the
QRS complex generally will be wider than normal and the direction
and amplitude of the R and T waves may be abnormal. An ECG
depicting idioventricular rhythm is shown in Fig. 14-4. The heart
rate estimated from this rhythm strip is slow, 38 beats/minute, the
QRS-interval is long, 0.12 second, and the QRS morphology is abnormal and characteristic of idioventricular beats.

It must be appreciated that this hierarchy of SA nodal, AV nodal, and
ventricular pacemakers serves an important function in providing the
heart with a backup system should the principal pacemaker(s) fail.
While slow AV nodal and idioventricular rhythms are abnormal, automaticity in such hearts should not be further suppressed (e.g., by
drugs). Complete cessation of cardiac activity, *cardiac standstill*,
could result.

THE ECTOPIC FOCUS. While the heart beat normally arises from within
the SA node and, as has been described, can also arise from within
the AV node and the Purkinje network, beats that can arise from
electrical events initiated within such sites are called "ectopic
beats," and the site of origin, which may be so small as to involve a
single or only a few cells, is called an "ectopic focus." The exact
anatomic location of such ectopic foci can be determined with some
degree of precision, but the electrophysiologic events occurring

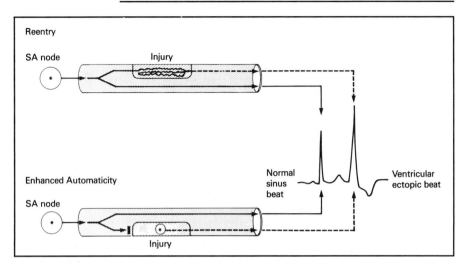

Fig. 14-5 : Schemes depicting the generation of ectopic beats by reentry and by enhanced automaticity.

therein are still unclear because it has not been technically possible to record from such foci during their activity. Thus, at present, our hypotheses about impulse formation within ectopic foci are based upon a variety of indirect observations.

It would seem that activity can be generated from ectopic foci in two distinctly different ways. In one case the focus generates impulses in a manner that is dependent on a prior external electrical event in another region of the heart. The initiating beat (which may be either a normal sinus beat or an ectopic beat) enters the ectopic focus where it is delayed in some manner until the surrounding tissue recovers from the initiating activity. Electrical depolarizing activity then emerges from the ectopic focus to stimulate the now excitable surrounding tissue. Not surprisingly, this phenomenon is called "reentry" and the arrhythmias generated in this manner are called "reentrant arrhythmias." Many arrhythmias in man seem to be generated in this manner.

Alternatively, there are examples of ectopic activity that are apparently the result of enhanced automaticity. This activity is not associated with preceding electrical events, but rather occurs independently. In these cases, the ectopic focus may represent one or more neighboring cells with enhanced automaticity that functions not unlike a misplaced, fast-firing, SA node that competes with other pacemakers for expression. *Accelerated idioventricular rhythm*, a distinct but not too common arrhythmia in man, is probably an example of this.

Figure 14-5 shows how ectopic beats might arise due to reentry and to enhanced automaticity. With respect to reentry (top of figure), the normal sinus beats are initiated within the SA node due to its automaticity (asterisk) and conducted over the heart in the normal manner (solid line) giving rise to normal sinus beats (to the right). In the presence of myocardial injury (shaded area) the impulses reaching the injury (dashed line) are delayed due to a slowing of conduction in the area (wavy line) and/or because they are forced along a circuitous route. Under appropriate conditions they reemerge into normal tissue to reactivate the heart in a manner dependent on the exact location of the injury (ectopic focus) and produce an aberrant or ectopic beat (far right). The abnormal beat shown has the general characteristics of an ectopic beat arising from a ventricular focus. In cases of enhanced automaticity (bottom of figure) a highly automatic ectopic focus develops in a region of injury where conditions are such that it is protected from depolarization by normally initiated impulses but can itself activate the heart to produce ectopic beats. Notice that the morphology of the abnormal beat gives no clue as to the possible mechanism for its production.

Cardiac Arrhythmias and Their Treatment

Since the term *cardiac arrhythmia* is used to refer to a wide variety of disturbances in either the initiation or the conduction of the heart beat, arrhythmias can be conveniently classified on these bases. Because the defects represent conditions where events occur either too slowly or too rapidly, there are four major categories of arrhythmia (Table 14-1): those representing defects where impulse initiation is too slow (the bradyarrhythmias) or too fast (the tachyarrhythmias), or where conduction through part of the heart is too slow or too fast.

Since arrhythmias are the consequence of a wide variety of underlying diseases (e.g., ischemic heart disease, electrolyte disturbances, drug toxicity), treatment should at all times be directed towards these basic disturbances. In addition, there are, however, more specific measures for controlling arrhythmias.

Drugs

A wide variety of drugs are used in the treatment of cardiac arrhythmias, but in general they fall into three groups: (1) those drugs that modify the control of cardiac function by the autonomic nervous system, (2) the naturally occurring and semisynthetic agents known collectively as the "cardiac glycosides" or "digitalis," and (3) a group of drugs known as "antiarrhythmic agents." It should be noted that not all drugs used to treat arrhythmias are considered antiarrhythmic agents, and that antiarrhythmic agents are not used to treat all arrhythmias.

AUTONOMIC AGENTS. Drugs that interact with the autonomic nervous system can selectively control certain arrhythmias by virtue of their ability to suppress or stimulate impulse formation and/or conduction in the heart. Among these agents, the anticholinergic drugs, such as atropine, stimulate the heart by blocking the inhibitory effect of the

Table 14-1 : Classification of major cardiac arrhythmias

Classification	Individual arrhythmias	Specific treatment(s)
Defects in initiation of the heart beat	Bradyarrhythmias	
	Sinus bradycardia	Atropine, electrical pacing
	Sinus arrhythmia	Usually no therapy
	Nodal rhythm	Atropine, electrical pacing
	Idioventricular rhythm	Atropine, electrical pacing
	Ventricular standstill	Chest thump, cardiac massage and intravenous epinephrine, electrical pacing
	Tachyarrhythmias	
	Sinus tachycardia	Propranolol
	Atrial premature beats	Usually no therapy
	Paroxysmal atrial tachycardia	Increase vagal tone, propranolol, verapamil, electrical pacing, cardioversion
	Atrial flutter	Cardioversion, cardiac glycoside, propranolol
	Atrial fibrillation	Cardioversion, cardiac glycoside, propranolol, quinidine, verapamil
	Nodal premature beats	Usually no therapy
	Nodal tachycardia	Increase vagal tone, propranolol, verapamil, electrical pacing, cardioversion
	Ventricular premature beats	Quinidine, procainamide, lidocaine, disopyramide
	Ventricular bigeminy	Quinidine, procainamide, lidocaine, disopyramide
	Ventricular tachycardia	Quinidine, procainamide, lidocaine, disopyramide
	Ventricular flutter	Quinidine, procainamide, lidocaine, disopyramide
	Ventricular fibrillation	Electrical defibrillation
Defects in conduction of the heart beat	States of impaired conduction	
	Sinoatrial block	Usually no therapy
	Atrioventricular block	Vagolytic drugs, sympathomimetic amines, electrical pacing
	Intraventricular block	No specific treatment(s)
	States of enhanced conduction	
	Short P-R interval in the Wolff-Parkinson-White syndrome	Surgery, propranolol, no therapy
	Short P-R interval in the Lown-Ganong-Levine syndrome	Surgery, propranolol, no therapy

arrhythmic agents and has proven effective in the suppression of, and prevention of, life-threatening ventricular tachyarrhythmias. Verapamil is also distinctly different from all other agents. It is often referred to as a "calcium channel blocker" because it strongly inhibits calcium-carried membrane currents in cardiac cells.

As seen in Table 14-2, the effectiveness of these antiarrhythmic agents against tachyarrhythmias can be described, at best, as "often effective." Patients with these arrhythmias do not uniformly respond favorably to treatment—drug-resistant arrhythmias are common. As a result, patients are often treated in sequence with several drugs, in trial-and-error fashion, seeking an effective treatment.

Drug-induced adverse or toxic effects are a continuous problem when treating patients with these agents. This reflects the basic nature of these drugs as a group, and in addition reflects the use of maximally tolerated doses as a consequence of their relative ineffectiveness, especially in some patients. Quinidine, procainamide, and disopyramide produce undesirable depressant effects upon the heart; especially prominent are impairments in conduction. In fact, the width of the QRS is often monitored during treatment to prevent overdosing. In addition to these cardiac depressant effects, quinidine can also cause gastrointestinal side effects. Moreover, a syndrome resembling lupus erythematosus is not uncommon after chronic use of high doses of procainamide. Quinidine, procainamide and disopyramide all have vagolytic actions; however, disopyramide also produces anticholinergic side effects, especially dry mouth, urinary hesitancy, visual disturbances, and constipation. The principal adverse effects of lidocaine are generally preceded by tingling of the lips, and involve the central nervous system—lightheadedness, muscular twitching, and convulsions. Phenytoin causes a different spectrum of central nervous system effects—nystagmus, ataxia, slurred speech, visual disturbances, and behavioral changes. Bretylium causes bothersome postural hypotension, and verapamil causes hypotension, bradycardia, and depression of intracardiac conduction and cardiac contractility.

As a consequence of the failure of these drugs to be widely effective, considerable effort is now being directed towards developing new agents that may be even more effective. However, because these newer agents now in clinical trial are not widely available, their description is beyond the scope of this chapter. Nevertheless, reports of the clinical trials being conducted on these agents, especially amiodarone, aprindine, ethmozin, mexelitine, and tocainide, are not uncommon.

Reflexly-induced vagal stimulation

Cardiac arrhythmias can also be controlled by a variety of nondrug means. Because of the marked depressant effects of the vagus nerve upon supraventricular electrical function, some supraventricular tachyarrhythmias can be terminated by measures that increase vagal tone. Intravenous infusions of pressor agents have already been described as one means of reflexly turning on the vagus nerve. Carotid sinus massage is another. When properly done, massage stimulates carotid sinus baroreceptors and reflexly increases vagal tone, depressing the automaticity, excitability, and conductibility of supraventricular structures. In patients with certain arrhythmias this may normalize cardiac rhythm. Vagal activity can also be increased by other means, notably Valsalva's maneuver and gagging.

CARDIOVERSION. Some tachyarrhythmias can be terminated electrically. Such *cardioversion* involves placing large electrodes on the skin of the back and the chest and then applying a brief but strong direct current shock between the electrodes. Shocks of appropriate size will completely depolarize all of the cells of the heart, and normal sinus rhythm usually resumes shortly thereafter. Cardioversion is somewhat more complicated in patients who have been treated with a cardiac glycoside because severe glycoside-related cardiotoxicity may become manifest after conversion.

Electrical pacing

In some patients with arrhythmias it may be advisably or necessary to pace the heart electrically using an electronic pacemaker to deliver stimuli of appropriate magnitude to the atria and/or ventricles by electrode-tipped catheters threaded into the heart via the venous circulation. For this purpose there are many electrical pacemakers available commercially. In general they fall into two categories: those for temporary pacing utilizing a pulse generator located outside the body; and those for long-term, chronic use where the impulse generator and power source are planted subcutaneously. Some of these pacemakers stimulate the heart at a constant fixed rate at all times, while the output of others is controlled by circuits sensing the presence or absence of P waves or R waves and responding accordingly.

Temporary and/or permanent pacemakers are used in the treatment of patients with severe bradyarrhythmias, where heart rate must be maintained at more reasonable levels. They are also used for patients with conduction defects that might progress to complete failure of all cardiac activity, and under certain conditions to suppress or prevent the appearance of some tachyarrhythmias.

Surgery

The possibility of surgically terminating drug-resistant, severe or life-threatening ventricular tachyarrhythmias is presently receiving considerable attention. In patients with rapidly discharging ventricular ectopic foci producing tachyarrhythmias, the electrical activity of both the epicardial and endocardial surfaces of the ventricles can be recorded before and/or during open-heart surgery in order to deter-

Fig. 14-6 : Sinus bradycardia.

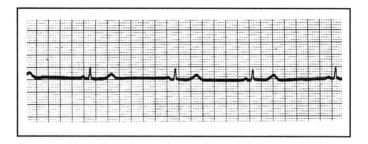

mine the exact site of origin of the ectopic beats. After being located, the ectopic focus can then be removed surgically or destroyed by freezing. The initial results with this surgical approach for controlling ventricular tachyarrhythmias have been encouraging, but its role in treating these arrhythmias is far from established.

Arrhythmias Due Primarily to Defects in Initiation of Electrical Activity

Bradyarrhythmias

The following is a brief description of major bradyarrhythmias and the means by which they are treated (Table 14-1). These arrhythmias are characterized by failure of normal impulse formation within the SA node and by the failure of automatic pacemakers to develop as expected within the AV node or ventricles.

SINUS BRADYCARDIA. Persons in normal sinus rhythm generally have a heart rate in the range of 60–100 beats/minute. In *sinus bradycardia* the heart beat is initiated and conducted normally, except that the heart rate is slow, less than 60 beats/minute. In the example given in Figure 14-6 the rate is about 43 beats/minute and the Q-T interval is long but normal for a slowly beating heart.

If the heart rate of patients with sinus bradycardia slows excessively or if symptoms develop, the rate can be increased by the administration of anticholinergic agents. Intravenously administered atropine is most widely used for this purpose.

SINUS ARRHYTHMIA. Some ECGs may exhibit what resembles normal sinus rhythm except that there are obvious cyclical variations in the P-P intervals. This is called "sinus arrhythmia," (Fig. 14-7) and the cyclical variations are related to respiration, with shorter intervals corresponding to inspiration. In the tracing shown in Fig. 14-7 the variation in cycle length is readily apparent; the R-R intervals are 0.70, 0.86, 0.64, 0.82, and 0.70 seconds, respectively. While sinus arrhythmia may cause concern in some patients who are aware of their irregular heart beat, it rarely has hemodynamic consequences or merits treatment.

Fig. 14-7 : Sinus arrhythmia.

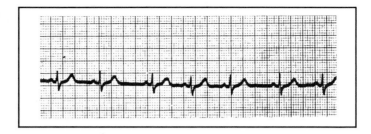

Fig. 14-8 : Nodal rhythm with inverted P waves.

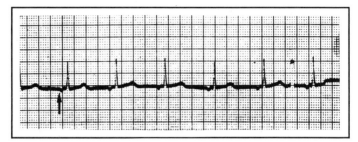

NODAL RHYTHM AND IDIOVENTRICULAR RHYTHM. Two other examples of bradyarrhythmias have already been given— *nodal rhythm* (Fig. 14-3) and *idioventricular rhythm* (Fig. 14-4). Nodal rhythm usually results when for some reason the SA node becomes inactive and pacemaker activity shifts down to the AV node. In the example of nodal rhythm shown in Fig. 14-4, no distinct P waves are seen. However, inverted P waves may occur in some cases. This is the case in the example shown in Fig. 14-8. When the pacemaker is located within the AV node it activates the ventricle in the normal, antegrade manner producing a normal QRS complex and T wave. At the same time, this AV nodal pacemaker can also activate the atria in a retrograde manner. This latter sequence produces an inverted P wave because the atria are activated in a manner that is the reverse of the normal pathway of activation.

From Fig. 14-8 it will be appreciated that if both the inverted P wave and the normal ventricular complex result from the same pacemaker, then activity of that pacemaker must have preceded the earlier of the two events (i.e., inscription of the inverted P wave), occurring at about the relative time indicated by the arrow before the first fully recorded beat. It should also be appreciated that the relative positions of the inverted P wave and the ventricular complex in the ECG will be related to the position of the pacemaker relative to the atria and the ventricles. If the pacemaker is located relatively close to the atria, the inverted P wave will clearly precede the ventricular complex, whereas if the pacemaker is located relatively close to the ventricles, the inverted P wave may be lost in the ventricular complex (see Fig. 14-3). These conditions have been referred to as "high nodal rhythm" and "low nodal rhythm," respectively. If the AV node

Fig. 14-9 : Sinus tachycardia.

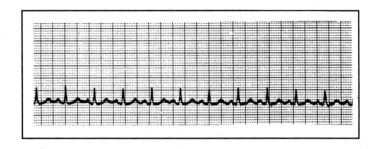

also fails, the pacemaker shifts again to the Purkinje fibers of the ventricle, resulting in idioventricular rhythm (see Fig. 14-4).

Treatment of both nodal and idioventricular rhythm is directed towards reestablishing the activity of both the SA and AV nodes and may involve reducing vagal tone by the use of atropine. Electrical pacing may be necessary.

CARDIAC ASYSTOLE. If cardiac automaticity is sufficiently depressed, for whatever reasons, the pacemaking capability of the SA node, AV node, and ventricular Purkinje system may all be abolished and *cardiac asystole*, total lack of activity, may result. This is a catastrophic event requiring immediate correction. Under these conditions, cardiac rhythm may be restored by a sharp blow to the chest or by cardiac massage plus mechanical ventilation and intracardiac or intravenous injection of epinephrine or isoproterenol. Again, electrical pacing may be necessary.

Tachyarrhythmias

In general, the tachyarrhythmias are a group of conditions all tending to increase heart rate. The individual arrhythmias reflect aberrant impulse formation within the SA node, the atria, the AV node and the ventricles.

SINUS TACHYCARDIA. The simplest of the tachyarrhythmias is *sinus tachycardia* (Fig. 14-9). In this condition, the only abnormality is that the heart rate is too fast, exceeding 100 beats/minute; the Q-T intervals are relatively short, although normal for rapidly beating hearts.

Sinus tachycardia is often an expression of hyperactivity of the sympathetic nervous system in response to a variety of underlying problems, which may include anxiety, pain, infection, fever, hypovolemia, congestive heart failure, hyperthyroidism, etc. Treatment is generally directed at these problems and not at the SA node per se. However, if required, the heart rate can be lowered by beta-adrenergic receptor blocking agents like propranolol.

NORMAL SINUS RHYTHM WITH PREMATURE ATRIAL CONTRACTIONS. Abnormal beats can arise from ectopic foci located within the atria. In the ECG shown in Fig. 14-10, the arrows above the tracing indi-

Fig. 14-10 : Normal sinus rhythm with premature atrial contractions.

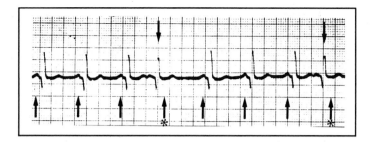

cate two *premature atrial contractions* (PACs), also known as "atrial premature beats," "atrial ectopic beats," or "atrial extrasystoles." These beats are called "premature" because they occur sooner than would be expected based upon the underlying normal sinus rhythm, and "atrial contractions" because they arise from ectopic foci within the atria and not from the SA node. PACs are characteristically followed by a long interval before the next beat occurs, the so-called compensatory pause.

The nature of the events occurring during the tracing shown in Fig. 14-10 is more readily understood if one focuses on the timing of the P waves of the normal sinus beats. Unadorned arrows have been placed in the figure below such P waves, and where the PACs occur, arrows with asterisks have been placed at the mid-point between the P waves of the preceding and following normal sinus beats. The resultant row of arrows thus indicates when the atria are, or should be, activated by the SA node if its rhythmicity remained undisturbed. One can see that the first three beats are normal sinus beats and that the PAC arises clearly ahead of schedule. In fact, the ventricle was already excited by the PAC at the time the next scheduled sinus beat was due; accordingly it was not expressed. As can be seen, the compensatory pause after the PAC represents the time spent waiting for the SA node to initiate the next normal sinus beat.

Despite the presence of P waves, two aspects of the tracing in Fig. 14-10 suggest that these ectopic beats arise in the atria and not in the SA node. First, the P wave morphology is different, being both smoother and more rounded. In addition, the presence of a PAC did not disturb the underlying rhythmicity of the SA node (the bottom row of arrows). The tracing is consistent with the presence of an ectopic atrial focus competing with the SA node for control over the atria.

Somewhat as an aside, it is worth noting that the interval between each of the PACs in Fig. 14-10 and the preceding normal beats is identical. In long rhythm strips from persons with PACs such intervals are characteristically quite constant and the PAC is said to be "coupled" to the preceding beat. Because of this, such PACs are generally felt to be reentrant in nature, reflecting the reemergence

Fig. 14-11 : Atrial tachycardia.

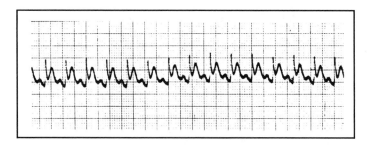

from the ectopic atrial focus of delayed activity from the preceding normal beat.

Although PACs are not uncommon, and they are of interest with respect to the electrophysiological basis for their production, such ectopic beats usually have little or no hemodynamic consequence and generally require no treatment.

ATRIAL TACHYCARDIA. Atrial ectopic foci similar to those producing PACs can produce other tachyarrthythmias. Figure 14-11 shows an *atrial tachycardia* where the heart rate is 167 beats/minute and where the QRS complex and T waves are merging. Such rhythms are often expressed at rates of 150–250 beats/minute.

At times it may be difficult to distinguish between sinus tachycardia, where impulses arise rapidly from the SA node, and atrial tachycardia, where impulses arise rapidly from the ectopic atrial focus. In general, however, atrial tachycardias can be identified because they tend to produce much higher heart rates, because they often manifest abnormal P waves and/or because their expression follows characteristic patterns. With respect to the latter, atrial tachycardias take two forms. In the less common form, the ectopic activity generally develops and speeds up to dominate the rhythm. More commonly, the arrhythmia has a sudden onset and then terminates spontaneously and abruptly; accordingly it is given the name *paroxysmal atrial tachycardia* (PAT). In some cases of PAT, each atrial contraction is conducted to the ventricles in the manner shown in Fig. 14-11. In other cases there may be a failure of some impulses to penetrate the AV node. In the resultant *AV block*, the ventricle may respond to every other atrial beat (2 : 1 block) or every third beat (3 : 1 block), etc. It should be realized that under these conditions AV block is a physiologic mechanism that protects the ventricle against excessive stimulation from above. The 1 : 1 conduction of high atrial rates to the ventricle could be intolerable.

With respect to treatment, individual attacks of PAT can usually be terminated by procedures that increase vagal tone (for example, carotid sinus massage, Valsalva's maneuver, gagging, neostigmine,

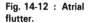

Fig. 14-12 : Atrial flutter.

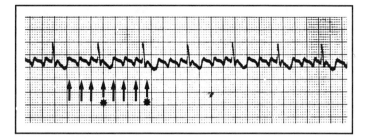

pressor agents, and/or cardiac glycosides), by propranolol, verapamil, and by atrial pacing or cardioversion. The reappearance of the arrhythmia can sometimes be prevented by prophylaxis with digitalis, quinidine, and/or propranolol.

ATRIAL FLUTTER. Another similar atrial tachyarrhythmia is atrial flutter. It is characterized by a faster atrial rate than atrial tachycardia, about 300 beats/minute; by larger, "saw-tooth" flutter waves; and by some degree of AV block that protects the ventricle from the high atrial rate. In the example shown in Figure 14-12 the atrial rate is about 300 beats/minute (P-P intervals are about 0.20 second) and the ventricular rate is about 75 beats/minute (R-R intervals are about 0.80 second); there is a 4 : 1 AV block.

Tracings such as these can often be confusing unless care is taken to identify all of the flutter waves. In this figure, each QRS complex is preceded by three flutter waves and these have been indicated by long arrows. On closer examination, however, what may be another flutter wave is seen superimposed on the S-T segment of each ventricular beat as indicated by short arrows with asterisks. That these are also flutter waves is indicated by the fact that they occur midway between two clearly defined flutter waves, where one would expect a flutter wave were the ectopic pacemaker truly rhythmic, and by their shape, which closely resembles that of other flutter waves.

Cardioversion is the treatment of choice for this arrhythmia; alternatively cardiac glycosides or propranolol may be used to control ventricular rate if needed.

ATRIAL FIBRILLATION. Atrial fibrillation (AF) is an atrial tachyarrhythmia that represents a somewhat different situation. In AF, all of the cells of the atria are undergoing asynchronous electrical activity producing small-amplitude undulations throughout the ECG. Depending on the penetration of this asynchronous atrial activity through the AV node, the ventricular rate may be normal, slow, or rapid. Figure 14-13 shows three cases of AF: in the top tracing (Panel A) the ventricular rate is 94 beats/minute; in the middle tracing (Panel B) the rate is 50 beats/minute; and in the bottom tracing (Panel C) the rate is 168 beats/minute.

Fig. 14-13 : Atrial fibrillation with normal ventricular rate (A), low ventricular rate (B), and high ventricular rate (C).

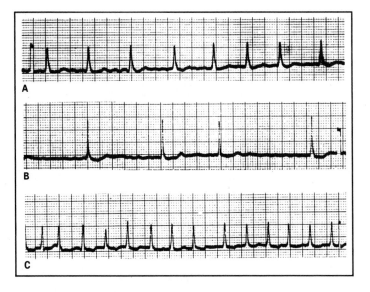

Fig. 14-14 : Nodal tachycardia.

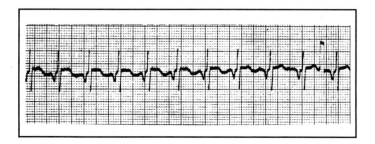

AF is generally terminated by cardioversion if rapid reversion to sinus rhythm is needed. Otherwise, if the ventricular rate is rapid, the cardiac glycosides, propranolol, or verapamil can effectively slow the ventricular rate and, on occasion, revert the fibrillation to normal sinus rhythm. If these fail, quinidine alone may produce reversion to normal sinus rhythm.

PREMATURE NODAL CONTRACTIONS AND NODAL TACHYCARDIA. The AV node can also generate tachyarrhythmias. It can give rise to *premature nodal contractions*, that is, premature beats not preceded by normal P waves but having otherwise normal QRS configuration, and it can give rise to *nodal tachycardias* such as that shown in Figure 14-14, where the heart rate is 120 beats/minute. Care must be observed in distinguishing between the slow nodal rhythm that results normally from depression of the SA node (see Figs. 14-3, 14-8) and the more rapid nodal tachycardia where the heart rate may be 100–150 beats/minute.

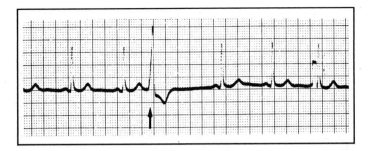

Because the AV node, like the atria, is densely innervated by the vagus, treatment of nodal tachycardias is the same as for paroxysmal atrial tachycardias. Atrial tachycardias and nodal tachycardias share certain features, so it has become commonplace in recent years to group these together and refer to them as "supraventricular tachycardias." These similarities make it probable that there is a reentrant basis for their generation. In addition, the treatments to which they respond are similar.

NORMAL SINUS RHYTHM WITH PREMATURE VENTRICULAR CONTRACTIONS. As in the atria and AV node, ectopic foci located within the ventricle can generate a family of ventricular tachyarrhythmias. Premature ventricular contractions (PVCs), also known as "ventricular premature beats," "ventricular ectopic beats," or "ventricular extrasystoles," are in many ways characteristic of such arrhythmias. Fig. 14-15 is a strip of normal sinus rhythm with one grossly abnormal beat—a PVC. As can be seen, this beat is premature because it occurs earlier than the next beat was expected, and is followed by a compensatory pause. Because they are initiated at ectopic foci, PVCs follow an abnormal conduction path, activating the ventricles in an anomalous manner and producing ECG complexes characterized by a wide QRS, prominent Q wave or R wave, and sometimes a large T wave. Since the focus of origin of a PVC can be anywhere within the ventricles, and since the pathway of ventricular activation will vary with the site of origin, PVCs assume a multitude of shapes and sizes each reflecting their site of origin. Electrophysiologic methods are available for locating these ectopic foci, but a description of these procedures is not necessary for the present purpose.

When PVCs occur singly, each following a normal sinus beat, the interval between the normal beat and the PVC is usually constant and the PVC is said to be "coupled" to the normal beat. When PVCs occur singly and infrequently, and when they are not closely coupled, they usually have minimal hemodynamic consequence and generally do not require treatment. A different situation exists, however, when the PVC is closely coupled to the normal beat; that is, the abnormal beat is initiated before the normal beat is terminated, as shown by the arrow in Fig. 14-16. While not true for the example

Fig. 14-16 : The R-on-T phenomenon: Normal sinus rhythm with a premature ventricular contraction falling on the T wave of a normal beat.

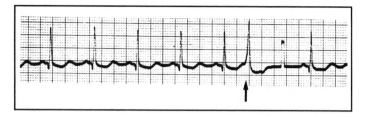

Fig. 14-17 : Ventricular bigeminy.

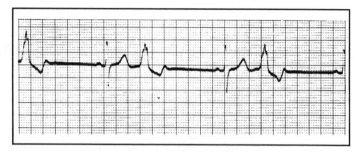

Fig. 14-18 : Normal sinus rhythm with premature ventricular contractions arising in pairs or couplets.

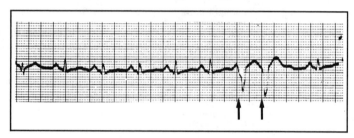

shown, under these conditions the 2-beat complex may lead immediately to ventricular tachycardia, flutter, or fibrillation (see below). This is referred to as the "R-on-T phenomenon" because it seems related to the R wave of the PVC falling on the T wave of the preceding beat. This seems to apply similarly to cases where the R wave of the ectopic beat also falls on the T wave of a preceding ectopic beat as well as a preceding normal sinus beat. To prevent the occurrence of more severe arrhythmias, patients with closely coupled or R-on-T PVCs are often treated with antiarrhythmic agents such as quinidine, procainamide, or lidocaine.

PVCs do not always appear singly. They often alternate with normal sinus beats in a seemingly stable condition called "ventricular bigeminy" (Fig. 14-17). At other times, each third beat or fourth beat may be a PVC; these rhythms are referred to as "ventricular trigeminy" and "ventricular quadrigeminy," respectively. PVCs may also arise in pairs or couplets (Fig. 14-18), and PVCs arising from different foci can occur concurrently (Fig. 14-19). While all of these permutations may be rather well tolerated, they may be harbingers of more severe arrhythmias and can be treated with quinidine, procainamide, or lidocaine.

Fig. 14-19 : Normal sinus rhythm with premature ventricular contractions arising from different foci.

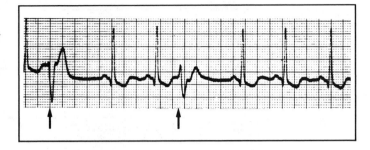

Fig. 14-20 : Normal sinus rhythm with an episode of ventricular tachycardia.

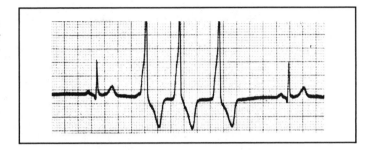

Fig. 14-21 : Ventricular flutter.

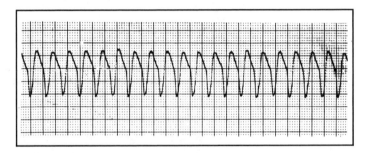

VENTRICULAR TACHYCARDIA. Although the definition is somewhat arbitrary, ventricular tachycardia (VT) is generally described as a run of three or more ventricular ectopic beats occurring at R-R intervals equivalent to a rate of 100 beats/minute or higher. Figure 14-20 shows one such episode of VT that was sustained at a rate equivalent to 109 beats/minute for three beats. Such rhythms usually compromise cardiac function severely and are often life-threatening. Depending on the urgency of the situation, treatment may include precordial thump followed by cardioversion or therapy with intravenous lidocaine; if this proves ineffective, intravenous procainamide may be useful.

VENTRICULAR FLUTTER. Ventricular flutter is an arrhythmia akin to VT except that the ventricular rate is faster, about 200 beats/minute, and the ventricular complexes are smoother and more symmetrical. It is treated in the same manner as VT. Figure 14-21 is a case of ventricular flutter with a rate of 215 beats/minute.

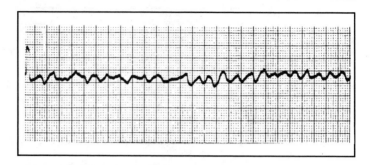

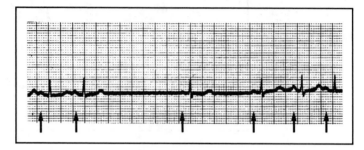

VENTRICULAR FIBRILLATION. Like atrial fibrillation, ventricular fibrillation (VF) is a chaotic state of the ventricles with completely asynchronous electrical activity (Fig. 14-22). The transition from other cardiac rhythms into VF occurs rapidly, often abruptly; during VF, cardiac output falls, and death generally ensues unless the situation is immediately corrected by electrical defibrillation and / or other resuscitative measures.

Arrhythmias Due Primarily to Defects in the Conduction of Electrical Activity

Impaired conduction

There are three locations in the heart prone to develop conduction disturbances. These are in or around the SA node, within the AV node, and within the specialized conduction system of the ventricle.

SA BLOCK. Figure 14-23 shows an ECG illustrating normal sinus rhythm with intermittent SA block. At first glance it appears that the SA node is firing irregularly. However, upon closer examination it will be seen that all of the P-P intervals are common multiples: the interval between beats 1 and 2 is 0.56 second; between beats 2 and 3 is 1.84 seconds (or 3 × 0.613 second); between beats 3 and 4 is 1.20 seconds (or 2 × 0.60 second); between beats 4 and 5 is 0.68 second; and between beats 5 and 6 is 0.56 second. It would seem that the SA node was firing at intervals of about 0.60 second (100

Fig. 14-24 : First-de-
gree AV block.

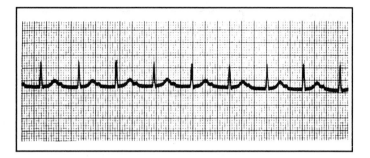

Fig. 14-25 : Second-
degree AV block with
2 : 1 block.

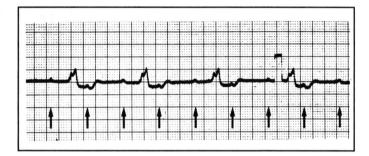

beats/minute) but that between beats 2 and 3 this activity twice
failed to conduct to the atria, and this happened once again between
beats 3 and 4; i.e., there was an intermittent blockade of conduction
from the SA node to the atria. Such a block is often called an "exit
block" since the electrical impulse fails to "exit" from the SA node.

AV BLOCK. Impairment of conduction through the AV node is custom-
arily divided into three categories depending on the severity of the
defect. In *first-degree AV block* (Fig. 14-24) there is no complete
block of transmission through the node but rather only a slowing of
conduction. This is reflected in a P-R interval of 0.30 second, which
is longer than normal (i.e., > 0.20 second).

In contrast to first-degree heart block where all supraventricular impulses reach the ventricle (albeit a little later than normally), in *sec-
ond-degree AV block*, some but not all impulses reach the ventricle.
Figure 14-25 is an example of 2 : 1 block where every other P wave
(shown by arrows) is followed by a ventricular complex (ignore the
"notch" in the QRS). Depending on circumstances, higher degrees
of block (e.g., 3 : 1, 4 : 1) can also occur.

Figure 14-26 shows another variant of second degree AV block. In
this case, the P-R interval progressively lengthens until one impulse
fails to reach the ventricle (at arrows) and the mechanism resets and
repeats; every third impulse is lost. This variant of second degree AV
block is called the "Wenckebach phenomenon."

Fig. 14-28 : Morphology of sinus beats in the preexcitation syndromes.

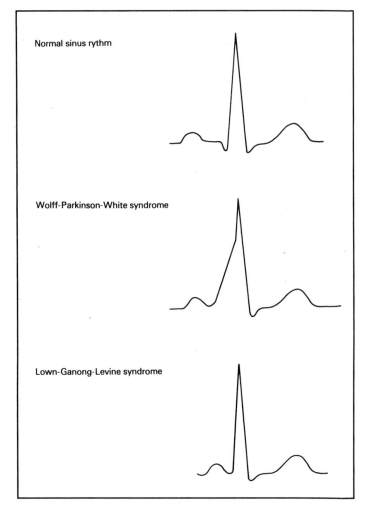

Normal sinus rythm

Wolff-Parkinson-White syndrome

Lown-Ganong-Levine syndrome

The tachycardias in the W-P-W syndrome respond to treatment with antiarrhythmic agents, presumably because of favorable changes in the slowing of conduction and/or the refractory periods of one or both of the two conduction pathways. In general, however, the tachycardias frequently respond to treatment with propranolol; they can also be terminated by cardioversion. Prophylaxis can be provided by quinidine and procainamide. Although difficult, the syndrome can be corrected by surgical disruption of the accessory pathways.

Lown-Ganong-Levine Syndrome Figure 14-28 also illustrates the form of pre-excitation characteristic of the Lown-Ganong-Levine syndrome. The P-R interval is short, as it is in the W-P-W syndrome, but the delta wave is missing and the QRS is of normal configuration. In cases such as this the bypass fibers probably lead from the atria to the common bundle, so that ventricular activation is normal but premature. Patients with this syndrome are also subject to the same tachyarrhythmias as those with the W-P-W syndrome and are treated similarly.

Perspective

The arrhythmias that have been presented were selected because they are either common or because they represent disturbances illustrative of certain kinds of electrophysiological defects. They are but a few of the many arrhythmias that can occur. In addition to the large number of individual arrhythmias, analysis of cardiac rhythm is often more complex because two or more defects coexist. Moreover, in practice, the exact nature of the rhythm disturbances that occur in some patients is not always readily apparent even to the experienced electrocardiographer. A thorough understanding of the selected disturbances described herein should provide an appropriate background for coping with the more complex disturbances in cardiac electrical activity.

Suggested Readings

Anderson JL et al: Antiarrhythmic drugs: Clinical pharmacology and therapeutic uses. *Drugs* 15:271, 1978.

Bigger JT, Hoffman BF: Antiarrhythmic drugs, in Gilman AG, Goodman LS, Gilman A (eds): *Goodman and Gilman's The Pharmacological Basis of Therapeutics*, ed 6. New York, Macmillan, 1980.

Gallagher JJ et al: The preexcitation syndromes. *Prog Cardiovasc Dis* 20:285, 1978.

Hoffman BF, Rosen MR: Cellular mechanisms for cardiac arrhythmias. *Circ Res* 49:1, 1981.

Marriot JL: *Practical Electrocardiography*, ed 5. Baltimore: Williams & Wilkins, 1972.

Mudge GH Jr: *Manual of Electrocardiography*. Boston, Little, Brown, 1981.

Weiss IW: *Essentials of Heart Rhythm Analysis*. Philadelphia, Davis, 1973.

15 : Peripheral and Cerebrovascular Disease

Clinicians commonly focus their attention on the sequelae of arteriosclerotic obstruction of the coronary arterial tree. However, peripheral vascular disease is of equal frequency and importance. In addition, an understanding of the pathophysiology of peripheral vascular disease increases ones' perception of disease mechanisms involved in coronary artery disease.

Peripheral Vascular Fluid Dynamics

Blood moves through the circulation as a result of kinetic and potential energy given to it by the pumping action of the heart. Because of friction in the human circulation, energy is lost as heat. Energy losses in the circulation are the result of two factors: frictional energy losses resulting from blood viscosity (Poiseuille's law) and inertial energy losses resulting from changes in blood flow velocity and/or direction. Poiseuille's law states that the pressure difference along a tube carrying a viscous fluid is directly proportional to the velocity of flow, the length of the tube, and the viscosity of the fluid in the tube and inversely proportional to the fourth power of the radius of the tube:

Pressure difference along a tube
$$= \frac{8 \times \text{mean velocity of fluid flow} \times \text{tube length} \times \text{fluid viscosity}}{\pi \times (\text{radius of the tube})^4}$$

From this equation has come the universally recognized relationship of pressure = flow × resistance (see Chap. 8). Resistance in this latter formula is related to viscosity, tube length, and radius in the Poiseuille equation with radius contributing the most significant resistive element.

Inertial energy losses are particularly important in occlusive vascular disease where blood must flow around and through obstructive lesions.

Despite viscous and inertial energy losses, blood flow through stenotic vascular lesions is surprisingly *un*impaired until very severe narrowing (> 80% reduction of luminal diameter) of the affected vessel develops (Fig. 15-1). The explanation for this seeming paradox lies in the fact that flow velocity increases in a region of decreasing vessel diameter (Bernoulli's law). Flow is thereby maintained as

267

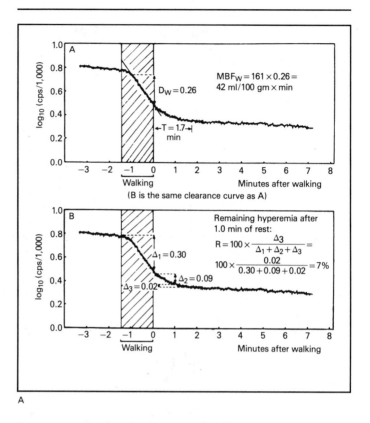

A

Fig. 15-1 : A. A xenon 133 clearance curve from the gastrocnemius muscle obtained during and after a standardized walking test in a normal individual. A small injection of radioactive xenon 133 is placed in the middle of the gastrocnemius muscle. The xenon is washed out of the muscle by blood flow and a scintillation detector placed over the muscle shows a large blood flow occurring in the muscle during walking (maximum blood flow during walking [MBF_w]), a brief period of post-exercise hyperemia (T), and a small residual hyperemia (R) after 1.0 minute of rest. The normal value for R is less than 25%. The calculations for deriving muscle blood flow and reactive hyperemia are shown above the figures. (From Alpert JS et al: Evaluation of arterial insufficiency of the legs; a comparison of arteriography and the ^{133}Xe walking test. *Cardiovasc Res* 2:161, 1968, with permission of the authors and publisher.) B. A xenon 133 clearance curve obtained during and after a standardized walking test in a leg with a distal arterial occlusion (femoral artery). Washout of xenon is recorded from the gastrocnemius muscle. The curve shows moderate blood flow during walking (MBF_w) and larger blood flow after walking (MBF_H). Blood flow during exercise is definitely less than in the normal leg shown in Fig. 15-1A. The time (T_H) from the cessation of walking to the commencement of hyperemic muscle blood flow is relatively short. There is prolonged post-exercise hyperemia (T) and the remaining hyperemia (R) is greater than 25%. Calculations of muscle blood flow and remaining hyperemia are shown on the figures. (From Alpert JS et al: Evaluation of arterial insufficiency of the legs; a comparison of arteriography and the ^{133}Xe walking test. *Cardiovasc Res* 2:161, 1968, with permission of the authors and publisher.)

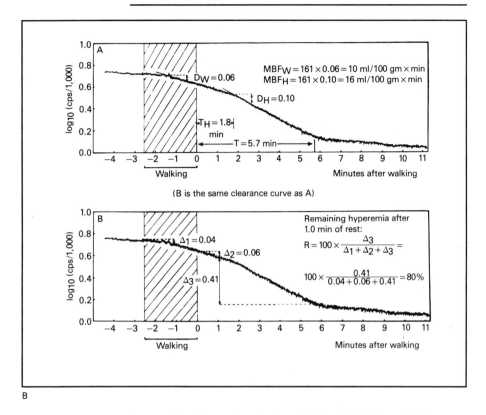

(B is the same clearance curve as A)

B

long as it continues in a laminar fashion. With increasingly severe stenosis, flow velocity becomes so great that turbulence results with marked increases in inertial energy losses. At that point (stenosis ≥ 80%), inertial energy losses become so great that blood flow decreases (see Fig. 12-7). These fluid dynamic principles are useful in understanding why patients with moderately severe atherosclerotic arterial narrowings (< 70% diameter reduction) in the peripheral circulation are frequently asymptomatic. Fluid dynamic principles also predict that stenoses in series produce cascades of turbulence that rob kinetic energy from the circulation, thereby decreasing the forces that keep blood flowing.

Obliterative Arterial Disease of the Lower Extremities

Obliterative arterial disease of the lower extremities, like coronary artery disease, is a manifestation of generalized atherosclerosis. Obliterative arterial disease of the legs is a common entity paralleling arteriosclerotic coronary artery disease in incidence. In addition, the pathophysiologic abnormalities of peripheral arterial disease resemble those seen in coronary artery disease (see Chap. 2). Stenotic or occluded regions in the arterial system to the lower extremities impede the normal flow of blood to the muscles and skin of the legs. As with coronary artery disease, exercise results in increased muscle metabolic demand. Arterioles in the muscles dilate in response to into the venous circulation. Such free-floating thrombi travel with the blood flow and arrive in the pulmonary circulation as pulmonary emboli (see Chap. 16).

Venous thrombosis that eventually leads to pulmonary embolism almost invariably begins in the veins of the calf. A surprisingly large percentage of patients (as high as 50–60%) admitted to general medical or surgical floors of a hospital develop small regions of venous thrombosis in the veins of the calf. In most of these individuals, venous thrombosis is localized and remains in calf veins with eventual resolution and without embolization to the lung. In a small number of these patients, venous thrombosis propagates proximally into the large veins of the thigh and pelvis. These latter patients frequently experience episodes of pulmonary embolism as venous thrombus is released from thigh veins. Thrombosis frequently begins in venous valve pockets.

Rarely, thrombosis extends throughout the entire venous system of an extremity. When this occurs, blood flow leaving that extremity is impaired and venous and capillary congestion develops. Such congestion, in turn, hinders arterial inflow to the affected limb: ischemia and even necrosis ensue. Episodes of venous thrombosis frequently damage venous valves. The result is increased back pressure transmitted from the affected veins to communicating venules and capillaries. Increased venular and capillary pressure, in turn, result in increased transudation of fluid from the intravascular to the extravascular space (Starling's law of capillary filtration) leading to edema of the surrounding tissues. The commonest cause of leg and foot edema is inadequate venous function (venous insufficiency) secondary to structural inadequacy of venous valves.

Varicose veins are also the result of structural inadequancy of venous valves and walls. Such structural defects are frequently inherited, but they may be the result of episodes of venous thrombosis or infection. Injury to or absence of adequate venous valves leads to increased pressure on the wall of the vein with resultant marked dilatation. Varicose veins are rarely of hemodynamic significance and their eradication is almost invariably the result of cosmetic concern.

Venous thro sis is usually treated with some form of anticoagulation: heparin and warfarin anticoagulants prevent propagation of venous thrombus, allowing local fibrinolytic and reparative processes to dissolve existing venous thrombus. Fibrinolytic enzymes (streptokinase, urokinase) may be administered intravenously, thereby dissolving venous thrombi. On occasion, a vein containing thrombus is ligated or an intravascular filter is inserted proximally, thereby preventing pulmonary embolization of venous thrombi.

Dissecting Aneurysm or Hematoma of the Aorta

Cleavage of the aortic wall by blood with the potential for aortic rupture is known as a "dissecting aneurysm" or "dissecting hematoma of the aorta." This condition is highly lethal with more than 90% of untreated, affected individuals dying within a few days of the onset of dissection.

Three factors interact in the predisposition to and the occurrence of aortic dissection. The first factor is a congenital weakness in the aortic wall. This weakness, usually called "cystic medial necrosis" by pathologists, is an almost universal finding in pathological sections of aortas obtained at the time of surgery or post-mortem examination in patients with aortic dissection. In some patients, cystic medial necrosis or degeneration is part of the Marfan syndrome, a generalized disorder of connective tissue, but most patients with dissection demonstrate no other finding of Marfan syndrome. It seems likely that aortic dissection can only occur upon the appropriate substrate of degenerative disease of the aortic medial layer. However, it has been suggested that cystic medial necrosis is the result of normal reparative processes that occur in response to small zones of damage in the aortic wall that are, in turn, the result of daily hemodynamic stresses.

The occurrence of cystic medial necrosis of the aorta in a particular patient does not guarantee that aortic dissection will occur in that individual. Two further factors are necessary: (1) an intimal tear to *initiate* the process of dissection and (2) hemodynamic forces to propagate the dissecting hematoma within the aortic medial layer (Fig. 15-3).

Intimal tears occur mostly in the ascending aorta just above the aortic valve and in the descending aorta, just distal to or at the origin of the left subclavian artery. Intimal tears occur at these two sites because of the pendulumlike motion of the heart suspended as it is from the aorta and great vessels. Each cardiac cycle results in significant side-to-side cardiac motion with the resultant wall stress concentrated in the ascending aorta. This constant minor trauma of daily hemodynamic events combined with atherosclerotic damage to the aortic intima results in aortic intimal disruption, the initiating factor in dissecting aortic aneurysms.

Once an intimal tear has occurred, certain hemodynamic conditions must be met in order for a dissecting hematoma to propagate through the aortic medial layer. It is commonly said that elevated blood pressure is an important contributing factor in the propagation of aortic dissection. Wheat, however, has shown with in vitro models of the aortic wall that elevated blood pressure per se does not result in propagation of a dissection [12] . Wheat and his co-workers have

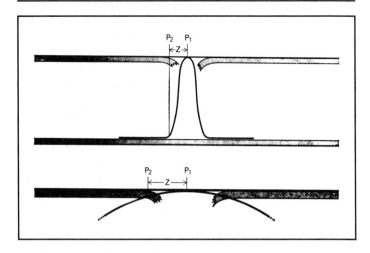

Fig. 15-4 : Steepness of the aortic pulse wave is a factor in propagating dissecting aneurysms of the aorta: in the schematic diagram depicted above, P_1 and P_2 are pressures exerted on the aortic wall at these two points; Z, constant and finite, equals the length of the torn intima and media. The driving force exerted on the torn intima is equal to P_1 minus P_2. If the pressure curve can be flattened (curve at the bottom), the driving force is reduced over a greater distance, Z. This reduces the force that propagates the aortic dissection. See text for a description of techniques employed to reduce this driving force. (From Wheat MW Jr et al: Management of acute dissecting aneurysms of the aorta. *Hospital Practice* 4(6):31, 1969, with permission of the authors and publisher.)

associated with a very large quantity of blood flow to the brain: 50 ml/100 gm of brain tissue per minute. Intellectual, sensory, or motor stimulation of the brain is associated with increased blood flow to the specific brain regions involved in the action undertaken. Brain cells are extremely sensitive to ischemia, with dysfunction occurring within a few seconds after cessation of blood flow. Irreversible neuronal injury can occur within 3–4 minutes of cessation of blood flow.

Atherosclerosis commonly affects the four major blood vessels supplying the brain: the two carotid arteries and the two vertebral arteries. Transient episodes of neurologic dysfunction, known as "TIAs" (transient ischemic attacks), appear to be the result of small platelet or platelet and fibrin thrombi that embolize to small brain arteries from the surface of complicated atherosclerotic plaques projecting into the lumen of major arteries supplying the brain. Episodes of focal brain ischemia are followed by reactive hyperemia in the same region. Drugs that inhibit platelet aggregation decrease or abolish TIAs by preventing the development of platelet thrombi.

Acute cerebral infarction or stroke is due to thrombosis of an atherosclerotic artery or embolism of a thrombus into the cerebral circulation from the heart or great vessels. A number of common cardiac conditions are associated with intracardiac thrombi that can and of-

Table 15-1 : Common cardiac conditions associated with intracardiac thrombi that can embolize to the brain

Myocardial infarction
Mitral stenosis
Atrial fibrillation (from any cause)
Sick sinus syndrome with atrial arrhythmias
Cardiomyopathy
Cardiac tumors
Mitral valve prolapse (rarely)

ten do embolize to the brain with resultant cerebral infarction (Table 15-1). Thrombi that cause embolic strokes are usually larger than those that produce TIAs. Moreover, the thrombi that produce embolic strokes are usually red thrombi containing platelets, fibrin, and red cells as compared to the white thrombi of TIAs that are composed predominantly of platelets.

The ischemic brain region affected by a stroke can be shown to have decreased blood flow with a zone of surrounding reactive hyperemia. Normal brain-blood vessel autoregulatory mechanisms are paralyzed by a stroke and blood flow to the affected regions varies directly with the level of systemic arterial blood pressure. Administration of a systemic vasodilating drug to patients with stroke results in arteriolar dilatation in normal areas of the brain. This can lead to increased flow in normal regions at the expense of decreased flow in the ischemic zone, the so-called intracerebral steal phenomenon.

Another interesting but rare condition involving a circulatory steal is the so-called subclavian steal. In this condition, both carotid arteries and one vertebral artery are occluded, usually as a result of atherosclerosis. Thus, the entire cerebral circulation is dependent on a single vertebral artery and the anastomotic circle of Willis. If the subclavian artery that gives rise to the single patent vertebral artery is appropriately stenotic or occluded, work by the muscles of the upper extremity on that side "steal" the subclavian arterial blood flow away from the patent vertebral artery. At such times patients may develop transient neurological abnormalities or syncope that resolves when arm work ceases.

During recovery from an acute cerebral infarction, cerebral blood flow and autoregulatory mechanisms gradually return toward normal although a small zone of abnormal perfusion usually persists. Surgery or vasodilating drugs administered at this point and seeking to improve cerebral circulatory capacity do not benefit the zone of infarcted brain tissue that has long since ceased to function.

Suggested Readings

deWolfe VG: Assessment of the circulation in occlusive arterial disease of the lower extremities. *Mod Conc Cardiovasc Dis* 45:91–95, 1976.

Weale FE: Hemodynamics of incomplete arterial obstruction. *Br J Surg* 51:689–693, 1964.

Delius W, Erikson U: Correlation between angiographic and hemodynamic findings in occlusions of arteries of the extremities. *Angiology* 3:201–210, 1969.

Carter SA: Response of ankle systolic pressure to leg exercise in mild or questionable arterial disease. *N Engl J Med* 287:578–582, 1972.

Bloor K: Natural history of arteriosclerosis of the lower extremities. *Ann R Coll Surg Engl* 28:36–52, 1961.

May AG, De Weese JA, Rob CG: Hemodynamic effects of arterial stenosis. *Surgery* 53:513–524, 1963.

Dahn I, Lassen NA, Westling H: On the mechanism of delayed hyperemia in the calf muscles in obliterative arterial disease. *Cardiovasc Res* I:145–149, 1967.

Alpert JS, Larsen OA, Lassen NA: Evaluation of arterial insufficiency of the legs; A comparison of arteriography and the 133Xe walking test. *Cardiovasc Res* 2:161–169, 1968.

Barnes RW: Hemodynamics for the vascular surgeon. *Arch Surg* 115:216–223, 1980.

Wu KK, Barnes RW, Hoak JC: Platelet hyperaggregability in idiopathic recurrent deep vein thrombosis. *Circulation* 53:687–691, 1976.

Stein PD, Evans H: An autopsy study of leg vein thrombosis. *Circulation* 35:671–681, 1967.

Wheat MW: Treatment of dissecting aneurysms of the aorta: Current status. *Prog Cardiovasc Dis* 16:87–101, 1973.

Simpson CF, Taylor WP: Effect of hydralazine on aortic rupture induced by B-aminopropionitrite in turkeys. *Circulation* 65:704–708, 1982.

Anagnostopoulos CE, Prabhakar MJS, Kittle CF: Aortic dissections and dissecting aneurysms. *Am J Cardiol* 30:263–273, 1972.

Cook P, James I: Cerebral vasodilators. *N Engl J Med* 305:1508–1512, 1560–1564, 1981.

Byer JA, Easton JD: Therapy of ischemic cerebrovascular disease. *Ann Intern Med* 93:742–756, 1980.

McHenry LC Jr: Cerebral blood flow measurement and regulation in man. *Curr Conc Cerebrovasc Dis* 11:1–4, 5–8, 1976.

Kontos HA: Mechanisms of regulation of the cerebral microcirculation. *Curr Conc Cerebrovasc Dis* 10:7–12, 1975.

Ingvar DH: Functional landscapes in the brain in normals and in patients with brain disorders. *Curr Conc Cerebrovasc Dis* 12:1–4, 1977.

16 : Pulmonary Embolism, Pulmonary Hypertension, and Acute Cor Pulmonale

Pulmonary hypertension, elevated pressure in the pulmonary artery, resembles systemic arterial hypertension in a number of ways. First, pulmonary hypertension can result from a variety of pathologic entities. Second, patients with pulmonary hypertension are frequently asymptomatic despite the presence of marked elevation in pulmonary arterial pressures for many years. Third, pulmonary hypertension produces pressure overload of that ventricle (right) that must generate the required elevated pulmonary arterial systolic pressure (Table 16-1). Right ventricular systolic wall tension is increased in patients with pulmonary hypertension. This pressure overload of the right ventricle leads to hypertrophy, dilatation, and eventually failure (elevated right ventricular filling pressure and reduced cardiac output).

The right ventricle is hypertrophied during uterine life when pulmonary vascular resistance is high and the right ventricle must pump considerable quantities of blood to the systemic circulation via the ductus arteriosus. Right ventricular hypertrophy normally regresses during early postnatal development since pulmonary vascular resistance falls to normal levels soon after birth. Right ventricular hypertrophy and elevated pulmonary vascular resistance may persist in individuals with certain forms of congenital heart disease, for example, ventricular septal defect, patent ductus arteriosus, and transposition of the great arteries. In such individuals, right ventricular pressure overload may be well tolerated for decades. However, in the normal adult, the development of pulmonary hypertension during adult life presents the relatively thin-walled right ventricle with a pressure overload. The right ventricle tolerates pressure overload less well than the thicker-walled left ventricle.

Systemic arterial hypertension is easily detected by means of the universally available blood pressure cuff. Unfortunately, no such simple, noninvasive device exists for determining pulmonary hypertension. Thus, pulmonary hypertension is often first discovered by cardiac catheterization at a time when right ventricular hypertrophy, dilatation, and failure are present.

Cor pulmonale is an old term commonly employed by clinicians to refer to right ventricular hypertrophy and / or dilatation secondary to

**Table 16-1 : Comparison between
pulmonary arterial and systemic arterial hypertension**

Pulmonary hypertension	Systemic hypertension
Multiple etiologies	Multiple etiologies
Long asymptomatic period despite marked pressure elevation	Long asymptomatic period despite marked pressure elevation
Right ventricle affected; eventually leads to cor pulmonale (right ventricular hypertrophy, dilatation, and failure)	Left ventricle affected; eventually leads to left ventricular hypertrophy, dilatation, and failure
Leads to dilatation of the pulmonary artery	Leads to dilatation of the aorta
Not a risk factor for coronary artery disease	A definite risk factor for coronary artery disease
No simple, noninvasive method available to detect pulmonary hypertension	Simple, noninvasive method available to detect pulmonary hypertension

pulmonary hypertension. Two forms of cor pulmonale exist: acute and chronic. Acute cor pulmonale results from a sudden increase in pulmonary arterial pressure such as that which results from pulmonary embolism. Chronic cor pulmonale results from long-standing pulmonary hypertension that is mild at its onset and gradually increases in severity with time. Chronic cor pulmonale is discussed in Chap. 8.

**Acute Cor
Pulmonale**

A sudden increase in pulmonary vascular resistance, e.g., as a result of an episode of pulmonary embolism (impaction of intravascular thrombi in the pulmonary vascular bed), produces a marked increase in right ventricular work. The right ventricle must pump blood at a higher pressure in order to overcome the increased pulmonary vascular resistance caused by the intravascular pulmonary thromboemboli. Right ventricular systolic pressure and work as well as right ventricular systolic wall tension increase. The increase in right ventricular pressure work occurs suddenly: there is no time for right ventricular hypertrophy to develop: the right ventricle dilates (Starling mechanism) in order to meet the increased work demands. If pulmonary vascular resistance is sufficiently increased, right ventricular failure develops.

Normally, the pulmonary circulation presents a low vascular resistance to blood flow from the right ventricle. In addition, the pulmonary vascular bed has enormous reserve (see Chap. 8). Therefore, the cross-sectional area of the normal pulmonary vasculature must be reduced by more than one-half before any rise in pulmonary vascular resistance or pressure is observed. For example, the removal of one lung does not result in pulmonary hypertension in the remaining lung provided that the remaining vasculature is normal (see Chap. 8).

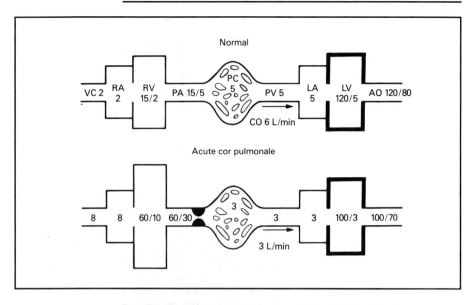

Fig. 16-1 : Hemodynamic changes occurring in patients with acute cor pulmonale secondary to pulmonary embolism. The sudden increase in pulmonary resistance which occurs secondary to the episode of pulmonary embolism results in marked right ventricular systolic and pulmonary arterial hypertension. Right ventricular and pulmonary arterial systolic pressure rises to approximately 60 mm Hg. The right ventricle (RV) dilates and right ventricular diastolic pressure also increases. Increases in right ventricular diastolic pressure are transmitted to the right atrium (RA) and central veins, which also demonstrate an increase in pressure. Distal to the pulmonary embolic obstruction, there is decreased blood flow and consequently left heart pressures fall. Specifically, pulmonary capillary (PC), pulmonary venous (PV), left atrial (LA), and left ventricular (LV) diastolic pressures fall. The decrease in left ventricular loading results in decreased left ventricular systolic pressure. Right ventricular decompensation results in a decreased right ventricular stroke volume that, of course, causes a decrease in left ventricular stroke volume. VC = vena cava; PA = pulmonary artery; CO = cardiac output; AO = aorta.

With loss of more than 50% of the cross-sectional area of the pulmonary vascular bed marked circulatory changes develop. Pressure in the pulmonary arteries rises in response to the increase in pulmonary vascular resistance. The normal right ventricle can generate a maximum of 60–70 mm Hg systolic pressure in the face of an acute increase in pulmonary vascular resistance. If pulmonary hypertension has previously been present, the right ventricle can generate 70–100 mm Hg or more in response to an acute increase in pulmonary vascular resistance (Fig. 16-1).

The sudden rise in right ventricular systolic pressure work may result in marked right ventricular dilatation with consequent deterioration in right ventricular function. In the latter situation, right ventricular diastolic pressure (= right atrial mean pressure) rises and stroke volume declines (Fig. 16-1). Systemic venous pressure increases secondary to the elevation in right atrial pressure. Falling stroke volume

churning, pumping action of the right ventricle breaks the venous thrombi into multiple pieces that are distributed throughout the pulmonary circulation according to the distribution pattern of pulmonary blood flow, i.e., more travel to the lower lobe than to the upper lobe. Emboli usually lodge in both lungs. The initial effect of pulmonary embolism is usually total blockade of blood flow through the affected vessel. Pulmonary arterial pressure increases as a result of the increase in pulmonary vascular resistance. The increase in pulmonary arterial pressure pushes the thrombus further down the vascular tree. Gradually, the thrombus is compressed along the wall of the affected pulmonary artery and a small amount of blood flow is reestablished through the vessel. Further resolution of the thrombus depends on activation of the intrinsic fibrinolytic system. Complete dissolution of pulmonary thromboemboli takes approximately two weeks in individuals without heart or lung disease; resolution takes considerably longer and may be incomplete in patients with heart or lung disease.

Pulmonary infarction results when the obstructing embolus completely interrupts pulmonary blood flow to a lung segment for a considerable amount of time. The pulmonary parenchyma infarcts but bronchial collateral circulation is sufficient to maintain the viability of the fibrous skeleton of the lung, the bronchi, and the muscular pulmonary arteries. Pulmonary infarction usually occurs when an embolism obstructs middle-sized or smaller pulmonary arteries (Table 16-2). Obstruction of one of the two main pulmonary arteries does not lead to infarction of the entire lung because bronchial collateral flow for the entire lung is able to maintain viability of the pulmonary parenchyma. Infarction is more likely to occur in patients with left ventricular failure and pulmonary venous hypertension in whom the collateral circulation from bronchial arteries is compromised by pulmonary venous congestion.

When pulmonary thromboembolism is sufficiently massive so that more than 50% of the pulmonary vascular bed is obstructed, acute cor pulmonale may result (Table 16-2). Acute dyspnea results whenever pulmonary thromboemboli lodge in the pulmonary circulation. This may be the only symptom associated with an episode of pulmonary embolism if (1) the quantity of thromboembolism is insufficient to produce the degree of pulmonary vascular obstruction required for acute cor pulmonale and 2) the type of pulmonary arterial obstruction is such that pulmonary infarction is *not* produced. Acute dyspnea and the associated tachypnea are the result of a reflex set into motion by stimulation of nerve endings in the pulmonary vasculature by the impacting thromboemboli and the resultant pulmonary arterial hypertension.

Essentially all patients with pulmonary embolism demonstrate some degree of pulmonary arterial hypertension regardless of the magni-

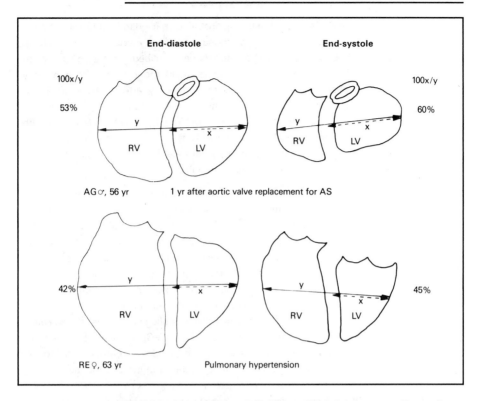

Fig. 16-3 : Demonstration of the "reverse Bernheim phenomenon" at cardiac catheterization. Right and left ventricular silhouettes at end-diastole and at end-systole have been traced from cineangiograms obtained at the time of cardiac catheterization. The upper panel is a tracing from a patient with normal right and left ventricular function 1 year following aortic valve replacement for aortic stenosis. The lower panel is from a patient with severe pulmonary hypertension. The relative position of the intraventricular septum is assessed by a derived variable that relates left ventricular diameter (x) to left + right ventricular diameter (y). A quotient x divided by y × 100 is derived and is shown for end-diastole and end-systole. The percentages in the left and right hand columns show that left ventricular diameter represents a much smaller percentage of total heart diameter in the patient with pulmonary hypertension than in the control patient who is status post aortic valve replacement for aortic stenosis (AS). In the patient with pulmonary hypertension (lower panel) the septum is displaced toward the left ventricular cavity thereby demonstrating the reverse Bernheim phenomenon. The septum is displaced toward the left at end-diastole as well as at end-systole. Moreover, the septum in the patient with pulmonary hypertension is vertical and straight at end-diastole and exhibits a slight convexity toward the left ventricle at end-systole. In contrast, the septum in the control patient is convex toward the right ventricle both at end-diastole and end-systole. LV = left ventricle; RV = right ventricle. (From Krayenbuehl HP et al: Left ventricular function in chronic pulmonary hypertension. *Am J Cardiol* 41:1150, 1978, with permission of the authors and publisher.)

tude of the thromboembolic insult. Larger quantities of thromboembolic material produce pulmonary arterial hypertension by mechanical obstruction of the pulmonary vascular bed. Smaller quantities of pulmonary thromboembolism result in modest rises in pulmonary arterial pressure secondary to pulmonary arterial vasoconstriction that in turn is caused by the hypoxemia that invariably accompanies episodes of pulmonary embolism. The hypoxemia associated with pulmonary embolism is the result of abnormal ventilation-perfusion patterns and intrapulmonary right-to-left shunting of blood that develops following pulmonary embolism.

Pulmonary embolism can depress left ventricular function modestly via three mechanisms. First, the arterial hypoxemia associated with pulmonary thromboembolism can lead to myocardial ischemia in patients with arteriosclerotic coronary artery disease. Second, dilatation of the right ventricle in patients with acute cor pulmonale can lead to abnormal left ventricular filling characteristics, i.e., decreased compliance. The dilated right ventricle pushes the interventricular septum into the left ventricular cavity thereby decreasing its filling capacity and altering left ventricular diastolic compliance, the so-called reverse Bernheim phenomenon (Fig. 16-3). Finally, obstruction of pulmonary blood flow leads to decreased left ventricular filling (reduced preload) with a resultant decrease in systolic function.

Suggested Readings

Dalen JE et al: Pulmonary angiography in experimental pulmonary embolism. *Am Heart J* 72:509, 1966.

Dalen JE et al: Resolution rate of acute pulmonary embolism in man. *N Engl J Med* 280:1194, 1969.

Dalen JE, Alpert JS: Natural history of pulmonary embolism. *Prog Cardiovasc Dis* 17(4):259, 1975.

Dalen JE et al: Pulmonary embolism, pulmonary hemorrhage and pulmonary infarction. *N Engl J Med* 296:1431, 1977.

Hyland JW et al: Behavior of pulmonary hypertension produced by serotonin and emboli. *Am J Physiol* 205:591, 1963.

Alpert JS et al: Pulmonary hypertension secondary to minor pulmonary embolism. *Chest* 73:795, 1978.

Mathur VS et al: Pulmonary angiography one to seven days after experimental pulmonary embolism. *Invest Radiol* 2:304, 1967.

McIntyre KM, Sasahara AA: Hemodynamic and ventricular responses to pulmonary embolism. *Prog Cardiovasc Dis* 17:175, 1974.

Stein PD et al: Right coronary blood flow in acute pulmonary embolism. *Am Heart J* 77:356, 1969.

Appendix A : Measurement of Heart Function: Invasive and Noninvasive Measures of Myocardial Contractile Function

Clinicians employ a wide range of diagnostic techniques to explore abnormalities of structure and function in the cardiovascular system. Two broad categories of techniques exist: invasive and noninvasive. Invasive techniques involve the placement of hollow plastic tubes filled with saline inside the body in different locations within the cardiovascular system. Noninvasive techniques are performed only on the surface of the body and consist of methods to examine cardiac or vascular function by recording electrical, mechanical, or anatomic events or alterations in the cardiovascular system.

Cardiac Catheterization: An Invasive Technique

Cardiac catheterization is an invasive, but low-risk, diagnostic technique. It provides the physician with very accurate and hence useful information concerning the state of the patient's heart and cardiovascular system. It requires considerable skill on the part of the operator as well as cooperation on the part of the patient. Cardiac catheterizations are performed in special laboratories designed specifically for that use. Two kinds of information are obtained from a cardiac catheterization. Physiologic data consists of pressures from the various heart chambers as well as cardiac output or blood flow pumped from the heart per minute. The second type of information obtained at cardiac catheterization is anatomic. Anatomic data is obtained by injecting radiopaque contrast material into various cardiac chambers and following ejection (clearance) of this contrast material by means of x-ray movies or serial x-ray films (angiography). Both types of information are critical in an accurate assessment of a particular patient. Physiologic data without anatomic information or vice versa seriously hampers the cardiologist's ability to assess the patient's pathological condition, as well as the heart's response to that particular condition.

Procedure of cardiac catheterization

Patients are brought to the cardiac catheterization laboratory in the fasting state, having received a mild tranquilizer before arriving. Cardiac catheterization is carried out under conditions of strict sterility similar to those found in an operating room. The first step in cardiac catheterization is careful sterilization and draping of the sites of entry for the cardiac catheters. There are a number of different approaches that the catheterizing cardiologist can take in advancing catheters into the various heart chambers.

In order to evaluate a patient's heart fully, one needs to record pressures from the right heart, that is the right atrium, right ventricle, and the pulmonary artery, as well as from the left heart, left atrium, and left ventricle. Access to the two sides of the heart is usually obtained by using two cardiac catheters. One catheter is introduced into a vein and advanced into the right side of the heart while another catheter is introduced into an artery and is advanced against the flow of blood, that is, in a retrograde fashion to the left side of the heart.

The routes usually followed for introducing the cardiac catheters are as follows: Right-sided cardiac catheterizations are performed by introducing the catheter into a femoral or antecubital vein. Left-sided catheterizations are performed by introducing the catheter into the femoral or brachial artery. All catheter manipulations occur with the heart and great vessels visualized by fluoroscopy so that one can see the passage and the direction of the cardiac catheters. Pressures in the different heart chambers can be measured by means of the cardiac catheter because these tubes are hollow. They are filled with saline and connected to a sensitive manometer that measures the small pressure changes occurring at the end of the catheter and transmitted through the hollow tube filled with saline to the manometer itself. Cardiac output or flow is determined by a number of different techniques. The commonest technique employed is the Fick technique, which depends on the difference in oxygen content between blood samples from the pulmonary artery and those taken from a systemic artery; the patient's total body oxygen consumption is measured as well.

Another popular technique for measuring cardiac output is the indicator dilution technique in which a small amount of harmless green dye is injected into the pulmonary artery; its appearance rate in a peripheral artery is then measured. Cardiac output can also be calculated from careful measurements made from angiograms of the patient's left ventricle during injections of x-ray contrast medium.

Angiographic studies are usually performed with injections of contrast medium into the left ventricle and aortic root. Occasionally, angiographic studies of the right ventricle and pulmonary artery are performed as well.

On occasion, the patient is exercised while cardiac pressures and flows are measured. This is done in order to see the response of the patient's heart to exercise stress. Other stresses also occasionally employed include isometric hand grip, isoproterenol infusion, rapid pacing of the heart, and infusion of a volume load such as dextran or saline.

Specific Abnormal Findings in Various Cardiac Disease States

Pericardial disease

In thickening of the pericardium or with a collection of fluid in the pericardial space, the normal filling of the right and left ventricles is impaired. This interferes with the heart's ability to pump the normal volume of blood into the pulmonary artery and aorta. When the heart is restricted in attaining its full potential for filling, cardiac output as well as all systolic pressures are reduced. During diastole, the heart fills rapidly to its maximum capacity because of the restricting influence of the layer of pericardial fluid or the thickened pericardium itself. Thus, the pressure tracing of a patient with constrictive pericarditis or pericardial effusion causing tamponade will demonstrate an early diastolic pressure rise in the right and left ventricles. Cardiac output is frequently reduced and pressures in the right atrium, left atrium, both ventricles, and the pulmonary artery are all equal during diastole.

Anatomic (angiographic) studies demonstrate the thickened pericardial wall or layer of pericardial fluid. These examinations consist of the injection of angiographic contrast medium into either the atrial or ventricular chambers. If an effusion or pericardial thickening exists, one notes the considerable thickness of the heart shadow that still exists beyond the edge of the ventricular cavity as outlined by the x-ray contrast material. Difficulties can be encountered in differentiating between constrictive pericarditis and certain restrictive myocardial diseases which may have similar physiologic and anatomic abnormalities.

Valvular heart disease

Valvular heart disease is also investigated with physiologic and anatomic techniques. Patients with valvular stenoses can be identified at catheterization because pressure increases in the heart chamber directly beyond the stenotic cardiac valve. Thus, in stenosis of the mitral valve, pressure in the left atrium rises. A pressure tracing recorded simultaneously from the left atrium and left ventricle will demonstrate a considerable difference in these two pressures during diastole. This pressure difference is called a "gradient." Its existence is in marked contrast to the essentially superimposable pressure tracings that one obtains in normal subjects. Patients with stenosis of the aortic valve demonstrate a pressure gradient between the left ventricle and the aorta during systole. These pressure differences or gradients across valves are used to estimate the severity of valvular stenosis. Using the hydraulic Gorlin formula, one can calculate the orifice size of a stenotic valve in square centimeters if one knows the gradient across the valve, the cardiac output, and the heart rate.

Insufficiency of heart valves can be suggested in the pressure tracings from those heart chambers that lie just behind the leaky valve. Thus, marked mitral regurgitation results in large increases in the left atrial pressure during systole when regurgitation of blood is occurring from left ventricle to left atrium (V waves). In aortic insufficiency, regurgitation occurs during diastole. Since there is no ventricular contraction during diastole, there are no V waves in the left ventricular diastolic tracing. However, the large volume of blood regurgitating into the left ventricle during diastole causes the pressure in the left ventricle to rise markedly towards the end of diastole. Confirmation of valvular insufficiency and its quantitation depends upon angiographic techniques. Contrast medium is injected into the heart chamber that lies in front of the valve in question and regurgitation of blood is actually visualized. Thus, in mitral insufficiency, contrast material is injected into the left ventricle: one actually sees the regurgitation of blood and angiographic dye into the left atrium during each systole. A quantitative estimate of the volume of regurgitant blood can be made by examining the angiograms of the left ventricle and left atrium made during contrast medium injection. Occasionally, the pulmonic and tricuspid valves are also insufficient and the techniques described above apply equally well to these valves.

Coronary heart disease

Coronary heart disease can be accurately evaluated by cardiac catheterization. The physiologic variables measured tell the cardiologist about the function of the heart with coronary vascular lesions. Such patients are occasionally exercised or electrically paced in order to see the response of the heart to these forms of stress.

Of critical importance in the evaluation of coronary heart disease is the coronary angiogram and the left ventricular angiogram. During coronary angiography, radiographic contrast material is injected selectively into the two coronary arteries and cineangiograms are taken. This enables the cardiologist to delineate the extent of coronary atherosclerosis that is narrowing the lumens of the coronary blood vessels. Injection of contrast material into the left ventricle shows the cardiologist the ventricular contractile pattern. In patients who have not suffered a myocardial infarction, the contractile pattern of the left ventricle is vigorous and symmetrical. Patients who have suffered one or more myocardial infarctions, however, demonstrate areas of the left ventricular wall that contract poorly. These hypokinetic or akinetic zones represent areas of scar secondary to the infarction. In evaluating patients with coronary heart disease, it is important to know not only whether narrowings or obstructions exist in the coronary arterial system, but also whether there has been damage to the left ventricular wall from myocardial infarction causing alterations in cardiac pressures and output.

Myocardial diseases

Primary myocardial disease is demonstrated at catheterization by ruling out pericardial, valvular, and coronary heart diseases. Once all these other entities have been eliminated and cardiac function has been demonstrated to be abnormal, one can only explain the abnormalities demonstrated by postulating primary abnormalities of the cardiac muscle itself. Physiologically, one notes that diastolic pressures in the ventricles are elevated. Moreover, angiography demonstrates dilatation of the ventricular chambers involved (usually both ventricles). In addition, it is usually noted during angiography that the pattern of contraction of the ventricle is quite abnormal, with markedly reduced vigor of each contraction. Occasionally, myocardial biopsy is performed using a special catheter biotome.

Intracardiac defects: Shunts

Intracardiac shunts (holes or defects in the heart), such as atrial septal defect or ventricular septal defect, are demonstrated by physiologic and angiographic techniques. Physiologically, shunts are demonstrated by means of a technique known as the "diagnostic run." This technique takes advantage of the fact that shunts of oxygenated blood from the left side of the heart to the right side of the heart (atrial septal defect, ventricular septal defect, or patent ductus arteriosus) markedly increase the oxygen content of the venous blood present on the right side of the heart. Thus, by measuring the oxygen content in samples of blood from the pulmonary artery, right ventricle, right atrium, and superior and inferior venae cavae, one can determine the place in the heart where the oxygenated blood is arriving. In this way, one determines the level at which the shunt is located. In right-to-left shunts, resulting from severe resistance to blood flow in the pulmonary circulation (pulmonary vascular obliterative disease or Eisenmenger reaction), marked oxygen desaturation will be noted in arterial blood samples since venous blood from the right side of the heart is shunting over to the left side. To confirm left-to-right and right-to-left shunts, one employs serial injections of green dye into different locations in the cardiovascular system with sampling of the flow pattern of this dye in different chambers of the heart. For example, in a patient with atrial septal defect and a right-to-left shunt, green dye is injected into the right atrium; a small amount of dye shunts across the defect and arrives at a peripheral arterial sampling site earlier than the major part of the injectate of green dye that has followed the normal circulatory path (through the right ventricle, pulmonary artery, pulmonary capillaries, left atrium, left ventricle, and aorta). Thus, one sees a small early appearing hump on the right atrial to brachial arterial dye curve. This proves the existence of a right-to-left shunt. Similar reasonings and dye curve inscriptions confirm the existence of left-to-right shunts as well. By varying the sites of injection and sampling, one can accurately locate the intracardiac shunt. In addition, injection of angiographic contrast material into various heart chambers can actually visualize blood shunting through an intracardiac defect.

Arterial and venous
disease

Arterial stenoses or occlusion and venous obstruction by thrombi can be readily visualized by peripheral vascular angiography. A catheter is placed in the vessel to be assessed in the vicinity of the suspected pathological alteration. Contrast medium is then injected and x-ray pictures are obtained. Large segments of arterial and venous systems can be visualized by this technique.

Complications of
Cardiac
Catheterization

Although cardiac catheterization is a low-risk procedure, it does entail a definite small risk to the patient. It is only undertaken, therefore, when definite benefit to the patient can result from the information obtained. Complications include sustained arrhythmias, emboli from clots that can form on the tips of catheters and break off, and perforations of the heart by the cardiac catheter. Moreover, allergic reactions can occur to the contrast material injected during angiographic studies. Fortunately, complications are rare. In appropriate hands, mortality from cardiac catheterization should be 1 in 300 patients or less. Minor complications occur in a small percentage of patients. These less important complications include loss of pulse in one limb, transient arrhythmias, perforation without sequelae, and minor allergic reactions to contrast material. Less important complications include nausea and vomiting related to angiographic contrast material administration. All of these latter problems are usually rapidly reversible and the patient's life is not threatened.

In summary, cardiac catheterization represents the cardiologist's keenest diagnostic tool. It enables one to evaluate accurately the function of a patient's heart with respect to the integrity of the cardiac chambers, the ability of the heart to contract vigorously and forcefully, and the function and anatomy of the valves and blood vessels of the heart. Without cardiac catheterization, there could be no cardiac surgery since clinical diagnoses are more than occasionally incorrect. Most patients undergoing cardiac surgery should have cardiac catheterization for definitive diagnosis before surgery is undertaken. The small risk which the catheterization represents is definitely justified in terms of the important information obtained.

Table A-1 : Cardiac diseases or abnormalities that may be demonstrated by electrocardiography

Arteriosclerotic coronary artery disease with or without myocardial infarction
Fibrosis, infarction, or other form of interruption of the conduction system
Arrhythmias
Pericarditis with or without tamponade
Left and/or right ventricular hypertrophy
Electrolyte (mineral) imbalance

Noninvasive Techniques

Electrocardiography

An electrocardiogram (ECG) is a recording of the cardiac electrical current (voltage, potential). Recordings are obtained from the skin by attaching metal electrodes to a variety of sites on the surface of the body (arms, legs, chest). The ECG records cardiac electrical activity generated in the atria, the ventricles, and the specialized conducting tissue within the heart (see Chap. 14). Electrocardiography can demonstrate abnormalities in myocardial mass, coronary arterial perfusion, conducting tissue function, and cardiac rhythm. The ECG can be recorded in one plane (scalar electrocardiography) or in "three dimensions" (vectorcardiography). The latter technique is infrequently used. Electrocardiography is useful in the diagnosis of a variety of cardiac diseases (Table A-1). Abnormalities of cardiac rhythm may be recorded with routine scalar electrocardiography or with a technique known as "ambulatory electrocardiographic monitoring." The latter technique employs small paper electrodes that are glued to the skin for 24 hours. The electrodes are connected to a small, battery-powered tape recorder that records all of the patient's heart beats during a normal day's activities. When the 24-hour monitoring period is completed, the tape recording is analyzed by a computer that detects and prints out all arrhythmias. This technique enables the physician to "catch" brief periods of arrhythmia that would otherwise go unnoticed if only simple scalar electrocardiography were employed.

The scalar ECG is often recorded during and after a period of exertion. Patients are often exercised to exhaustion with careful electrocardiographic monitoring during and after exercise. Such exercise tolerance (or "stress") tests are commonly employed in the diagnosis of arteriosclerotic coronary artery disease. Ischemia, induced by exercise, produces specific, reversible changes in the ECG.

Echocardiography

Echocardiography is a technique for visualizing a variety of cardiac structures by means of reflected ultrasound. The principle that lies behind the imaging of cardiac anatomical details is the same as that employed in sonar imaging of underwater objects such as fish or submarines. A single quartz crystal transducer sends and receives rapid, high-frequency, ultrasound pulses. Electronic circuitry con-

Table A-2 : Cardiac diseases that may be demonstrated by echocardiography

Stenosis of all four cardiac valves
Regurgitation of all four cardiac valves (not as accurate as in the
    identification of stenotic valves)
Mitral valve prolapse*
Cardiomyopathy
Pericardial effusion*
Cardiac tumors*
Infectious endocarditis
Congenital heart disease
Dissection of the aorta
Stenosis of the left main coronary artery

* Echocardiography is the most accurate diagnostic modality for identifying this condition.

verts the reflected ultrasound into images that are displayed either on
a strip of paper (plotted against time) or on a television screen (two-
dimensional image). All four cardiac valves and chambers can be
examined as well as the pericardial space and a segment of the ascending aorta. A short segment of the left main coronary artery can
also be visualized. A variety of cardiovascular diseases can be identified by echocardiography (Table A-2). Some pathologic entities are
identified more readily by echocardiography than by any other diagnostic modality including cardiac catheterization.

*Phonocardiography
and pulse tracings*

Simultaneous recordings of heart sounds (phonocardiography), carotid arterial and jugular venous pulsations, apical impulse, and the
ECG can be useful to the physician in the noninvasive evaluation of
patients with myocardial, pericardial, and valvular heart disease. Calculated indices known as "systolic time intervals" can be derived
from such recordings. Systolic time intervals reflect the status of
overall left ventricular function. Abnormalities of carotid arterial,
jugular venous, and apical impulse recordings correlate with the
presence of a variety of cardiac diseases with specific patterns associated with certain pathological entities. For example, the patient with
severe aortic stenosis has a slowly rising carotid arterial pulse tracing, a normal jugular venous pulse tracing, and a sustained (and
often enlarged) apical impulse. A patient with cardiomyopathy may
have markedly abnormal systolic time intervals and normal carotid
arterial, jugular venous, and apical impulse recordings.

*Radiographic and
nuclear techniques*

RADIOGRAPHIC MEDICAL TECHNIQUES. Chest roentgenography and
electrocardiography are the two commonest noninvasive diagnostic
techniques employed in patients with cardiovascular disease. The
routine posteroanterior (PA) chest x-ray discloses information about
specific cardiac chamber and great vessel enlargement. Pericardial
and valvular calcification may also be detected on the PA chest film,
but fluoroscopy is a more sensitive technique for observing intracar-

diac calcification of coronary arteries, valves, or pericardium. Pulmonary venous and capillary hypertension secondary to left ventricular failure or mitral stenosis produces changes in the appearance of the pulmonary vasculature and parenchyma; elevated central venous pressure secondary to right ventricular failure results in azygous vein enlargement on the PA chest x-ray. Oblique views (right and left anterior oblique) of the heart, lungs, and great vessels are occasionally obtained in order to delineate specific cardiac chambers in a more complete and detailed fashion.

NUCLEAR MEDICAL TECHNIQUES. Three nuclear medical techniques are commonly employed in cardiovascular diagnostic evaluation: the radioventriculogram, the thallium-201 exercise test, and the technetium-99m pyrophosphate myocardial scan.

The *radioventriculogram* (radionuclide angiography) is a technique for assessing left and right ventricular function, quantitating valvular regurgitation and detecting left-to-right or right-to-left shunts. A radioactive isotope of technetium (^{99m}Tc) is attached to serum albumin or red blood cells and is injected intravenously. A nuclear camera (gamma ray detector) is positioned over the patient's precordium and radioactivity is quantitated in the various cardiac chambers during a number of preselected intervals throughout systole and diastole. Computer analysis of the collected data results in an accurate assessment of left and right ventricular ejection fraction. Appropriate manipulation of the technique and acquired data yields an accurate measure of intracardiac shunt flow and valvular regurgitation. The variables measured by radionuclide angiography correlate highly with similar parameters obtained invasively by means of cardiac catheterization. Radionuclide angiography can be performed during exercise as well as at rest, thereby furnishing the physician with a quantitative estimate of ventricular function during exercise.

The *thallium-201 exercise test* is a variant of the standard electrocardiographic exercise test. Patients exercise on a bicycle or treadmill according to a predetermined protocol of gradually increasing exercise demand. The electrocardiographic response is monitored continuously. At peak exercise, a small quantity of radioactive thallium-201 is injected intravenously. Thallium-102 is a potassium analog and as such is avidly taken up by the myocardium in proportion to the blood flow. Areas of myocardium that are poorly perfused during exercise (ischemic zones) receive little or no thallium-201 and they appear as zones of low radioactivity during exercise ("cold spots") on the gamma camera picture of the heart. Ischemic cold spots disappear in subsequent resting gamma camera pictures of the heart as blood flow reaches ischemic areas. The thallium-201 exercise test is a highly accurate noninvasive technique for detecting ischemia secondary to arteriosclerotic coronary artery disease. If the myocardium has been replaced by tissue that does not take up thallium-201 (scar tissue, tumors, sarcoid granulomas), cold spots are observed on the resting cardiac image.

The *technetium-99m pyrophosphate myocardial scan* is a technique for detecting freshly necrotic myocardium. Technetium-99m is bound to pyrophosphate and is injected intravenously. The technetium-99m pyrophosphate complex is taken up by irreversible, acutely injured myocardium. Such imaging is usually the result of a myocardial infarction. Normal myocardium does not take up the pyrophosphate complex. Thus, the gamma camera picture of the heart demonstrates a zone of increased radioactivity ("hot spot") only when recent myocardial necrosis is present.

Peripheral vascular tests

A variety of noninvasive techniques exist for detecting abnormal peripheral arterial and venous function. Most of these tests measure the adequacy of blood flow in these vessels.

Plethysmographic techniques (impedance, strain gauge, water tank) measure blood flow in a limb during and after a short period of venous occlusion. Arterial and venous patency can be assessed by this technique. Doppler techniques employ high-frequency sound waves to quantitate and even visualize flowing blood on either the arterial or venous side of the circulation. Significant arterial stenoses and venous thromboses are readily detected.

A number of nuclear medical techniques have been devised to assess the adequacy of arterial and venous blood flow. Arterial patency is assessed by injecting small quantities of a radioactive isotope (xenon, iodine, krypton) into a muscle supplied by the artery to be tested. Exercise or occlusion-induced hyperemia is then produced and the clearance of the radioisotope is then followed with a gamma camera. Clearance is proportional to the adequacy of arterial blood flow. Venous thrombosis can be detected by administering radioisotope labelled fibrinogen intravenously. The fibrinogen-isotope complexes are incorporated into recent intravascular thrombi. Gamma camera pictures of the extremities demonstrate increased counts over extremities with venous thrombosis.

Appendix B : Study Questions

Chapter 1

1. The central underlying theme in most patients with heart failure is:
   a. inadequate myocardial function
   b. excessive peripheral demand
   c. abnormal pulmonary function
   d. abnormal renal function

2. Cardiac performance depends on all but one of the following variables. Identify the *incorrect* response.
   a. intrinsic myocardial contractility
   b. preload
   c. arterial oxygen tension
   d. afterload

3. The most difficult property of cardiac function to define is:
   a. cardiac output
   b. left ventricular wall tension
   c. intrinsic myocardial contractility
   d. myocardial blood flow

4. The cardiovascular response to exercise includes all but one of the following events. Identify the *incorrect* response.
   a. arteriolar vasodilatation in exercising skeletal muscle
   b. arteriolar vasoconstriction in skin, nonexercising muscle, kidney, and splanchnic beds
   c. beta-adrenergic stimulation of the heart
   d. increased venous return
   e. increased arterial carbon dioxide tension

5. All but one of the following alterations occur in patients with heart failure. Identify the *incorrect* response.
   a. ventricular dilatation
   b. bradycardia
   c. decreased cardiac output
   d. depressed ejection fraction
   e. decreased ventricular compliance

6. In most forms of heart failure abnormal energy production is not the major cause of reduced myocardial contractility.
   a. true
   b. false

7. The major abnormality in failing myocardium is impairment of intracellular calcium regulation by sarcoplasmic reticulum.
   a. true
   b. false

8. One of the following alterations in autonomic nervous system function in patients with heart failure is incorrect. Identify the *incorrect* response.
   a. Norepinephrine concentration is markedly reduced in myocardial samples from animals and patients with heart failure.
   b. Circulating and urinary excretion of norepinephrine is increased in patients with heart failure.
   c. Exercise leads to minimal changes in plasma norepinephrine levels in patients with heart failure.
   d. Failing myocardium is hypersensitive to the effects of infused exogenous norepinephrine.
   e. Parasympathetic nervous stimulation of the heart produces less than the expected decrease in heart rate in patients with heart failure.

9. All of the following except one are true about peripheral vascular responses to heart failure. Identify the *incorrect* response.
   a. There is increased resting and exercise blood flow to skin, kidneys, and nonexercising muscles.
   b. Peripheral arterioles demonstrate a decreased capacity for vasodilatation in heart failure.
   c. Peripheral arterioles have an increased salt and water content in heart failure patients and animals.
   d. Blood flow increases to exercising muscles despite the heart failure state.

10. All but one of the following is a compensatory response of the cardiovascular system to heart failure. Identify the *incorrect* response.
    a. decreased ventricular compliance
    b. the Starling mechanism
    c. increased circulating norepinephrine levels
    d. cardiac hypertrophy

Chapter 2

1. All but one of the following are determinants of myocardial oxygen consumption. Identify the *incorrect* response.
   a. intracardiac systolic pressure
   b. ventricular diameter
   c. ventricular wall thickness
   d. heart rate
   e. myocardial blood flow

2. The product of heart rate and blood pressure (tension time index) is directly proportional to myocardial oxygen consumption.
   a. true
   b. false

3. Myocardium has a limited ability to generate adenosine triphosphate (ATP) by anaerobic metabolic reactions.
   a. true
   b. false
4. Which of the following metabolic products is produced by ischemic myocardium?
   a. glucose
   b. lactate
   c. fatty acids
   d. creatine phosphate
5. All but one of the following affects myocardial blood flow. Identify the *incorrect* response.
   a. autoregulation
   b. myocardial oxygen consumption
   c. mechanical compression of coronary blood vessels
   d. peripheral arterial smooth muscle tone
   e. autonomic nervous system activity
6. The process that leads to the development of an atherosclerotic lesion consists of all but one of the following. Identify the *incorrect* response.
   a. presence of a circulating anticoagulant
   b. platelet and fibrin deposition in an area of endothelial injury
   c. arterial smooth muscle cell migration and proliferation
   d. deposition of cholesterol and other lipids in an area of repetitive endothelial injury
   e. fibrotic and calcific response to cell necrosis
7. Collateral blood flow in the myocardium is frequently adequate to satisfy resting but not exercise cardiac metabolic demands.
   a. true
   b. false
8. All but one of the following occur within myocardial cells with the onset of ischemia. Identify the *incorrect* response.
   a. decline in intracellular levels of high energy phosphate compounds
   b. metabolism of lactate and pyruvate to produce ATP
   c. preferential use of glucose as a metabolic substrate
   d. breakdown of glycogen stored in myocardial cells
   e. intracellular acidosis and lipid accumulation
9. Each of the following alterations in myocardial performance occurs during ischemia except for one. Identify the *incorrect* response.
   a. marked depression of myocardial contractile performance develops within 10–15 seconds of the onset of ischemia
   b. eventual cessation of myocardial contraction with continuing ischemia
   c. increased myocardial compliance
   d. increased myocardial stiffness

10. Myocardial ischemia resulting in the symptom of angina pectoris can be the result of (a) a decrease in myocardial blood flow with a constant myocardial oxygen consumption (inadequate supply) or (b) an increase in myocardial oxygen consumption with constant myocardial blood flow (excessive demand).
   a. true
   b. false

11. How much of a reduction in coronary arterial luminal cross sectional area is necessary before a marked decrease in resting coronary blood flow occurs?
   a. 50%
   b. 60%
   c. 70%
   d. 80%
   e. 90%

12. During exercise a luminal diameter reduction of 50–60% of a coronary artery can result in impairment in the normal increase in coronary arterial blood flow.
   a. true
   b. false

Chapter 3

1. Individual myocardial cells differ in their ability to resist ischemia.
   a. true
   b. false

2. All but one of the following events occurs in myocardial cells that have been injured by ischemia. Identify the *incorrect* response.
   a. loss of maintenance of the sodium-potassium ionic gradient across the cell membrane
   b. increase in intracellular sodium and water content
   c. loss of creatine phosphokinase
   d. loss of mitochondrial and lysosomal integrity
   e. increased pumping of potassium intracellularly

3. All but one of the following ultrastructural alterations occurs in myocardial cells injured by ischemia. Identify the *incorrect* response.
   a. increased distinctness of tight junctions
   b. swollen sacs in the sarcoplasmic reticulum
   c. greatly enlarged mitochondria with few cristae
   d. thinning and fractionation of the myofilaments
   e. alterations in nuclear structure

4. Myocardial contractile activity slowly decreases over 30–40 minutes after interruption of myocardial oxygenation.
   a. true
   b. false

5. Ischemic myocardial cells demonstrate marked impairment of diastolic myocardial function (relaxation).
   a. true
   b. false

6. The greater the period of ischemia, the longer it takes for myocardial contractility and relaxation to return to normal.
   a. true
   b. false

7. All but one of the following statements are true. Identify the *incorrect* statement.
   a. Myocardial ischemia is associated with diminution or cessation of contractile activity in a localized, affected zone of myocardium.
   b. Uninvolved areas of the ventricle contract normally while ischemic regions either fail to contract (akinesis), or bulge passively during systole (dyskinesis).
   c. Myocardial zones surrounding an ischemic region often demonstrate increased contractile function (hyperkinesis).
   d. In zones of myocardium with normal myocardial blood flow, compensatory hyperdynamic wall motion is frequently noted.
   e. Overall systolic ventricular wall motion and hence contractile function is related to the percentage of the ventricle involved by the ischemic process.

8. When __% or more of the left ventricle ceases to function, adequate systemic blood pressure cannot be maintained and shock (inadequate tissue perfusion) develops.
   a. 10
   b. 20
   c. 30
   d. 40

9. The quantity of myocardium that is infarcted in animal experiments involving coronary occlusion and subsequent reperfusion is a function of the duration of the occlusive phase of the experiment: small amounts of myocardial necrosis result with 2 hours or less of occlusion; progressively larger amounts of myocardium are lost as occlusion time extends to 6–8 hours.
   a. true
   b. false

10. Cessation of regional contractile function in patients with myocardial infarction coupled with an increase in myocardial stiffness accompanying ischemia or infarction results in increased ventricular filling pressure that is transmitted during diastole to the left atrium, pulmonary veins, and pulmonary capillaries.
   a. true
   b. false

11. Identify the two commonest compensatory mechanisms of the cardiovascular system that are activated in a patient with acute myocardial infarction.
    a. sympathetic nervous system
    b. parasympathetic nervous system
    c. ventricular dilatation (Starling mechanism)
    d. bronchodilatation
    e. renal hyperperfusion

12. Mean aortic blood pressure should remain above _____ mm Hg in patients with acute myocardial infarction because coronary autoregulation is lost at levels of blood pressure below this point.
    a. 20–30
    b. 30–40
    c. 40–50
    d. 50–60
    e. 60–70

13. All but one of the following findings have been shown in experimental animals in which an intervention decreased infarct size. Identify the *incorrect* response.
    a. Propranolol decreases myocardial oxygen consumption.
    b. Nitroglycerin decreases myocardial oxygen consumption and increases coronary blood flow.
    c. Isoproterenol decreases myocardial oxygen consumption.
    d. Coronary artery reperfusion increases myocardial blood flow.

14. Some individuals develop coronary arterial occlusion from coronary thrombosis without developing myocardial infarction.
    a. true
    b. false

15. Some individuals develop total occlusion of a coronary artery secondary to coronary artery smooth muscle spasm. Such an occlusion may result in a myocardial infarction.
    a. true
    b. false

Chapter 4

1. One third of all deaths in the United States are a direct result of coronary heart disease.
    a. true
    b. false

2. During the 10-year period from 1968 to 1978 mortality from all causes decreased in the United States. Heart disease mortality, and particularly coronary heart disease mortality, fell more than any other disease category.
    a. true
    b. false

3. In patients suffering acute myocardial infarction, ___ percent of deaths occur within the first 24 hours after the onset of symptoms.
   a. 20
   b. 40
   c. 65
   d. 85
   e. 95

4. The majority of deaths from coronary heart disease occur suddenly before medical attention can be given to the patient.
   a. true
   b. false

5. Many studies show that levels of risk factors can be significantly modified in a favorable direction thereby resulting in definite, marked decreases in coronary heart disease morbidity and mortality.
   a. true
   b. false

6. A number of risk factors have been shown to be related to coronary heart disease risk and as such are known to be causative of coronary atherosclerosis.
   a. true
   b. false

7. All but one of the following risk factors have been consistently linked to the development of cardiovascular disease. Identify the *incorrect* response.
   a. hypertension
   b. smoking
   c. residence in a cold climate
   d. elevated serum cholesterol
   e. diabetes

8. All but one of the following risk factors have been shown to be highly related to the development of cardiovascular disease. Identify the minor risk factor.
   a. water hardness
   b. smoking
   c. hypertension
   d. elevated serum cholesterol
   e. heredity

9. Available data indicate that death from all causes is approximately _____ times as high among cigarette smokers as among nonsmokers.
   a. two
   b. three
   c. four
   d. five

10. The majority of excess deaths in patients who smoke cigarettes are the result of mortality from cardiovascular disease, in particular, sudden death and myocardial infarction.
    a. true
    b. false

11. There is a direct relationship between the number of cigarettes smoked and the risk of cardiac disease: the more one smokes the greater the risk of heart disease.
    a. true
    b. false

12. Unlike the risk of smoking and lung cancer, for which risk appears to be cumulative and expressible in number of pack years of smoking, the risk of coronary artery disease seems to be related to the current level of smoking and to be reversible when smoking is discontinued.
    a. true
    b. false

13. A favorable high-density lipoprotein (HDL) to total cholesterol ratio is:
    a. 4.5 or less to 1
    b. 6.0 or less to 1
    c. 8.0 or less to 1
    d. 2.0 or less to 1

14. Do interventions that lower serum cholesterol reduce coronary heart disease mortality rate in a population?
    a. Definitely yes.
    b. Definitely no.
    c. The data are not yet satisfactory for a definitive answer.

15. All but one of the following personality traits are characteristic of the so-called type A personality. Identify the *incorrect* response.
    a. aggressive
    b. constantly striving
    c. lack of time urgency
    d. ambitious
    e. competitive

16. The combination of birth control pills and cigarette smoking markedly increases a female patient's risk for thromboembolism, stroke, and myocardial infarction.
    a. true
    b. false

17. There is no definitive proof that the consumption of coffee or tea increases the risk of cardiovascular disease.
    a. true
    b. false

18. Risk factors for coronary heart disease appear to be additive such that individuals with several risk factors have a much

greater chance of developing coronary heart disease as compared with individuals with only a single risk factor.

a. true
b. false

Chapter 5

1. All of the below are known causes of valvular heart disease except one. Identify the *incorrect* response.
   a. Marfan syndrome
   b. rheumatic fever
   c. carcinoid disease
   d. myxomatous degeneration
   e. Klinefelter syndrome

2. The most reasonable pathophysiologic sequence leading to mitral stenosis in individuals who have acute rheumatic fever is:
   a. myxomatous change in the mitral valve
   b. inflammation leading to abnormal flow patterns across the mitral valve with resultant increased stress on the leaflets
   c. antibody mediated destruction of collagen crossbridges
   d. streptococcal toxin-induced lysis of elastin fibers

3. Stenotic valves have a pressure gradient across them.
   a. true
   b. false

4. The normal mitral valve area during diastole is:
   a. 1–2 cm²
   b. 1–3 cm²
   c. 4–5 cm²
   d. 5–6 cm²
   e. variable depending on body surface area

5. In mitral stenosis cardiac output is maintained at the expense of increased left atrial pressure.
   a. true
   b. false

6. In individuals without valvular heart disease left ventricular diastolic pressure is approximately equal to:
   a. left atrial pressure
   b. pulmonary capillary wedge pressure
   c. pulmonary arterial diastolic pressure
   d. all of the above

7. In patients with mitral stenosis, the major burden of the increased work is borne by the:
   a. right ventricle
   b. left atrium
   c. right atrium
   d. left ventricle

8. In mitral stenosis the left ventricle is:
   a. enlarged

b. atrophic

c. unaffected

9. Blood flow through a narrowed cardiac valve is determined by three of the following four factors. Identify the *incorrect* response.

   a. the pressure gradient across the valve

   b. the cardiac output

   c. the period of time allowed for the blood to flow across the valve

   d. the mass of the valvular leaflets

10. Pregnancy aggravates the hemodynamic abnormalities associated with mitral stenosis because the gravid state results in a decrease in heart rate and cardiac output.

    a. true

    b. false

11. In patients with mitral regurgitation, the volume of regurgitant blood flow across the mitral valve is dependent on all but one of the following factors. Identify the *incorrect* response.

    a. pulmonary capillary wedge pressure

    b. size of the mitral valve orifice during systole

    c. left ventricular systolic pressure

    d. left atrial pressure

    e. left ventricular systolic ejection time

    f. heart rate

12. In patients with mitral regurgitation the left ventricle ejects blood: (1) through the aortic valve to the systemic circulation, and (2) through the mitral valve into the left atrium.

    a. true

    b. false

13. The left ventricle tolerates pressure overload better than it tolerates volume overload.

    a. true

    b. false

14. Which of the following valvular lesions result in volume overload of the heart and which of the following lesions result in pressure overload of the heart?

    a. mitral stenosis

    b. tricuspid regurgitation

    c. aortic regurgitation

    d. aortic stenosis

15. Mitral regurgitation tends to perpetuate itself because left atrial dilatation pulls the posterior mitral leaflet further away from the anterior leaflet.

    a. true

    b. false

16. One of the below is not a cause of pressure overload left ven-

tricular hypertrophy. Identify the lesion that does *not* lead to pressure overload left ventricular hypertrophy.

a. aortic stenosis
b. mitral regurgitation
c. systemic hypertension
d. coarctation of the aorta
e. supraaortic stenosis

17. Aortic stenosis produces left ventricular hypertrophy that is greater than left ventricular dilatation while aortic regurgitation produces left ventricular dilatation that is greater than left ventricular hypertrophy.

a. true
b. false

18. Angina pectoris in patients with aortic stenosis in the absence of coronary arterial obstruction is the result of:

a. coronary spasm
b. excessive myocardial metabolic demand
c. coronary embolization
d. arterial hypoxemia

19. Syncope in patients with aortic stenosis is the result of all but one of the following. Identify the *incorrect* response.

a. coexistent severe mitral regurgitation
b. episodic arrhythmias
c. reflex or exercise induced vasodilatation
d. ventricular tachycardia or fibrillation

20. Bradycardia increases aortic regurgitant flow in patients with aortic insufficiency by increasing the period of time during which regurgitation occurs.

a. true
b. false

21. In aortic regurgitation each left ventricular contraction must eject the normal stroke volume *minus* the regurgitant volume.

a. true
b. false

22. Widened pulse pressure in patients with aortic stenosis is the result of the larger than normal stroke volume and the decreased resistance during diastole secondary to the large runoff of blood backwards into the left ventricle.

a. true
b. false

23. Left ventricular myocardial compliance in patients with aortic insufficiency is usually:

a. increased
b. decreased
c. initially increased then decreased
d. variable depending on size of aortic regurgitant orifice

24. The bounding pulses observed in patients with aortic insufficiency are the result of the markedly widened aortic pulse pressure.
    a. true
    b. false

25. Aortic regurgitation of sudden onset (acute aortic regurgitation) is quite similar in its pathophysiology to chronic aortic regurgitation.
    a. true
    b. false

26. A recording of right atrial pressure from a patient with tricuspid regurgitation usually demonstrates large regurgitant waves (V) similar to those that occur in the left atrial pressure tracing of patients with mitral regurgitation.
    a. true
    b. false

27. The electrocardiogram of patients with pulmonic stenosis usually demonstrates:
    a. left ventricular hypertrophy
    b. right ventricular hypertrophy
    c. left atrial enlargement
    d. anteroseptal myocardial infarction
    e. inferior myocardial infarction

Chapter 6

1. The classification of cardiomyopathy includes all but one of the following forms. Identify the *incorrect* response.
    a. hypertrophic
    b. congestive
    c. restrictive
    d. anemic

2. Abnormal myocardial hypertrophy is the hallmark of hypertrophic obstructive cardiomyopathy.
    a. true
    b. false

3. In patients with hypertrophic obstructive cardiomyopathy the hypertrophic process is apparently related to zones of disarrayed, disorganized, and bizarrely formed myocardial cells that work together rather than in opposition.
    a. true
    b. false

4. Left ventricular diastolic function (compliance) in patients with hypertrophic obstructive cardiomyopathy is:
    a. abnormally reduced
    b. abnormally increased
    c. normal

5. All but one of the following conditions result in abnormally reduced left ventricular diastolic function (compliance). Identify the condition with normal or increased compliance.
   a. aortic regurgitation
   b. aortic stenosis
   c. hypertrophic obstructive cardiomyopathy
   d. ischemic heart disease
   e. restrictive cardiomyopathy

6. In patients with hypertrophic obstructive cardiomyopathy and a dynamic (changing) gradient across the left ventricular outflow tract, interventions that increase left ventricular cavity size _____ the degree of outflow tract obstruction.
   a. increase
   b. decrease

7. All but one of the following measures of left ventricular contractility are usually abnormally reduced in patients with congestive cardiomyopathy. Identify the *incorrect* response.
   a. dp/dt
   b. V_{max}
   c. ejection fraction
   d. heart rate
   e. V^{cf}

8. Patients with congestive cardiomyopathy usually die from all but one of the following complications. Identify the *incorrect* complication.
   a. intractable heart failure
   b. malignant ventricular arrhythmias
   c. cardiac rupture
   d. arterial or venous embolism

9. Approximately 100 ml of fluid can be accommodated in the pericardial space without an increase in intrapericardial pressure. However, small amounts of additional fluid beyond that volume produce large increases in pressure in the pericardial space.
   a. true
   b. false

10. All but one of the following physical findings occur in patients with cardiac tamponade. Identify the *incorrect* response.
    a. pulsus paradoxus
    b. elevated jugular venous pressure
    c. tachycardia
    d. wide pulse pressure

11. The hemodynamic hallmark of cardiac compression or constriction is marked difference in right heart diastolic pressures.
    a. true
    b. false

1. In patients with atrial septal defect (ASD), blood samples from all but one of the following cardiac chambers will demonstrate abnormally increased oxygen saturation. Identify the *incorrect* chamber.
   a. right atrium
   b. right ventricle
   c. left ventricle
   d. pulmonary artery

2. The left-to-right shunt in patients with ASD occurs because right ventricular compliance is greater than left ventricular compliance.
   a. true
   b. false

3. The development of pulmonary vascular disease and pulmonary hypertension in patients with ASD can result in shunt reversal with resultant arterial hypoxemia.
   a. true
   b. false

4. In patients with ASD and a left-to-right shunt, the right ventricle is subjected to:
   a. volume overload
   b. pressure overload
   c. no overload at all

5. All of the following statements about ventricular septal defect (VSD) are true except for one. Identify the *incorrect* statement.
   a. During uterine life there is little flow across the atrial septal defect because of high pulmonary vascular resistance and high right ventricular systolic pressure.
   b. Left ventricular systolic pressure postpartum is usually much higher than right ventricular systolic pressure producing a net left-to-right shunt of blood across the VSD.
   c. In patients with VSD, increased blood oxygen saturation occurs in the right atrium.
   d. The development of pulmonary vascular disease during adult life in patients with VSD can result in right-to-left shunting of blood and resultant arterial hypoxemia.

6. The quantity of blood that shunts across a VSD is determined by all but one of the following variables. Identify the *incorrect* variable.
   a. pulmonary vascular resistance
   b. size of the defect
   c. left ventricular systolic pressure
   d. right ventricular systolic pressure
   e. left atrial pressure

7. Patients with patent ductus arteriosus (PDA) and Eisenmenger syndrome shunt desaturated blood to:
   a. the fingers

b. the head

c. primarily the left carotid artery

d. the descending aorta

8. The more severe the narrowing in the aorta in patients with coarctation of the aorta, the greater will be the obstruction to normal aortic blood flow and the larger will be the pressure gradient across the obstruction.

   a. true

   b. false

9. An obstructive coarctation of the aorta produces systemic arterial _____ proximal to the narrowed region of the aorta and arterial _____ distal to the coarctation.

   a. hypertension

   b. hypotension

10. Individuals with congenital heart disease who reside at altitude (5,000 feet elevation or higher) have a reduced chance of developing pulmonary vascular disease than persons residing at sea level.

   a. true

   b. false

11. All but one of the following are manifestations of Eisenmenger syndrome. Identify the *incorrect* response.

   a. elevated red blood cell count

   b. clubbing of fingernails and toenails

   c. increased renal secretion of erythropoeitin

   d. arterial hypoxemia

   e. increased systemic blood pressure

Chapter 8

1. Flow through the pulmonary circulation is determined by all but one of the following factors. Identify the *incorrect* response.

   a. pressure

   b. viscosity

   c. cross sectional diameter of the vascular bed

   d. ventricular preload

2. Pulmonary artery end-diastolic pressure is approximately equal to left ventricular end-diastolic pressure.

   a. true

   b. false

3. Pulmonary vascular resistance is approximately __% of the resistance across the systemic vascular bed.

   a. 10

   b. 25

   c. 50

   d. 70

4. In the upright position, pulmonary blood flow increases in a linear fashion from the lowermost lung segments to the uppermost lung segments.

a. true

b. false

5. All but one of the following conditions can result in "passive" pulmonary hypertension. Identify the *incorrect* response.

   a. chronic obstructive pulmonary disease

   b. mitral stenosis

   c. mitral regurgitation

   d. myocardial infarction

   e. congestive cardiomyopathy

6. In patients with chronic obstructive pulmonary disease, pulmonary vascular resistance increases secondary to vasoconstriction in the pulmonary circuit from alveolar hypoxia and acidemia.

   a. true

   b. false

7. Patients with primary pulmonary hypertension can demonstrate all but one of the following pathological findings in their pulmonary arterioles. Identify the *incorrect* response.

   a. intimal thickening

   b. smooth muscle hypertrophy

   c. lysis of the adventitia

   d. intimal fibrosis

   e. arteritis with necrosis

8. All but one of the following are causes of precapillary pulmonary hypertension. Identify the *incorrect* response.

   a. primary pulmonary hypertension

   b. diffuse interstitial lung disease

   c. chronic obstructive pulmonary disease

   d. atrial septal defect with Eisenmenger reaction

   e. mitral stenosis

9. In "reactive" pulmonary hypertension, the pulmonary artery diastolic to pulmonary capillary wedge pressure gradient is _____ mm Hg or greater and the pulmonary capillary wedge pressure is elevated.

   a. 0–4

   b. 5–10

   c. 10–20

   d. 20–30

10. Factors involved in determining the rate of fluid movement across the capillary wall and into the interstitial space include all but one of the following. Identify the *incorrect* response.

    a. capillary pressure

    b. arterial pressure

    c. interstitial pressure

    d. capillary filtration coefficient

    e. intracapillary colloid osmotic pressure

11. Pulmonary edema is characterized by two stages: the first stage is characterized by interstitial edema with increased lymphatic

flow and the second stage is characterized by alveolar edema
that results when interstitial fluid spills over into the alveoli.

a. true
b. false

12. All but one of the following statements are true about cor pulmonale. Identify the *incorrect* statement.

a. Pulmonary arterial hypertension may be caused by intrinsic
lung disease of the interstitium, tracheobronchial tree, alveoli, or pulmonary vascular tree.

b. Pulmonary arterial hypertension must be present and is the
cause of right ventricular enlargement.

c. Neither congenital heart disease nor acquired disease of the
left side of the heart can be implicated as the cause for the
pulmonary hypertension.

d. Mitral stenosis is a common cause of cor pulmonale.

13. The five-year prognosis for patients with cor pulmonale secondary to chronic obstructive pulmonary disease is excellent.

a. true
b. false

Chapter 9

1. A 66-year-old man with congestive heart failure is begun on indomethacin for acute gouty arthritis. One week later he is found to
have developed bilateral pedal edema. The following lab values
are obtained at a time when he is producing 800 ml urine/day.

BUN = 54 mg/dl (25 mg/dl before indomethacin)
Serum creatinine = 1.5 mg/dl (0.9 mg/dl before indomethacin)

The indomethacin is stopped and one week later, the edema is
gone and renal function returns to normal. Explain the edema
formation and change in renal function which occurred while on
indomethacin.

2. A 72-year-old man is begun on hydrochlorothiazide for treatment
of mild cardiac failure with edema. One month later he is brought
to the emergency room with mental confusion. On exam he is
found to have orthostatic hypotension and diminished skin turgor. Laboratory values include:

BUN = 100 mg/dl
Serum creatinine = 2.0 mg/dl
Serum sodium = 110 mEq/L
Serum potassium = 3.0 mEq/L

a. What is the likely explanation of his hyponatremia?
b. How do you explain his azotemia?
c. How would you treat the hyponatremia?

Chapter 10

1. The immediate cause of mean arterial blood elevation is an increase in either cardiac output or peripheral resistance or both.
   a. true
   b. false

2. Rare patients with clinical hypertension have an increase in peripheral vascular resistance due to arteriolar narrowing.
   a. true
   b. false

3. All the following statements expect one are true about pheochromocytoma. Identify the *incorrect* response.
   a. These tumors are characterized by a high basal and frequently superimposed paroxysmal secretion of norepinephrine and epinepherine.
   b. Pheochromocytomas are usually found in the adrenal medulla or as embryonal rests along the sympathetic ganglia.
   c. Sympathetic alpha-blocking agents (for example phentolamine) often cause hypertensive responses in patients with pheochromocytoma.
   d. Elevated plasma renin activity is found in 70% of patients with pheochromocytoma.
   e. Plasma volume is contracted on the average by 15% in patients with pheochromocytoma.

4. Juxtaglomerular cell tumors increase circulating levels of renin and angiotensin II and thereby produce vasoconstriction and resultant hypertension.
   a. true
   b. false

5. The reduction in the renal arterial lumen must be approximately __ % in order to activate the renin secretory mechanism.
   a. 20
   b. 40
   c. 60
   d. 80
   e. 95

6. Primary hyperaldosteronism is characterized by all but one of the following. Identify the *incorrect* response.
   a. autonomous high secreting adenoma of the adrenal gland
   b. accelerated exchange of hydrogen and potassium ions in the distal renal tubule
   c. decreased plasma and extracellular volume
   d. suppression of renal renin secretion

7. All but one of the following statements are true about patients with Cushing syndrome. Identify the *incorrect* response.
   a. Cortisol has intrinsic mineralocorticoid effects that produce sodium and water retention.
   b. Steroids inhibit the chemical reaction whereby renin is converted to angiotensin II.

    c. The renin angiotensin system is stimulated because hepatic synthesis of renin substrate is increased.

    d. The vascular effects of catecholamines are potentiated.

8. The sympathetic nervous system demonstrates heightened activity and/or sensitivity in patients with essential hypertension.

    a. true

    b. false

9. All patients with essential hypertension demonstrate increased levels of renin in their blood stream.

    a. true

    b. false

10. A number of animal and patient studies demonstrate the importance of the kidney in the development of essential hypertension.

    a. true

    b. false

11. All but one of the following probably play a role in the development of essential hypertension. Identify the *incorrect* response.

    a. abnormal hypothalamic function

    b. abnormal peripheral vascular smooth muscle response

    c. abnormal renal vascular smooth muscle response

    d. abnormal parasympathetic nervous system function

    e. abnormal sympathetic nervous system function

Chapter 11

1. Identify the two major cardiac compensatory responses to impaired myocardial function or excessive peripheral demand from the following list.

    a. increased sympathetic nervous stimulation of the heart

    b. peripheral arteriolar vasodilatation

    c. ventricular chamber dilatation and/or hypertrophy of the myocardium leading to increased myocardial mass

    d. increased peripheral venous pressure

2. Cardiac sympathetic and parasympathetic nervous function is increased in patients with heart failure.

    a. true

    b. false

3. In patients with advanced heart failure, cardiac output is depressed and systemic arteriovenous oxygen difference is increased at rest.

    a. true

    b. false

4. Vasoconstriction of arterioles and veins is found in all but one of the following organs in patients with heart failure. Identify the *incorrect* organ.

    a. stomach

    b. brain

    c. skin

d. kidney

e. spleen

5. The body's regulating mechanisms sense heart failure as if there had been a decrease in circulating blood volume such as might have occurred secondary to hemorrhage.

   a. true

   b. false

Chapter 12

1. All but one of the following symptoms can be present in patients with left ventricular failure. Identify the *incorrect* symptom.

   a. abdominal swelling

   b. orthopnea

   c. paroxysmal nocturnal dyspnea

   d. dyspnea on exertion

2. All but one of the following symptoms can be present in patients with right ventricular failure. Identify the *incorrect* response.

   a. peripheral edema

   b. abdominal swelling

   c. fatigue

   d. anorexia

   e. orthopnea

3. All but one of the following physical findings can be found in patients with left ventricular failure. Identify the *incorrect* physical findings.

   a. third heart sound

   b. fourth heart sound

   c. hepatomegaly

   d. rales over the lung fields

   e. pulsus alternans

4. All but one of the following physical findings may be found in patients with right ventricular failure. Identify the *incorrect* physical finding.

   a. fourth heart sound

   b. third heart sound

   c. hepatomegaly

   d. peripheral edema

   e. rales over the lung fields

5. All but one of the following may be found at cardiac catheterization in patients with heart failure. Identify the *incorrect* finding.

   a. elevated ventricular filling pressures

   b. depressed cardiac output

   c. reduced ventricular contractility

   d. increased myocardial compliance indices (decreased stiffness)

6. Individuals with effort-induced angina probably develop myocardial ischemia as the result of increased heart rate and blood pressure associated with effort.

a. true

b. false

7. Heart sounds are often loud or crisp in patients with myocardial ischemia or infarction.

a. true

b. false

Chapter 14

1. Cardiac arrhythmias include a large number of conditions characterized by disturbances in the heart's ability to initiate and conduct impulses in a normal fashion.

a. true

b. false

2. In the pacemaker hierarchy, heart cells in the sinoatrial node beat fastest and therefore initiate depolarization of the ventricles under normal conditions.

a. true

b. false

3. If the activity of the sinoatrial node is disrupted, subsidiary pacemaker cells take over the heart rhythm. All but one of the following rhythms can occur if the sinoatrial node ceases to function. Identify the *incorrect* response.

a. nodal rhythm

b. idioventricular rhythm

c. accelerated idioventricular rhythm

4. Abnormal cardiac rhythm arises as a result of either enhanced automaticity or reentry.

a. true

b. false

5. All but one of the following are bradyarrhythmias. Identify the *incorrect* response.

a. sinus bradycardia

b. nodal rhythm

c. cardiac asystole

d. atrial fibrillation

6. All but one of the following are tachyarrhythmias. Identify the *incorrect* response.

a. cardiac asystole

b. sinus tachycardia

c. ventricular tachycardia

d. atrial flutter

e. ventricular fibrillation

7. All but one of the following examples of impaired cardiac conduction are the result of interruption of normal conduction in the bundle branches. Identify the *incorrect* response.

a. left bundle branch block

b. right bundle branch block

c. Wolff-Parkinson-White syndrome

d. third-degree atrioventricular block

Chapter 15

1. All but one of the following terms are involved in the Poisseuille relationship, which defines the relation between pressure difference along a tube carrying a viscous fluid. Identify the *incorrect* term.

   a. velocity of fluid flow
   b. radius of the tube
   c. tube length
   d. viscosity
   e. red cell mass

2. The symptom of intermittent claudication is analogous to that of angina pectoris in that both are discomfort resulting from inadequate blood flow to a muscle.

   a. true
   b. false

3. The long delay period following cessation of exercise before reactive hyperemia develops in a distal muscle of a limb affected by arterial disease is the result of a phenomenon known as "proximal steal."

   a. true
   b. false

4. Compensatory collateral vessels increase in size in response to occlusive peripheral arterial disease and are able to supply sufficient blood flow to skeletal muscle during exercise to prevent the development of ischemia.

   a. true
   b. false

5. Ischemic gangrene of the lower extremities first involves the most _____ part of the circulatory bed.

   a. proximal
   b. distal

6. Venous thrombosis is the result of all but one of the following three factors. Identify the *incorrect* response.

   a. blood volume
   b. inflammation in the wall of the vein
   c. stagnant blood in the vein
   d. increased tendency of the blood to coagulate

7. Venous thrombosis that eventually leads to pulmonary embolism usually begins in the veins of the pelvis.

   a. true
   b. false

8. The percentage of patients admitted to general medical or surgical floors who develop at least small foci of venous thrombosis is __%.

   a. 10–20
   b. 20–30
   c. 30–40
   d. 40–50
   e. 50–60

9. Thrombosis frequently begins in venous valve pockets.
   a. true
   b. false

10. All but one of the following factors relate to predisposition and occurrence of aortic dissection. Identify the *incorrect* factor.
    a. congenital weakness in the aortic wall
    b. cardiac output
    c. aortic intimal tear
    d. hemodynamic forces propagating the dissecting hematoma within the aortic medial layer

11. Aortic intimal tears occur most commonly in two of the following sites. Identify these two areas.
    a. the ascending aorta just above the aortic valve
    b. the aortic arch just proximal to the brachiocephalic artery
    c. just distal to or at the origin of the left subclavian artery
    d. just proximal to the left carotid artery

12. Steepness (dp/dt) of the aortic pressure trace is more important than the presence of hypertension in determining propagation of an aortic dissecting aneurysm.
    a. true
    b. false

13. Transient episodes of neurologic dysfunction known as "TIAs" (transient ischemia attacks) are apparently the result of:
    a. cerebral arterial vasospasm
    b. small platelet or platelet and fibrin thrombi that embolize to small brain arteries
    c. emboli from left ventricular mural thrombi
    d. cholesterol emboli from ruptured aortic plaques

14. An ischemic brain region affected by a stroke can be shown to have decreased blood flow centrally with a zone of surrounding reactive hyperemia.
    a. true
    b. false

Chapter 16

1. Right ventricular hypertrophy during uterine life is the result of increased pulmonary vascular resistance.
   a. true
   b. false

2. All but one of the following are true about patients with acute cor pulmonale. Identify the *incorrect* response.

a. A sudden increase in pulmonary vascular resistance results from the episode of pulmonary embolism.

b. Increased pulmonary vascular resistance leads to a decrease in right ventricular work.

c. Right ventricular systolic wall tension is increased.

d. Right ventricular dilatation (Starling mechanism) develops.

3. A normal right ventricle can generate a maximum of _____ mm Hg systolic pressure in the face of an acute increase in pulmonary vascular resistance.

   a. 30–40

   b. 40–50

   c. 50–60

   d. 60–70

   e. 80–90

4. A sudden rise in right ventricular systolic pressure work often results in minimal right ventricular dilatation with consequent deterioration in right ventricular function.

   a. true

   b. false

5. All but one of the following can be present in a patient with acute pulmonary embolism. Identify the *incorrect* response.

   a. increased systemic venous pressure secondary to an elevation in right atrial pressure

   b. falling stroke volume

   c. heightened sympathetic nervous system activity

   d. decreased heart rate

   e. fall in arterial blood pressure

6. Normal right ventricular function in the face of an acute pressure workload depends on normal right ventricular myocardial blood flow.

   a. true

   b. false

7. The hemodynamic alterations that occur in patients with acute cor pulmonale are reversible.

   a. true

   b. false

8. Whether an episode of pulmonary embolism results in acute cor pulmonale, pulmonary infarction, or acute dyspnea depends on all but one of the following factors. Identify the *incorrect* factor.

   a. the condition of the bronchial circulation

   b. volume of the thromboembolic material

   c. preexisting right ventricular function

   d. preexisting pulmonary vascular resistance

   e. the site in the pulmonary circulation where the thromboemboli lodge

9. Thromboemboli originate in the veins of the lower extremities in 50% of cases of clinically detectable pulmonary embolism.

a. true
b. false

10. The churning, pumping action of the right ventricle breaks venous thrombi into multiple pieces that are distributed throughout the pulmonary circulation according to the distribution pattern of pulmonary blood flow, i.e., lower lobes greater than upper lobes.
    a. true
    b. false

11. Complete dissolution of pulmonary thromboemboli takes approximately _____ in individuals without heart or lung disease.
    a. 6 weeks
    b. 2 weeks
    c. 3 months
    d. 6 months
    e. 1 year

12. Patients with pulmonary infarction demonstrate necrosis of the pulmonary parenchyma. However, bronchial collateral circulation is sufficient to maintain the viability of the fibrous skeleton of the lung, the bronchi, and the muscular pulmonary arteries.
    a. true
    b. false

13. Pulmonary infarction usually occurs when embolism obstructs _____ pulmonary arteries.
    a. mainstem
    b. very small
    c. middle-sized
    d. bronchial

14. Pulmonary thromboembolism sufficiently massive to obstruct more than 50% of the pulmonary vascular bed often results in acute cor pulmonale.
    a. true
    b. false

15. Acute dyspnea and the associated tachypnea that accompany pulmonary embolism are the result of:
    a. reflexes set into motion by stimulation of nerve endings in the pulmonary vasculature by the impacting thromboemboli
    b. stimulation of the right ventricular endocardium
    c. activation of the sympathetic nervous system by fibrinolysis
    d. activation of the renin angiotensin system by the episode of acute pulmonary embolism

16. Essentially all patients with pulmonary embolism demonstrate some degree of pulmonary arterial hypertension regardless of the magnitude of the thromboembolic insult.
    a. true
    b. false

17. Small quantities of pulmonary thromboembolism result in modest rises in pulmonary arterial pressure secondary to pulmonary arterial vasoconstriction which in turn is caused by the hypoxemia that invariably accompanies episodes of pulmonary embolism.
    a. true
    b. false

Appendix C : Answers to Study Questions

Chapter 1

1. a
2. c
3. c
4. e
5. b
6. true
7. true
8. c
9. a
10. a

Chapter 2

1. e
2. true
3. true
4. b
5. d
6. a
7. true
8. b
9. c
10. true
11. e
12. true

Chapter 3

1. true
2. e
3. a
4. false
5. true
6. true
7. c
8. d
9. true
10. true
11. a, c
12. e
13. c

14. true
15. true

Chapter 4

1. true
2. true
3. d
4. true
5. false
6. false
7. c
8. a
9. a
10. true
11. true
12. true
13. a
14. c
15. c
16. true
17. true
18. true

Chapter 5

1. e
2. b
3. true
4. c
5. true
6. d
7. a
8. b
9. d
10. false
11. a
12. true
13. true
14. a. pressure overload
    b. volume overload
    c. volume overload
    d. pressure overload
15. true
16. b
17. true
18. b
19. a
20. true
21. false
22. false

23. c
24. true
25. false
26. true
27. b

Chapter 6

1. d
2. true
3. false
4. a
5. a
6. b
7. d
8. c
9. true
10. d
11. false

Chapter 7

1. c
2. true
3. true
4. a
5. c
6. e
7. d
8. true
9. a, b
10. false
11. e

Chapter 8

1. d
2. true
3. a
4. false
5. a
6. true
7. c
8. e
9. b
10. b
11. true
12. d
13. false

Chapter 9

1. The change in serum creatinine and the edema formation are likely to be due to functional renal impairment caused by indomethacin. This agent is a potent inhibitor of prostaglandin syn-

thesis (see text). Indomethacin and other nonsteroidal antiinflammatory drugs may also produce decreased renal function by inducing acute interstitial nephritis. The rapidity of recovery in this case suggests that blockade of prostaglandin synthesis led to a temporary decompensation of renal function which was readily reversed when the drug was stopped.

2. a. Although cardiac failure itself may be associated with impaired water excretion and hyponatremia, the clinical signs of hypovolemia in this patient indicate that the problem is likely to be due to diuretics. As described (see text), thiazides may cause hyponatremia by causing hypovolemia and impaired delivery of solute to the diluting segment while circulating antidiuretic hormone (ADH) is likely to be present, thus rendering the collecting duct permeable to water. Furthermore, thiazides impair the function of the diluting segment thereby raising the urinary osmolarity causing retention of solute-free water.

b. The azotemia is probably on the basis of hypovolemia (prerenal azotemia) as indicated by the severe elevation of the BUN and only a modest increase in the serum creatinine.

c. The hyponatremia may be corrected by administering either normal saline (thereby correcting the hypovolemia and restoring normal urinary dilution) or by giving hypertonic (3%) saline. In this patient the latter is preferable since the volume required to give additional NaCl is reduced and rapid correction of the hypotonicity of body fluids is indicated by the patient's depressed mental status.

Rapid correction of hyponatremia has been associated with neurologic defects thought to be due to central pontine myelinolysis. Hence, correction should be done slowly, for example, over 48 hours.

In patients with severe heart failure, administration of hypertonic saline may be precluded by pulmonary vascular congestion. In these cases, it is useful to give furosemide simultaneously and to replace the urinary losses of NaCl in addition to the calculated deficit.

Chapter 10

1. true
2. false
3. c
4. true
5. d
6. c
7. b
8. true
9. false
10. true
11. d

Chapter 11

1. a, c
2. false
3. true
4. b
5. true

Chapter 12

1. a
2. e
3. c
4. e
5. d
6. true
7. false

Chapter 14

1. true
2. true
3. c
4. true
5. d
6. a
7. c

Chapter 15

1. e
2. true
3. true
4. false
5. distal
6. a
7. false
8. e
9. true
10. b
11. a, c
12. true
13. b
14. true

Chapter 16

1. true
2. b
3. d
4. false
5. d
6. true
7. true
8. a
9. false
10. true

11. b
12. true
13. c
14. true
15. a
16. true
17. true

Index